Extraction and Analysis of Plant Active Ingredients

Extraction and Analysis of Plant Active Ingredients

Editor

Ernesto Reverchon

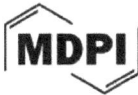 Basel • Beijing • Wuhan • Barcelona • Belgrade • Novi Sad • Cluj • Manchester

Editor
Ernesto Reverchon
University of Salerno
Fisciano, Italy

Editorial Office
MDPI
St. Alban-Anlage 66
4052 Basel, Switzerland

This is a reprint of articles from the Special Issue published online in the open access journal *Separations* (ISSN 2297-8739) (available at: https://www.mdpi.com/journal/separations/special_issues/extraction_analysis_plant_active_ingredients).

For citation purposes, cite each article independently as indicated on the article page online and as indicated below:

Lastname, A.A.; Lastname, B.B. Article Title. *Journal Name* **Year**, *Volume Number*, Page Range.

ISBN 978-3-0365-8502-4 (Hbk)
ISBN 978-3-0365-8503-1 (PDF)
doi.org/10.3390/books978-3-0365-8503-1

Contents

About the Editor

Ernesto Reverchon

Prof. Ernesto Reverchon is a Full Professor of Chemical Plants Design at the Department of Industrial Engineering of the University of Salerno, Italy. He has been the Head of the Department of Chemical and Food Engineering of University of Salerno (2002–2008); Coordinator of the PhD Studies in Chemical Engineering (1999–2006) and of PhD Studies in Industrial Engineering (2015–2018) at the Department of Industrial Engineering of the University of Salerno. He is among the top 20 World Scientists in Chemical Engineering. Among his research areas are (a) nutraceutical and pharmaceutical compounds extraction, (b) micro- and nano-particles production, (c) microcapsules, (d) membranes, scaffolds, and aerogels, and (e) nanosomes formation. He has also worked at the development of some industrial plants related to the applications of supercritical fluids in the nutraceutical and pharmaceutical field.

Preface

The extraction of active ingredients from vegetable matter is one of the most attractive research fields in the literature. A perspective that promotes this large interest is the possibility of identifying eco-friendly and innovative processes, active products, and materials. However, care must be taken in selecting process arrangements and extraction conditions to minimize the co-extraction of undesired compounds. The analysis of the composition of the extracted compounds by chromatography, mass spectrometry and related techniques, is a relevant step in determining the performance of the extraction process and the purity of the extracted compounds to be used for pharmaceutical applications.

This book includes 10 Research papers, 1 Communication, and 1 Review, and reports innovative extraction techniques and advanced analytical methods used for the recovery and the identification of high-added value compounds from vegetable matter.

Ernesto Reverchon
Editor

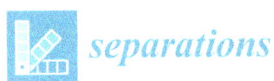

MDPI

Editorial

Extraction and Analysis of Plant Active Ingredients

Ernesto Reverchon * and Lucia Baldino

Department of Industrial Engineering, University of Salerno, Via Giovanni Paolo II, 132, 84084 Fisciano, Italy;
lbaldino@unisa.it
* Correspondence: ereverchon@unisa.it; Tel.: +39-08-996-4116

Citation: Reverchon, E.; Baldino, L. Extraction and Analysis of Plant Active Ingredients. *Separations* **2023**, *10*, 383. https://doi.org/10.3390/separations10070383

Received: 15 May 2023
Accepted: 31 May 2023
Published: 29 June 2023

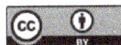
The extraction of active ingredients from vegetable matter is one of the most attractive research fields in the literature. An objective that promotes this large interest is the possibility of identifying eco-friendly and innovative processes, active products, and materials. However, care must be taken in selecting processes and extraction conditions to minimize the co-extraction of undesired compounds. The analysis of the composition of the extracted compounds by chromatography, mass spectrometry, and related techniques is a relevant step in determining the performance of the extraction process and the purity of the extracted compounds in order to use them for pharmaceutical applications.

This Special Issue includes 10 research papers, 1 communication, and 1 review, and reports innovative extraction techniques and advanced analytical methods used for the recovery of high-added-value compounds from vegetable matter.

In particular, Rehman et al. [1] studied the bronchodilator effect of *Achillea fragrantissima* essential oil (AFO) in guinea pigs' tracheas and the influence of drying on the quantity and composition of AFO using GC-MS and GC analyses. These authors found that AFO induced a strong relaxation to counteract the effects of carbachol (CCh) and showed bronchodilator effects predominantly due to anticholinergic and K^+ channel activation followed by weak Ca^{++} channels inhibition.

El Mansouri et al. [2] investigated the adsorption behavior of Eriochrome Black T (EBT) on waste hemp activated carbon (WHAC). The surface of the WHAC was modified by H_3PO_4 acid treatment. They concluded that the adsorption mechanism followed pseudo-second-order kinetics and the maximum removal of EBT by WHAC was in the range of 44–62% at pH 7, using an adsorbent dose of 10–70 mg, a contact time of 3 h, and an initial dye concentration of 10 mg L^{-1}.

Althurwi et al. [3] compared essential oils (EOs) prepared from the fresh and dried stems of *Commiphora gileadensis*. Although the components were quite similar, the amount of oil decreased from about 2.20 to 1.80% upon drying. The topical application of the *Commiphora gileadensis* chloroform extract promoted wound healing in rats.

Abdel-Kader et al. [4] designed a reverse-phase high-performance thin-layer chromatography (RP-HPTLC) protocol for the simultaneous determination of bioactive sesquiterpene coumarins feselol and samarcandin in the methanol extract of five *Ferula* species. The results indicated that *F. drudeana* contained the highest abundance of the more active samarcandin, whereas *F. duranii* had the largest quantity of the less active feselol.

In another work, Abdel-Kader et al. [5] developed and applied an HPTLC method that can simultaneously and effectively detect and quantify curcumin I, curcumin II, and curcumin III in fresh, dry rhizomes of *Curcuma longa* and in an herbal formulation of *C. longa* extracts.

Scognamiglio et al. [6] highlighted that supercritical fluid extraction coupled with fractional separation can represent a suitable alternative to isolate cuticular waxes from vegetable matter that preserves their natural properties and composition, without contamination with organic solvent residues. Operating in this way, they can be considered as a fingerprint of the vegetable matter, where C_{27}, C_{29}, and C_{31} were the most abundant compounds.

Zou et al. [7] developed a UHPLC-ESI-QTOF-MS/MS method to be an efficient strategy to annotate bioactive compounds, to reveal the difference in bioactive components of *Morus* spp. leaves, and to provide important information for the high-value production of *Morus* cultivars in the food and supplement fields.

Wang and Li [8] proposed an environmentally friendly method for the extraction of seven active coumarins from *Angelica dahurica (Hoffm.) Benth. & Hook.f. ex Franch. & Sav. (A. dahurica)* based on deep eutectic solvents (DESs). The DES system using a molar ratio of choline chloride, citric acid, and water of 1:1:2 showed the best extraction effect whereas the optimal extraction conditions were a liquid/solid ratio of 10:1 (mL/g), extraction time of 50 min, extraction temperature of 59.85 °C, and moisture content of 49.28%.

Givonetti et al. [9] investigated the SDS-PAGE profile of hempseed proteins; They compared different methods of extraction, two conditions to maintain low temperatures during seed grinding, and two solubilization buffers. TCA/acetone, MTBE/methanol, and direct protein solubilization of defatted hempseed flour resulted in the highest protein content.

Ilyas et al. [10] evaluated the immunomodulatory activity of various fractions of *Phyllanthus maderaspatensis*, column eluents of the ethyl acetate fraction, and their polyphenols. They found that the ethyl acetate fraction contained a high amount of catechin, quercetin, ellagic acid kaempferol, and rutin, which are involved in immunomodulation.

Rajasree et al. [11] measured the antioxidant activity of a methanolic extract of *Cucumis melo Linn* (MECM). The results showed the presence of various phytochemical constituents, such as carbohydrates, alkaloids, sterols, phenolic compounds, terpenes, and flavonoids, and suggested that MECM may serve as a putative source of natural antioxidants for therapeutic and nutraceutical applications.

Chiriac et al. [12] summarized the current advances in the state of the art for polyphenol identification and quantification. In particular, analytical techniques ranging from high-pressure liquid chromatography to hyphenated spectrometric methods were discussed, and they highlighted that the elucidation of the compound's structure is one of the most important steps for natural products research.

Author Contributions: Conceptualization, E.R.; writing—review and editing, L.B. and E.R. All authors have read and agreed to the published version of the manuscript.

Funding: This research received no external funding.

Acknowledgments: We thank all the authors who contributed to this Special Issue. We wish to acknowledge the efforts of the reviewers as they significantly contributed to the quality of this Special Issue.

Conflicts of Interest: The authors declare no conflict of interest.

References

1. Rehman, N.U.; Salkini, M.A.A.; Alanizi, H.M.K.; Alharbi, A.G.; Alqarni, M.H.; Abdel-Kader, M.S. *Achillea fragrantissima* Essential Oil: Composition and Detailed Pharmacodynamics Study of the Bronchodilator Activity. *Separations* **2022**, *9*, 334. [CrossRef]
2. El Mansouri, F.; Pelaz, G.; Morán, A.; Esteves Da Silva, J.C.G.; Cacciola, F.; El Farissi, H.; Tayeq, H.; Zerrouk, M.H.; Brigui, J. Efficient Removal of Eriochrome Black T Dye Using Activated Carbon of Waste Hemp (*Cannabis sativa* L.) Grown in Northern Morocco Enhanced by New Mathematical Models. *Separations* **2022**, *9*, 283. [CrossRef]
3. Althurwi, H.N.; Salkini, M.A.A.; Soliman, G.A.; Ansari, M.N.; Ibnouf, E.O.; Abdel-Kader, M.S. Wound Healing Potential of *Commiphora gileadensis* Stems Essential Oil and Chloroform Extract. *Separations* **2022**, *9*, 254. [CrossRef]
4. Abdel-Kader, M.S.; Alqarni, M.H.; Baykan, S.; Oztürk, B.; Salkini, M.A.A.; Yusufoglu, H.S.; Alam, P.; Foudah, A.I. Ecofriendly Validated RP-HPTLC Method for Simultaneous Determination of the Bioactive Sesquiterpene Coumarins Feselol and Samarcandin in Five *Ferula* Species Using Green Solvents. *Separations* **2022**, *9*, 206. [CrossRef]
5. Abdel-Kader, M.S.; Salkini, A.A.; Alam, P.; Alshahrani, K.A.; Foudah, A.I.; Alqarni, M.H. A High-Performance Thin-Layer Chromatographic Method for the Simultaneous Determination of Curcumin I, Curcumin II and Curcumin III in *Curcuma longa* and Herbal Formulation. *Separations* **2022**, *9*, 94. [CrossRef]
6. Scognamiglio, M.; Baldino, L.; Reverchon, E. Fractional Separation and Characterization of Cuticular Waxes Extracted from Vegetable Matter Using Supercritical CO$_2$. *Separations* **2022**, *9*, 80. [CrossRef]

7.   Zou, X.-Y.; He, Y.-J.; Yang, Y.-H.; Yan, X.-P.; Li, Z.-B.; Yang, H. Systematic Identification of Bioactive Compositions in Leaves of *Morus* Cultivars Using UHPLC-ESI-QTOF-MS/MS and Comprehensive Screening of High-Quality Resources. *Separations* **2022**, *9*, 76. [CrossRef]

8.   Wang, T.; Li, Q. DES Based Efficient Extraction Method for Bioactive Coumarins from *Angelica dahurica* (Hoffm.) Benth. & Hook.f. ex Franch. & Sav. *Separations* **2022**, *9*, 5.

9.   Givonetti, A.; Cattaneo, C.; Cavaletto, M. What You Extract Is What You Get: Different Methods of Protein Extraction from Hemp Seeds. *Separations* **2021**, *8*, 231. [CrossRef]

10. Ilyas, U.; Katare, D.P.; Naseef, P.P.; Kuruniyan, M.S.; Elayadeth-Meethal, M.; Aeri, V. Immunomodulatory Activity of *Phyllanthus maderaspatensis* in LPS-Stimulated Mouse Macrophage RAW 264.7 Cells. *Separations* **2021**, *8*, 129. [CrossRef]

11. Rajasree, R.S.; Ittiyavirah, S.P.; Naseef, P.P.; Kuruniyan, M.S.; Anisree, G.S.; Elayadeth-Meethal, M. An Evaluation of the Antioxidant Activity of a Methanolic Extract of *Cucumis melo* L. Fruit (F1 Hybrid). *Separations* **2021**, *8*, 123. [CrossRef]

12. Chiriac, E.R.; Chiţescu, C.L.; Geană, E.-I.; Gird, C.E.; Socoteanu, R.P.; Boscencu, R. Advanced Analytical Approaches for the Analysis of Polyphenols in Plants Matrices—A Review. *Separations* **2021**, *8*, 65. [CrossRef]

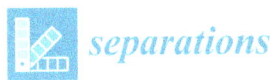

separations

MDPI

Article

Achillea fragrantissima Essential Oil: Composition and Detailed Pharmacodynamics Study of the Bronchodilator Activity

Najeeb Ur Rehman [1,*], Mohammad Ayman A. Salkini [2], Hatem M. K. Alanizi [3], Abdulrahman G. Alharbi [4], Mohammed H. Alqarni [2] and Maged S. Abdel-Kader [2,5]

[1] Department of Pharmacology and Toxicology, College of Pharmacy, Prince Sattam Bin Abdulaziz University, Al-Kharj 11942, Saudi Arabia
[2] Department of Pharmacognosy, College of Pharmacy, Prince Sattam Bin Abdulaziz University, Al-Kharj 11942, Saudi Arabia
[3] College of Pharmacy, Prince Sattam Bin Abdulaziz University, Al-Kharj 11942, Saudi Arabia
[4] Maternity and Children's Hospital, Ministry of Health, Al-Kharj 11942, Saudi Arabia
[5] Department of Pharmacognosy, Faculty of Pharmacy, Alexandria University, Alexandria 21215, Egypt
* Correspondence: n.rehman@psau.edu.sa; Tel.: +966-537-192-380

Abstract: The bronchodilator effect of the *Achillea fragrantissima* essential oil (AFO) was studied in guinea pigs' tracheas and the influence of drying on the quantity and composition of AFO was studied using GC-MS and GC analyses. AFO produced a complete and potent relaxation against carbachol (CCh), while lower potency and partial efficacy were observed against high K^+ (80 mM), thus producing dual inhibitory effects similar to dicyclomine. The anticholinergic-like action was further confirmed when pre-incubation tracheal tissues were used at lower concentrations with AFO displacing the CCh concentration-response curves (CRCs) to the right in a competitive manner similar to atropine. However, non-parallel shifts in CCh CRCs were observed with higher doses, similar to dicyclomine. Further confirmation of the CCB-like effect was obtained from the non-specific deflection of Ca^{++} CRCs toward the right using the pre-incubated tissues with AFO in Ca^{++} free medium, similar to verapamil. When AFO was tested against low K^+-mediated contractions to explore the possible involvement of additional antispasmodic mechanism(s), AFO interestingly showed a complete inhibition with a higher potency. This inhibition was found to be sensitive to tetraethylammonium (TEA) and 4-aminopyridine (4 AP), whereas glibenclamide (Gb) remained inactive. These results show that AFO possesses bronchodilator effects predominantly from its anticholinergic and K^+ channel activation followed by weak Ca^{++} channels inhibition.

Keywords: *Achillea fragrantissima* oil; GC-MS; bronchodilator; anticholinergic; Ca^{++} channel blocker; potassium channel opener; guinea pig trachea

Citation: Rehman, N.U.; Salkini, M.A.A.; Alanizi, H.M.K.; Alharbi, A.G.; Alqarni, M.H.; Abdel-Kader, M.S. *Achillea fragrantissima* Essential Oil: Composition and Detailed Pharmacodynamics Study of the Bronchodilator Activity. *Separations* 2022, 9, 334. https://doi.org/10.3390/separations9110334

Academic Editor: Stefania Garzoli

Received: 5 October 2022
Accepted: 17 October 2022
Published: 1 November 2022

Publisher's Note: MDPI stays neutral with regard to jurisdictional claims in published maps and institutional affiliations.

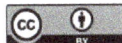

1. Introduction

Achillea fragrantissima is a flowering plant belonging to the Asteraceae family. *Achillea* is a genus that comprises approximately 100 species. Most family members of this genus are characterized by the biosynthesis of sesquiterpene lactones and flavonoids [1]. Members of the genus *Achillea* are well-known in traditional medicine. They are used for the treatment of many aliments such as stomach pain, menstrual disorders, bleeding, hemorrhoids, gastrointestinal tract inflammation, rheumatism, allergic rhinitis, and pneumonia. They are also useful during breast feeding and possess wound-healing potential [2] *A. fragrantissima* is popular in folk medicine for many Arab countries and is used for the management of some common health problems including diabetes, respiratory disorders, gastrointestinal disturbances, dysmenorrhea, eye infections, smallpox, fever, headaches, and fatigue [3–5]. *A. fragrantissima* is also used in Saudi Arabia as for its anticancer, antibacterial, antifungal, antimalarial, appetizer, treatment of respiratory problem, aphrodisiac, antispasmodic, and relaxant effects [6]. The plant extract as well as the isolated methoxylated flavonoids exhibit promising antitumor activities attributed to their antioxidant potential [7]. Studies of the essential oil of the plants collected from Jourdan revealed the presence of α-thujone (33.8%) and β-sesquiphellandrene (28.6%) as the principal constituents [8]. The volatile nature of the essential oil extracted from different medicinal plants is the most effective for treating respiratory diseases as their volatile nature can help in the delivery to the site intended to be treated [9]. The importance of essential oil use in bronchoconstriction can be estimated from the official inclusion of more than 25 essential oils in European Pharmacopoeia [10]. Among them, thyme, anise, eucalyptus, fennel, and peppermint are the mostly used in practice for addressing respiratory ailments such as bronchoconstriction [11].

The current study aims to quantitatively and quantitatively evaluate the effect of drying on *A. fragrantissima* oil (AFO). The brochodilator effect of AFO was evaluated with detailed pharmacodynamics explored in the isolated tracheal tissues of guinea pigs using an ex vivo experimental organ bath setup.

2. Materials and Methods

2.1. Plant Material

The plants of *Achillea fragrantissima* (Forssk.) Sch.Bip. were collected in February, 2021 from Faydat Alhayra (29°32′49.7″ N 43°22′47.6″ E), west of Rafha, North of Saudi Arabia and close to the border with Iraq. The plant was authenticated by the taxonomist Dr. Mohammad Atiqur Rahman, MAP-PRC, College of Pharmacy, King Saud University, Riyadh, Saudi Arabia. A voucher specimen (#18507) was preserved at the center's herbarium.

2.2. Chemicals

Carbamylcholine, verapamil, dicyclomine, atropine, glibenclamide, tetraethylammonium, and 4-aminopyridine were obtained from Merck (Rahway, NJ, USA) previously, Sigma-Aldric.

2.3. Preparation of AFO

A sample quantity of 250 g comprising the fresh plant and 100 g of shade dried aerial parts (acquired from 250 gm fresh stems after drying) of *A. fragrantissima* were used for AFO extraction for a time period of 5 h using hydrodistillation with Clevenger apparatus (Dolphin Instruments, Mumbai, India). The fresh plants were cut using a knife into small pieces (approximately 2 cm long), while the dried plants in the shade under controlled temperature were ground and used for AFO preparation. After the hydrodistillation process, the AFO layers were collected after separation and the water layers were extracted with diethyl ether; the ethereal layers were combined, dehydrated with sodium sulfate (anhydrous), and the ether layer was evaporated using a rotary evaporator to leave pure AFO. From this oil, 300 mg/mL stock solution in propylene glycol is produced for biological testing. Each experiment was performed in triplicate.

2.4. GC-MS Analysis

AFO samples of 5 ppm concentrations were prepared in MeOH. From each sample, 1 μL was injected for GC-MS analysis using an Agilent Model 7890 MSD GC-MS instrument (Agilent Technologies Inc., Santa Clara, CA, USA) equipped with an (30 m × 0.25 mm i.d., 0.25 μm coating) HP-5MS capillary column. The injections were performed via the Autosampler in the split-less mode in triplicates. The temperature program started at 60 °C and was unchanged for 10 min, then increased by 4 °C/min until it reached 220 °C, from which it was held for 5 min. Then, the temperature was increased by 10 °C/min to reach a final temperature of 290 °C and kept constant for 5 min with for a total run time of 67 min. Helium (99.999% purity) was the used carrier gas with a flow rate of 1.0 mL/min. Quadrupole mass spectroscopy analysis was recorded using the EI ionization mode set at 70 Ev. The range of mass detection was adjusted between 30 and 600 m/z. AFO compound identification was performed by comparing the obtained MS spectra with the library of the NIST 2017 (National Institute of Standards and Technology) data base. The results analysis and control were achieved using the MASSHUNTER software (Version B.04.xx, Agilent Technologies Inc., Santa Clara, CA USA).

2.5. GC Analysis

GC chromatograms were obtained using a GC Agilent 7890B equipped with the capillary column HP-5 19091J-413 (30 m × 0.25 mm) along with FID detector applying conditions used for GC-MS analysis. *n*-Alkanes series were used to calculate the relative retention index (RRI) applied for peak identification. The area for each peak was measured automatically to enable the quantification of the peaks (Figure 1).

A

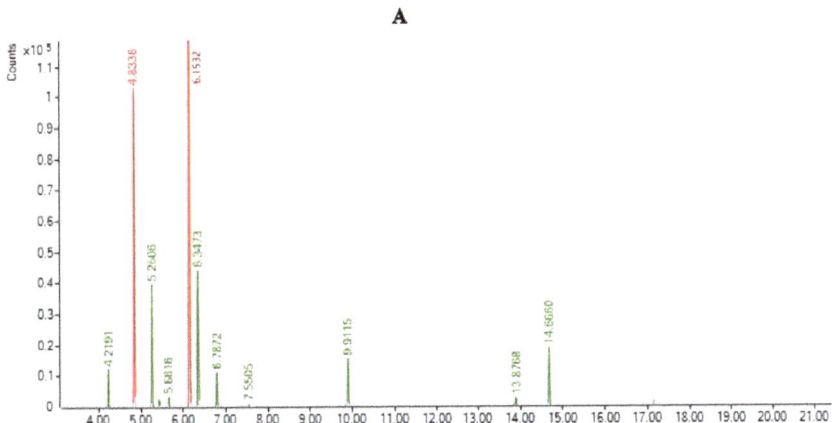

B

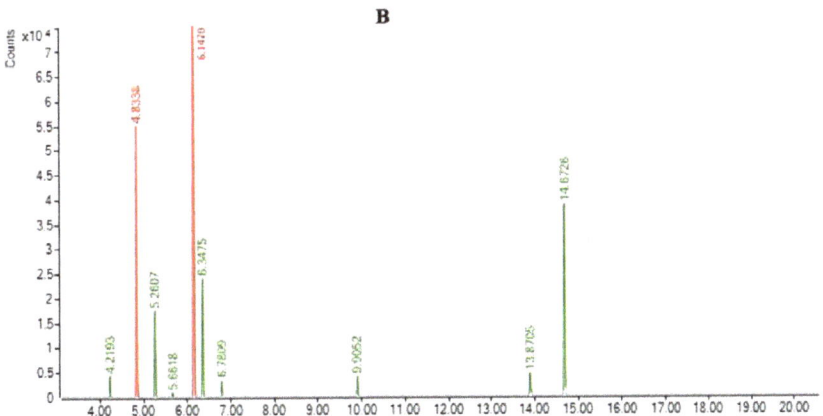

Figure 1. GC chromatogram of AFO obtained from fresh (**A**) and dried (**B**) plant samples.

2.6. Bronchoduilator Study

2.6.1. Animals

Experimental guinea pigs of 500–550 g weight of either gender were obtained from the King Saud University animal laboratory. All the animals received due care at the Animal Care center of the College of Pharmacy, PSAU, KSA where a standard temperature of 23–25 °C was maintained while a standard commercial diet and running water ad libitum was provided to all tested animals. Animal ethical guidelines for laboratory animals were followed during experimental assays with compliance to the guidance of the Institute of Laboratory Animal Resources, Commission on Life Sciences, National Research Council [12]. The ex vivo protocol followed in this study has been registered with reference number BERC-001-12-19 by Bio-Ethical Research Committee (BERC) at PSAU.

2.6.2. Isolated Tissue Preparation

Animals were humanely sacrificed by cervical dislocation. The tracheal tubes were removed and preserved in an ice-cold Krebs–Henseleit solution immediately. The composition of the Krebs–Henseleit solution was (mM) as follows: $NaHCO_3$ 25.0, NaCl 118.0, KH_2PO_4 1.2, KCl 4.7, $MgSO_4$ 1.2, glucose 11, and $CaCl_2$ 2.5 [13]. Carbogen (95% O_2: 5% CO_2) was passed through the solution that was maintained at 37 °C.

The accompanied connective tissue and fats were removed with care and the tracheas were cut into rings 2–3 mm wide. The rings were open opposite to the tracheal muscles and fitted together forming a tracheal chain [14]. The preparation under testing was mounted in the 20 mL tissue bath containing Kreb's solution at 37 °C with continuous aeration with carbogen (95% O_2 and 5% CO_2). A tension of 1 g was applied and kept constant throughout the experiment to each tracheal strip.

Soon after an hour stabilization period is provided to the tracheal tissues in an organ bath, the preparations were chemically contracted using a bronchoconstrictor drug; carbamylcholine (CCh, 1 µM) and potassium chloride having final bath concentrations of 80 mM and K^+-25 mM while the tissue tension was recorded using an emkaBATH data acquisition system (France) equipped with isometric force transducer. After getting stable bronchoconstriction, different concentrations of AFO as well as the used standard drugs were tested in a cumulative way to record the bronchial relaxant response [15].

2.6.3. Determination of the Possible Mechanisms of Action

To determine the involvement of antimuscarinic and Ca^{++} channels' inhibitor-like pharmacodynamics in the relaxant effect of AFO, the CCh-mediated CRC were obtained in the absence and presence of the pre-incubated tracheal tissues with two increasing doses of AFO; the results were compared with parallel experiments conducted using pre-incubated tissues with atropine, an anticholinergic [16]; dicyclomine, a dual inhibitor of muscarinic receptors; and Ca^{++} channels [17].

To confirm the inhibitory effect of AFO on Ca^{++} channels, the Ca^{++} CRCs were recorded in the absence and presence of pre-incubated tissues with the AFO in tracheal tissues previously made Ca^{++} free. The tracheal tissues were made Ca^{++} free by incubating tissues for an hour in a Ca^{++}-Krebs solution containing EDTA to chelate the intracellular stores of Ca^{++} [18]. The results were compared with parallel experiments conducted with standard drugs, dicyclomine and verapamil, known CCBs [19].

To assess the involvement of K^+ channels' opening-like effects, the spasmolytic effects of the test samples were explored on low K^+ (25 mM) [20]. After getting sustained contraction from low K^+, the test materials were added in a cumulative fashion to obtain the concentration-dependent relaxant responses. The relaxation of the tracheal tissue was demonstrated as the percentage of control contraction mediated by low K^+.

To characterize the specific type of K^+ channels' activation involved in the bronchodilator effect, the bronchodilator effects of the AFO was reproduced against low K^+-mediated contractions in the absence and presence of different K^+ channel antagonists such as tetraethylammonium (TEA, 1 mM), a nonselective K^+ channel blocker [21]; 4-aminopyridine (4-AP, 100 µM), a selective blocker of voltage sensitive K^+ channels [22]; and glibenclamide (Gb, 10 µM), a selective blocker of ATP-dependent K^+ channels [23].

2.7. Statistical Analysis

The recorded findings are presented as mean ± standard error of the mean while "n" represents the number of individual experiments repeated with EC_{50} (the median effective concentrations) with 95% confidence intervals (CI). A one-way analysis of variance and a

Dunnett's test were utilized to determine the bronchodilatation. $p < 0.05$ is considered to be statistically significant. Non-linear regression was applied to statistically analyze the CRCs using a GraphPad program (GraphPad, San Diego, CA, USA).

3. Results

3.1. Preparation of AFO and GC-MS Study

The fresh plants provided 0.694 g AFO from 250 g plant material, while the drying of the same weight resulted in 100 g dry plants that provided 0.545 g (Table 1). GC-MS analysis of the fresh and dry AFO enable the identification of the same nine components representing 98.219 and 99.732% of the AFO prepared from the fresh and dry plants, respectively (Table 2, Figure 2).

Table 1. Yield of AFO from the fresh and dried plant samples of *A. fragrantissima* *.

Condition	Weight (g)	Weight of Oil (g)	% w/w
Fresh	250	0.694 ± 0.021	0.28
Dried	100	0.545 ± 0.018	0.218 **

* Expressed values are the mean of triplicate determination (n = 3) ± standard deviations. ** The weights of the fresh plant samples were used to calculate the oil percentage.

Table 2. Components of fresh and dried plant samples AFO.

Name of Components	RT	RRI	Area%	
			Fresh	Dry
Yomogi alcohol	4.2191	1000	2.458	1.228
(+)-Santolina alcohol	4.8336	1038	25.643	21.711
artemisia ketone	5.2606	1061	9.949	7.209
α-Thujone	6.1470	1102	34.471	33.397
β-Thujone	6.3475	1110	11.939	10.704
Sabinol	6.7872	1143	3.052	1.268
Sabinyl acetate	9.9115	1291	4.582	1.585
Bicyclosesquiphellandrene	13.8768	1498	0.614	2.562
β-sesquiphellandrene	14.666	1525	5.511	20.068
Monoterpenes%			**92.094**	**77.102**
Sesquiterpenes			**6.125**	**22.63**
Total			98.219	99.732

The bold Monoterpenes and sesquiterpenes represent main groups of compounds.

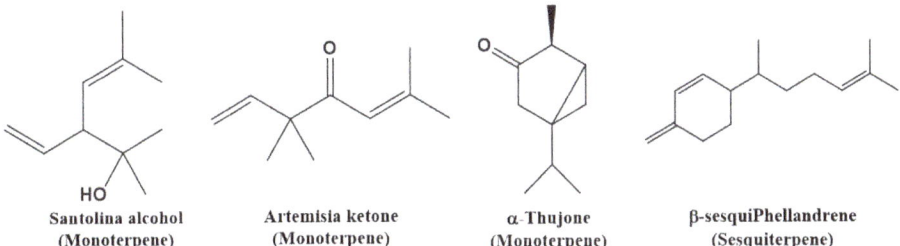

Figure 2. Chemical structure of some components of AFO.

3.2. Bronchodilator Activity

AFO caused concentration-dependent relaxation responses (Figure 3A) with complete relaxation against CCh with resultant EC_{50} values of 0.42 mg/mL (0.38–0.46, 95% CI, n = 4), while high K^+ was partially inhibited with a amaximum relaxation of 78% at the highest concentration of 5 mg/mL (Figure 3A). Similarly, dicyclomine also showed a higher potency against CCh compared to high K^+-mediated spasms with resultant EC_{50} values of 0.36 μM (0.32–0.45, 95% CI, n = 4) and 9.62 μM (8.68–10.24, 95% CI, n = 4), respectively (Figure 3B). Verapamil, on the other hand showed a significantly higher potency to inhibit high K$^+$ compared to CCh-evoked contractions with respective EC$_{50}$ values of 0.35 μM (0.28–0.43, 95% CI, n = 4) and 5.14 μM (4.26–6.42, 95% CI, n = 4) as shown in Figure 3C. The confirmation of the anticholinergic effect of AFO was processed by the CCh-mediated CRCs constructed in the absence and presence of AFO at a concentration of 0.1 and 0.3 mg/mL where the CRCs of CCh were shifted toward the right without an in-parallel manner or suppression at 0.1 mg/mL; the non-parallel shift was observed at 0.3 mg/mL with a suppression of the maximum response (Figure 4A). Similarly, dicyclomine (Figure 4B) also showed parallel and non-parallel shifts in CCh-mediated CRCs at the respective doses of pre-incubated tissues with 0.1 and 0.3 μM, whereas atropine, an anticholinergic drug, showed a parallel shift toward the right in CCh-CRCs at both doses of 0.01 and 0.03 μM pre-incubation (Figure 4C).

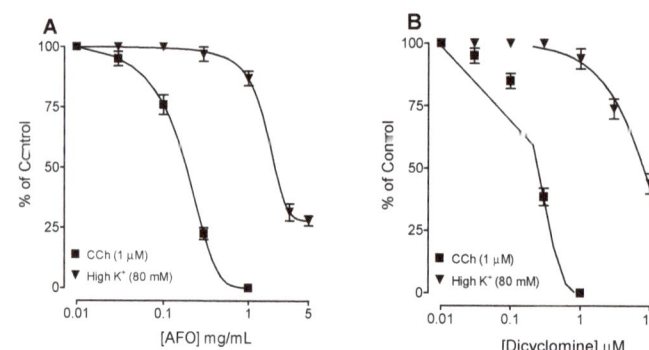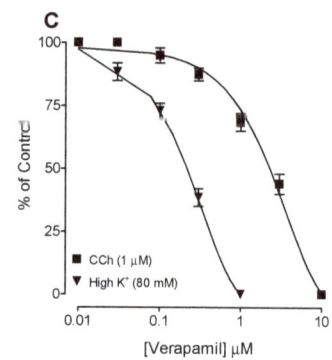

Figure 3. Concentration-dependent inhibitory effects of the (**A**) essential oil (AFO), (**B**) dicyclomine and (**C**) verapamil against carbachol (CCh; 1 μM) and high K$^+$ (80 mM)-induced contraction in isolated guinea pig tracheal preparations. Symbols represent mean ± SEM; n = 4.

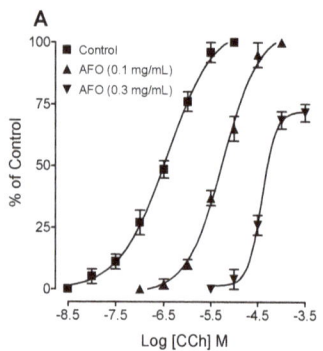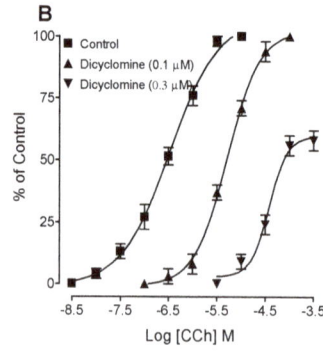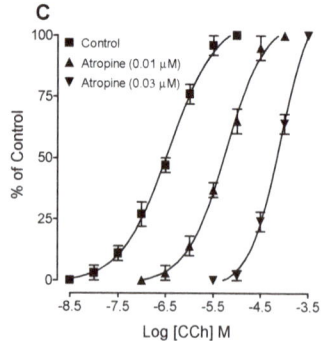

Figure 4. Concentration-response curves of carbachol (CCh) in the absence and presence of the increasing concentrations of the (**A**) essential oil (AFO), (**B**) dicyclomine and (**C**) atropine in isolated guinea pig tracheal preparations. Symbols represent mean ± SEM; n = 5.

The effect of AFO to inhibit Ca^{++} channels was further authenticated when the tracheal tissues pre-incubated with AFO (0.3 and 1 mg/mL) suppressed the Ca^{++}-mediated CRCs with a rightward shift constructed in a Ca^{++}-free medium (Figure 5A). Similarly, the standard drugs, dicyclomine (Figure 5B) and verapamil (Figure 5C), also showed suppression of the Ca^{++} CRCs with a rightward shift, as expected.

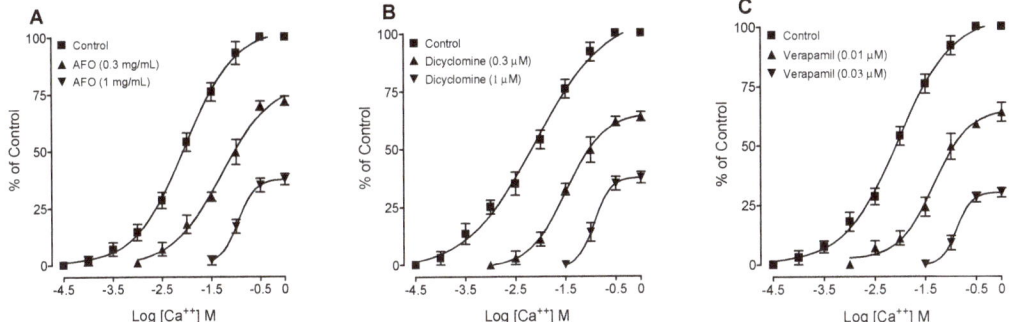

Figure 5. Concentration-response curves of Ca^{++} in the absence and presence of the increasing concentrations of the (**A**) essential oil (AFO), (**B**) dicyclomine and (**C**) verapamil in isolated guinea pig tracheal preparations. Symbols represent mean $\pm$ SEM; n = 5.

Previous studies established the fact that the spasmolytic effect of many medicinal plants may be mediated via K^+ channel opener activity, hence AFO was tested against evoked contractions in the isolated trachea with a low K^+ (25 mM). Interestingly, AFO led to significant relaxation in a concentration-dependent manner with resultant EC_{50} values of 0.26 mg/mL (0.22–0.29, 95% CI; n = 4) as shown in Figure 6A, whereas it failed to antagonize high K^+ (80 mM)-provoked contractions completely (Figures 3A and 6A). This inhibitory effect of AFO against low K^+ was not effected when the tissues were pre-incubated with glibenclamide (10 µM) (Figure 6B); TEA (1 mM) shifted the inhibitory response of AFO toward the right in a significant way (Figure 6C), whereas maximum inhibition was seen with 4-AP (100 µM) as shown in Figure 6D.

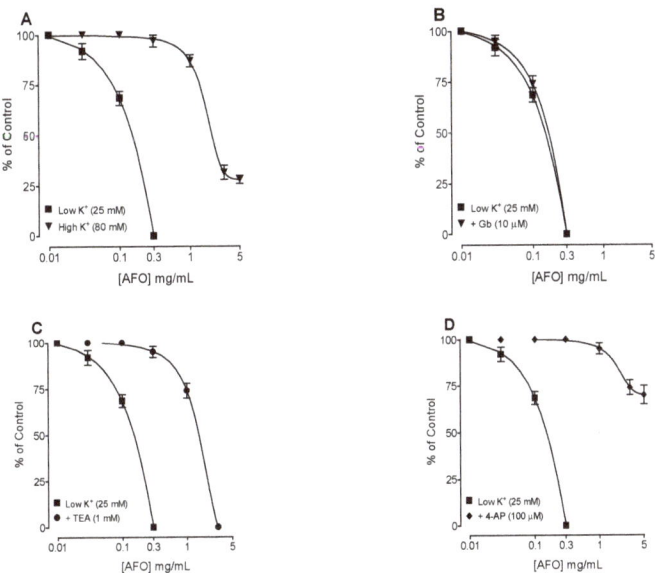

Figure 6. Concentration-dependent inhibitory effects of the essential oil (AFO) against (**A**) low K^+ and high K^+, and low K^+ in the presence of (**B**) glibenclamide (Gb; 10 µM), (**C**) tetraethylammonium (TEA; 1 mM) and (**D**) 4-aminopyridine (4-AP; 100 µM) in isolated guinea pig tracheal tissues. Symbols represent mean $\pm$ SEM; n = 4.

4. Discussion

The drying process resulted in a 21.5% loss of the AFO when compared with a fresh plant's yield (Table 1). There was no qualitative difference in the components present in the two AFO samples. The AFO is characterized by the absence of monoterpene hydrocarbons. All the seven identified monoterpenes were oxygenated (Table 2). Only two sesquiphellandrene derivatives could be detected in AFO prepared from the fresh and dry plants. In the AFO prepared from the fresh plants, the percentage of sesquiterpenes was 6.125, which increased to 22.63 in the AFO obtained from dry plant materials. This indicates that the loss in the lighter monoterpenes was greater than in the sesquiterpenes with a higher molecular weight (Figure 2) [24,25].

Among several airway diseases, asthma is the most common and is a major disabling syndrome that accounts for considerable deaths worldwide [26]. Asthma is one of the most important and common airways ailments, expressed as periodic wheezing following cough and chest rigidity mainly because of obstruction of the air passage [27]. The existing pharmacotherapy for the management of asthma has been classified into different classes, including bronchorelaxants, such as cholinergic-antagonists, β-receptor agonists, PDE-inhibitors, and anti-inflammatory drugs such as corticosteroids, mast cells stabilizers, leukotriene inhibitors, K^+ channel openers, and Ca^{++} channel inhibitors [28,29]. The drugs available are expensive (inhaler), beyond the access of laymen in the developing world, and have side-effects, particularly, if employed orally. Hence, less satisfaction is felt by many patients with the conventional medicines as patients need permanent therapy and believe that herbal medications are natural and can sometimes be taken without notifying their physician [30].

A. fragrantissima is a medicinal plant with a famous traditional history for its use in the treatment of bronchitis and bronchial asthma [3–6]. To date, no literature has been found to support these claims to the best of our knowledge. The current study aims to verify these traditional uses using isolated guinea pig tracheal tissues, a well-known ex vivo model in airways research [13,31]. The extracted essential oil from *A. fragrantissima* was tested for its possible tracheal smooth-muscle-relaxant effects against contractions provoked by carbamylcholine (CCh, 1 μM) and high K^+ (K^+-80 mM) in isolated tracheal preparations. Interestingly, AFO inhibited both types of evoked contractions with a selectively higher potency and efficacy against CCh, thus suggesting anti-muscarinic and Ca^{++} channel inhibition [32,33]. The anti-muscarinic and CCB-like actions of AFO were further confirmed, respectively, through CCh and Ca^{++} CRCs in the pre-incubated tracheal tissues with different concentrations of the AFO and the relevant standard drugs. A parallel shift of CCh curves without affecting the contractions' efficacy observed at the lower concentration of AFO is a known characteristic of the standard drug atropine, a competitive or specific muscarinic-receptor blocker [32], whereas the next higher dose of AFO exhibited a nonparallel shift in the CCh CRCs with a suppression of the efficacy, thus clearly pointing toward the involvement of non-specific inhibitory components similar to verapamil, a voltage-gated L-Type Ca^{++} antagonist [33]. The double inhibitory actions exhibited by AFO are strengthened by comparing them with the shift in the CCh CRCs obtained with dicyclomine [32], while verapamil, on the other hand, caused deflection of CCh CRCs rightward but also caused a non-parallel shift with a decrease in the efficacy at both concentrations. Atropine, as expected from competitive antagonists, deflected CCh CRCs in a parallel way toward a higher potency but caused no change in the efficacy [32]. The pretreatment of tissues with AFO shifted the Ca^{++} curves to the right accompanied by the suppression of maximum responses, similar to that caused by verapamil, confirming the Ca^{++} antagonistic effect. Interestingly, Ca^{++} antagonists are also useful in bronchoconstriction [34], besides the well-established role of anticholinergics in asthma [35].

According to previously conducted studies, it is experienced that plants with medicinal importance in bronchoconstriction also have an activation effect on K^+ channels [36], hence AFO was tested on low K^+-mediated contractions where it showed the highest potency compared to its anticholinergic and CCB-like effects. The inhibitory effects of AFO on contractions provoked by low K$^+$ (25 mM) at a higher potency and efficacy compared to its inhibitory effect on high K$^+$ indicate their predominant effect on K$^+$ channel activation, as substances that selectively inhibit the contractions provoked by K$^+$ (25 mM) at a higher potency and are denoted as potassium channel openers [37]. On the other hand, substances that inhibit the contractions resulting from low (25 mM) and high (80 mM) K$^+$ concentrations at a comparable potency are termed as Ca^{++} channel blockers [38,39]. These experiments undoubtedly differentiate between the potassium channel openers and calcium channel blocker classes from a mechanistic viewpoint. To explore the contributions of different types of potassium channels, AFO was applied to low K$^+$ (25 mM)-provoked contractions in tissues pretreated with different K$^+$ channel antagonists, namely glibenclamide, an ATP-dependent K$^+$ blocker [23]; TEA, a non-selective K$^+$ channel blocker [21]; and 4-AP, a voltage-sensitive K$^+$ channel antagonist [40]. The classes of potassium channel openers could have a potential clinical interest as they have the ability to induce vascular and nonvascular smooth muscle relaxation, including in the respiratory tract muscles [41]. These compounds can open the K$^+$ channels and consequently cause membrane hyperpolarization by increasing in K$^+$ efflux, thus causing a decrease in the intracellular free Ca^{++} leading to smooth muscle relaxation [42,43].

5. Conclusions

The process of drying led to some changes in AFO quantity and the relative percentages of the AFO components obtained from fresh and dried stems of *A. fragrantissima*. The drying process resulted in an increase of the sesquiterpenes and decrease of the monoterpenes' relative percentages. The AFO prepared from fresh and dried plants were free from monoterpene hydrocarbons.

Our study also shows that AFO possesses bronchodilator effects mediated predominantly through a muscarinic receptor blockade and triggers the activation of the voltage sensitive and non-specific types of K$^+$ channels followed by the partial involvement of Ca^{++} channel inhibition. This study supports the traditional use of AFO for the treatment of respiratory disorders with the potential of the essential oil to be developed as a remedy for the management of bronchial asthma.

Author Contributions: Conceptualization, M.S.A.-K., M.H.A. and N.U.R.; methodology, N.U.R., M.A.A.S., H.M.K.A., and A.G.A.; software, N.U.R., M.A.A.S., H.M.K.A. and A.G.A.; validation, N.U.R., M.A.A.S. and M.H.A. formal analysis, N.U.R., M.A.A.S., H.M.K.A. and A.G.A.; investigation, N.U.R., M.A.A.S., H.M.K.A. and A.G.A.; resources, M.S.A.-K., M.H.A. and H.M.K.A.; data curation, A.G.A., M.S.A.-K. and N.U.R.; writing—original draft preparation, N.U.R., M.H.A. and M.A.A.S.; writing—review and editing, M.S.A.-K. and N.U.R.; visualization, N.U.R., M.A.A.S., H.M.K.A. and A.G.A.; supervision, M.S.A.-K.; project administration, M.S.A.-K.; funding acquisition, M.S.A.-K. All authors have read and agreed to the published version of the manuscript.

Funding: This research received no external funding.

Institutional Review Board Statement: The study has been approved by Bio-Ethical Research Committee (BERC) at Prince Sattam Bin Abdulaziz University with reference number BERC-001-12-19 on 1 December 2019.

Data Availability Statement: Not applicable.

Acknowledgments: Authors of the paper are thankful to the Deanship of Scientific Research, Prince Sattam Bin Abdulaziz University, Al-Kharj, Saudi Arabia for supporting this research.

Conflicts of Interest: The authors declare no conflict of interest.

References

1. Vasisht, K.; Kumar, V. *Compendium of Medicinal and Aromatic Plants*; ICS-UNIDO: Trieste, Italy, 2004; Volume 1, p. 124.
2. Saeidnia, S.; Gohari, A.; Mokhber-Dezfuli, N.; Kiuchi, F. A review on phytochemistry and medicinal properties of the genus *Achillea*. *DARU J. Fac. Pharm. Tehran Univ. Med. Sci.* **2011**, *19*, 173–186.

3. Abdel-Azim, N.S.; Shams, K.A.; Shahat, A.A.; El Missiry, M.M.; Ismail, S.I.; Hammouda, F.M. Egyptian herbal drug industry: Challenges and future prospects. *Res. J. Med. Plant.* **2011**, *5*, 136–144. [CrossRef]
4. Rawashdeh, I.M. Genetic diversity analysis of *Achillea fragrantissima* (Forskal) Schultz Bip. Populations collected from different regions of Jordan using RAPD Markers. *Jordan J. Biol. Sci.* **2011**, *4*, 21–28.
5. Eissa, T.A.F.; Palomino, O.M.; Carretero, M.E.; Gómez-Serranillos, M.P. Ethnopharmacological study of medicinal plants used in the treatment of CNS disorders in Sinai Peninsula, Egypt. *J. Ethnopharmacol.* **2014**, *151*, 317–332. [CrossRef]
6. Available online: https://www.mosoah.com/health/alternative-and-natural-medicine (accessed on 10 October 2022).
7. Awad, B.M.; Abd-Alhaseeb, M.M.; Habib, E.S.; Ibrahim, A.K.; Ahmed, S.A. Antitumor activity of methoxylated flavonoids separated from *Achillea fragrantissima* extract in Ehrlich's ascites carcinoma model in mice. *J. Herbmed. Pharmacol.* **2020**, *9*, 28–34. [CrossRef]
8. Ahmed, W.; Aburjai, T.; Hudaib, M.; Al-Karablieh, N. Chemical Composition of Essential Oils Hydrodistilled from Aerial Parts of *Achillea fragrantissima* (Forssk.) Sch. Bip. and *Achillea santolina* L. (Asteraceae) Growing in Jordan. *J. Essent. Oil Bear. Plants* **2020**, *23*, 15–25. [CrossRef]
9. Harris, B. Technology, and Application. In *Handbook of Essential Oils*; Can Baser, K.H., Buchbauer, G., Eds.; CRC Press: Boca Raton, FL, USA; Taylor & Francis Group: New York, NY, USA, 2010; pp. 315–351.
10. Horváth, G.; Ács, K. Essential oils in the treatment of respiratory tract diseases highlighting their role in bacterial infections and their anti-inflammatory action: A review. *Flavour Fragr. J.* **2015**, *30*, 331–341. [CrossRef]
11. *European Pharmacopoea*, 5th ed.; Directorate for the Quality of Medicines of the Council of Europe: Strasburg, France, 2004; Volume 2, pp. 1004, 1108, 1570, 2206, 2534, 2569.
12. NRC (National Research Council). *Guide for the Care and Use of Laboratory Animals*; National Academy Press: Washington, DC, USA, 1996; pp. 1–7.
13. Venkatasamy, R.; Spina, D. Novel relaxant effects of RPL554 on guinea pig tracheal smooth muscle contractility. *Br. J. Pharmacol.* **2016**, *173*, 2335–2351. [CrossRef]
14. Holroyde, M. The influence of epithelium on the responsiveness of guinea-pig isolated trachea. *Br. J. Pharmacol.* **1986**, *87*, 501–507. [CrossRef]
15. Van-Rossum, J.M. Cumulative dose response curves. II. Technique for making of dose-response curves in isolated organs and the evaluation of drug parameters. *Arch. Int. Pharmacodyn. Ther.* **1963**, *143*, 299–330.
16. Goldberg, L.A.; Rucker, F.J. Opposing effects of atropine and timolol on the color and luminance emmetropization mechanisms in chicks. *Vis. Res.* **2016**, *122*, 1–11. [CrossRef] [PubMed]
17. Abdel-Kader, M.S.; Rehman, N.U.; Alghafis, M.A.; Al-Matri, M.A. Brochodilator Phenylpropanoid Glycosides from the Seeds of *Prunus mahaleb* L. *Rec. Nat. Prod.* **2022**, *5*, 443–453. [CrossRef]
18. Rehman, N.U.; Ansari, M.N.; Ahmad, W.; Ahamad, S.R. Dual inhibition of phosphodiesterase and Ca^{++} channels explain the medicinal use of *Balanites aegyptiaca* (L.) in hyperactive gut disorders. *Plants* **2022**, *11*, 1183. [CrossRef] [PubMed]
19. Palande, N.V.; Bhoyar, R.C.; Biswas, S.P.; Jadhao, A.G. Short-term exposure to L-type calcium channel blocker, verapamil, alters the expression pattern of calcium-binding proteins in the brain of goldfish, *Carassius auratus*. *Comp. Biochem. Physiol. C: Toxicol. Pharmacol.* **2015**, *176–177*, 31–43. [CrossRef] [PubMed]
20. Rehman, N.U.; Ansari, M.N.; Ahmad, W.; Samad, A. *In silico* and *ex vivo* studies on the spasmolytic activities of Fenchone using isolated guinea-pig trachea. *Molecules* **2022**, *27*, 1360. [CrossRef]
21. Cook, N.S. The pharmacology of potassium channels and their therapeutic potential. *Trend Pharmacol. Sci.* **1988**, *9*, 21–28. [CrossRef]
22. Satake, N.; Shibata, M.; Shibata, S. The inhibitory effects of iberiotoxin and 4-aminopyridine on the relaxation induced by beta1- and beta2-adrenoceptor activation in rat aortic rings. *Br. J. Pharmacol.* **1996**, *119*, 505–510. [CrossRef]
23. Frank, H.; Puschmann, A.; Schusdziarra, V.; Allescher, H.D. Functional evidence for a glibenclamide-sensitive K^+ channel in rat ileal smooth muscle. *Eur. J. Pharmacol.* **1994**, *271*, 379–386. [CrossRef]
24. Alqarni, M.H.; Salkini, A.A.; Abujheisha, K.Y.; Daghar, M.F.; Al-khuraif, F.A.; Abdel-Kader, M.S. Qualitative, quantitative and antimicrobial activity variations of the essential oils isolated from *Thymus Vulgaris* and *Micromeria Fruticosa* Samples Subjected to Different Drying Conditions. *Arab. J. Sci. Eng.* **2022**, *47*, 6861–6867. [CrossRef]
25. Althurwi, H.N.; Salkini, M.A.; Soliman, G.A.; Ansari, M.N.; Ibnouf, E.O.; Abdel-Kader, M.S. Wound Healing Potential of *Commiphora gileadensis* Stems Essential Oil and Chloroform Extract. *Separations* **2022**, *9*, 254. [CrossRef]
26. Dharmage, S.C.; Perret, J.L.; Custovic, A. Epidemiology of Asthma in Children and Adults. *Front. Pediatr.* **2019**, *7*, 246. [CrossRef] [PubMed]
27. Canning, B.J. Animal model of asthma and chronic obstructive pulmonary diseases. *Pulm. Pharmacol. Ther.* **2008**, *21*, 695. [CrossRef]
28. Mathewson, H.S. Anti-asthmatic properties of calcium antagonists. *Respir. Care* **1985**, *30*, 779–781.
29. Thirstrup, S. Control of airway tone: II-Pharmacology of relaxation. *Respir. Med.* **2000**, *94*, 519–528. [CrossRef] [PubMed]
30. Clement, Y.N.; Williams, A.F.; Aranda, D.; Chase, R.; Watson, N.; Mohammed, R.; Stubbs, O.; Williamson, D. Medicinal herb use among asthmatic patients attending a specialty care facility in Trinidad. *BMC Complement. Altern. Med.* **2005**, *5*, 3. [CrossRef]

31. Rehman, N.U.; Ansari, M.N.; Hailea, T.; Karim, A.; Abujheisha, K.Y.; Ahamad, S.R.; Imam, F. Possible tracheal relaxant and antimicrobial effects of the essential oil of Ethiopian *Thyme* specie (*Thymus serrulatus* Hoschst. Ex Benth.): A multiple mechanistic approach. *Front. Pharmacol.* **2021**, *12*, 615228. [CrossRef]
32. Arunlakhshana, O.; Schild, H.O. Some quantitative uses of drug antagonists. *Br. J. Pharmacol.* **1959**, *14*, 48–58. [CrossRef]
33. Gilani, A.H.; Khan, A.U.; Ali, T.; Ajmal, S. Mechanisms underlying the antispasmodic and bronchodilatory properties of *Terminalia bellerica* fruit. *J. Ethnopharmacol.* **2008**, *116*, 528–538. [CrossRef]
34. Twiss, M.A.; Harman, E.; Chesrown, S.; Hendeles, L. Efficacy of calcium channel blockers as maintenance therapy for asthma. *Br. J. Clin. Pharmacol.* **2002**, *53*, 243–249. [CrossRef]
35. Barnes, P.J. Drugs for asthma. *Br. J. Pharmacol.* **2006**, *147* (Suppl. 1), S297–S303. [CrossRef]
36. Rehman, N.U.; Khan, A.U.; Alkharfy, K.M.; Gilani, A.H. Pharmacological basis for the medicinal use of *Lepidium sativum* in airways disorders. *Evid.-Based Complement. Altern. Med.* **2012**, *2021*, 596524.
37. Gilani, A.H.; Khan, A.U.; Ghayur, M.N.; Ali, S.F.; Herzig, J.W. Antispasmodic effects of Rooibos tea (*Aspalathus linearis*) is mediated predominantly through K$^+$-channel activation. *Basic Clin. Pharmacol. Toxicol.* **2006**, *99*, 365–373. [CrossRef] [PubMed]
38. Khan, A.; Rehman, N.U.; AlKharfy, K.M.; Gilani, A.H. Antidiarrheal and antispasmodic activities of *Salvia officinalis* are mediated through activation of K+ channels. *Bangladesh J. Pharmacol.* **2011**, *6*, 111–116. [CrossRef]
39. Kishii, K.; Morimoto, T.; Nakajima, N.; Yamazaki, K.; Tsujitani, M.; Takayanagi, I. Effect of LP-805, a novel vasorelaxant agent, a potassium channel opener on rat thoracic aorta. *Gen. Pharmacol.* **1992**, *23*, 347–353. [CrossRef]
40. Okabe, K.; Kitamura, K.; Kuriyama, H. Feature of 4-aminopyridine sensitive outward current observed in single smooth muscle cells from the rabbit pulmonary artery. *Pflug. Arch.* **1987**, *409*, 561–568. [CrossRef]
41. Quest, U. Potassium channel openers: Pharmacological and clinical aspects. *Fund. Clin. Pharmacol.* **1992**, *6*, 279–293. [CrossRef]
42. Cunha, J.; Campestrini, F.; Calixto, J.; Scremin, A.; Paulino, N. The mechanism of gentisic acid-induced relaxation of the guinea pig isolated trachea: The role of potassium channels and vasoactive intestinal peptide receptors. *Braz. J. Med. Biol. Res.* **2001**, *34*, 381–388. [CrossRef]
43. Lenz, T.; Wagner, G. Potential role of potassium channel openers for the treatment of cardiovascular disease. In *Hypertension: Pathophysiology, Diagnosis and Management*; Laragh, J.H., Brenner, B.M., Eds.; Raven Press: New York, NY, USA, 1995; pp. 2953–2968.

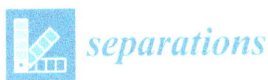 *separations*

Article

Efficient Removal of Eriochrome Black T Dye Using Activated Carbon of Waste Hemp (*Cannabis sativa* L.) Grown in Northern Morocco Enhanced by New Mathematical Models

Fouad El Mansouri [1,*], Guillermo Pelaz [2], Antonio Morán [2], Joaquim C. G. Esteves Da Silva [3], Francesco Cacciola [4,*], Hammadi El Farissi [5], Hatim Tayeq [6], Mohammed Hassani Zerrouk [7] and Jamal Brigui [1]

[1] Research Team: Materials, Environment and Sustainable Development (MEDD), Faculty of Sciences and Techniques of Tangier, BP 416, Tangier 90000, Morocco
[2] Chemical and Environmental Bioprocess Engineering Group, Natural Resources Institute, University of León, 24071 León, Spain
[3] Centro de Investigação Em Química (CIQUP), Instituto De Ciências Moleculares (IMS), Departamento De Geociências, Ambiente e Ordenamento Do Território, Faculdade De Ciências, Universidade Do Porto, Rua Do Campo Alegre S/N, 4169-007 Porto, Portugal
[4] Department of Biomedical, Dental, Morphological and Functional Imaging Sciences, University of Messina, 98125 Messina, Italy
[5] Laboratory of Environment and Applied Chemistry of the Natural Resources and Processes, Department of Chemistry, Faculty of Sciences, Mohamed First University, BP 524, Oujda 60000, Morocco
[6] MAE2D Laboratory, Polydisciplinary Faculty of Larache, Abdelmalek Essaadi University, Tetouan 93020, Morocco
[7] Environmental Technologies, Biotechnology and Valorisation of Bio-Resources Team, TEBVB, FSTH, Abdelmalek Essaadi University, Tetouan 93020, Morocco
* Correspondence: fouad.elmansouri@etu.uae.ac.ma (F.E.M.); cacciolaf@unime.it (F.C.); Tel.: +212-662-102-847 (F.E.M.); +39-090-676-6570 (F.C.)

Citation: El Mansouri, F.; Pelaz, G.; Morán, A.; Da Silva, J.C.G.E.; Cacciola, F.; El Farissi, H.; Tayeq, H.; Zerrouk, M.H.; Brigui, J. Efficient Removal of Eriochrome Black T Dye Using Activated Carbon of Waste Hemp (*Cannabis sativa* L.) Grown in Northern Morocco Enhanced by New Mathematical Models. *Separations* 2022, 9, 283. https://doi.org/10.3390/separations9100283

Academic Editor: Ernesto Reverchon

Received: 15 August 2022
Accepted: 29 September 2022
Published: 3 October 2022

Publisher's Note: MDPI stays neutral with regard to jurisdictional claims in published maps and institutional affiliations.

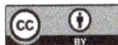

Highlights:

- The use of inexpensive, easily obtained, and ecological adsorbents.
- New bio-adsorbents were made for Colorant adsorption from an aqueous solution.
- EBT dye adsorption capacities ranged from 1.8 to 2.8 mg.g^{-1}.
- Adsorptions of EBT dye by the activated carbon of cannabis.
- This study provides cost effective and sustainable production of activated carbon.
- Application of mathematical modeling to develop new relevant mathematical models based on experimental results.

Abstract: In the present work, the adsorption behavior of Eriochrome Black T (EBT) on waste hemp activated carbon (WHAC) was examined. The surface of the WHAC was modified by H_3PO_4 acid treatment. The surface and structural characterization of the adsorbents was carried out using Fourier transform infrared spectroscopy (FTIR), and scanning electron microscopy (SEM) analysis. The effect of influential adsorption parameters (pH, contact time, dosage, and initial concentration) on the adsorption of EBT onto WHAC was examined in batch experiments; some adsorption parameters such as pH, concentration and dose were improved by new mathematical models. The adsorption behavior of EBT on the surfaces of WHAC was evaluated by applying different isotherm models (Langmuir, Freundlich, Temkin and Dubinin–Radushkevich) to equilibrium data. The adsorption kinetics was studied by using pseudo-first-order, pseudo-second-order, Elovich and intraparticle models on the model. Adsorption followed the pseudo-second-order rate kinetics. The maximum removal of EBT was found to be 44–62.08% by WHAC at pH = 7, adsorbent dose of 10–70 mg, contact time of 3 h and initial dye concentration of 10 mg.L^{-1}. The maximum adsorption capacities were 14.025 mg.g^{-1} obtained by calculating according to the Langmuir model, while the maximum removal efficiency was obtained at 70 mg equal to 62.08% for the WHAC. The adsorption process is physical in the monolayer and multilayer.

Keywords: cannabis waste; isotherms; Eriochrome black T; biosorbent; mathematical models

1. Introduction

Hemp or (*Cannabis sativa* L.), is an annual herbaceous plant, belonging to the family of Cannabaceae, and originating in Central Asia. Regardless of its origin, hemp is commonly grown and cultivated not only in Asian countries [1] but in Africa, Europe, Canada, and the United States, and is one of the oldest cultivated plants known to humans. Since 5000–4000 BC, [2], it has been used as a food and fiber source, as well as playing an important role in medical use. It contains several chemically bioactive compounds, such as cannabinoids, terpenoids, flavonoids, and alkaloids [3]. It contains more than 100 active chemical compounds well-known as 'cannabinoids' [4].

Waste is a major worldwide problem and produces severe ecological and socio-economic troubles. The exploitation of waste has become of vast scientific and industrial importance in order to reduce ecological harm, attain sustainability and progress, apropos a circular economy. Energy, fuels, and other value-added products can be recuperated from waste [5]. Moreover, owing to the fast growth in the quantity and nature of agricultural waste biomass, which comes from the growth of population and rigorous agricultural behaviors, these wastes are deemed as a consequential cause of pollution with an annual growth frequency of 5–10%. People produce about 150 billion metric tons of agricultural waste [6].

As a biological and ecological alternative, the application of agro-waste as precursors of materials with high adsorptive abilities is being explored [7]. Bio-adsorbents (bioproducts) are natural elements suitable for water treatment in view of the many benefits and remarkable characteristics of these assets. They are ample, inexhaustible, decomposable, and economic [8], moreover, they have macromolecular chains with various extremely reactive chemical functions [9]. In addition, adsorption is designed within the effective methods for the elimination of water contaminants because of its facility of function and the aptitude to eliminate various kinds of contaminants, providing larger application in water quality management [10].

Amid the diversity of adsorbents, activated carbon has been demonstrated to remain efficient in the elimination of contaminants from water and even in a gaseous atmosphere [11] Activated carbon, a commonly used adsorbent in industrial procedures, is constituted of a pored, consistent organization with a great surface area and displays radiation stability [12]. On the other hand, its application is restricted because it is expensive and very difficult to be regenerated [13,14]. Therefore, an investigation of the fabrication of activated carbon from inexhaustible, inexpensive native farming waste has won interest due to its reduced cost and extremely plentiful qualities [15,16]; in this context, certain of the farming wastes that have been investigated as an alternative source of activated carbon are barley seeds [17], orange peel [18], cassava peel [19], eucalyptus bark [20], coconut shells [21], hazel nuts [22], and tobacco steam [23].

Eriochrome Black T (EBT) is one of the colorants that are employed in water hardness resolution, in the production of paper and textiles, and also in the biomedical research field [24]. It was identified as a water pollutant which causes substantial damage to the environment. EBT is an organic azo colorant that is tolerant to natural treatment as most azo colorants are, due to their aromatic rings and sulfonate groups. Even at reduced amounts, it is not easily decayed by chemical or bacterial deterioration [25].

The overall objective of this study is to report the synthesis and characterization of hemp waste (*Cannabis sativa* L.) and its activated carbon. The as-synthesized materials were used as adsorbents for the removal of Eriochrome Black T dye in an aqueous solution. The effects of various experimental parameters on the adsorption of the dye were examined. The adsorption parameters (pH, concentration, and dose) were improved by new mathematical models obtained with a polynomial interpolation.

2. Materials and Methods

In the current study, activated carbon was geared up from residues of *Cannabis sativa* L. with the saturation of a chemical activating agent at reduced temperatures. We note there are only a few limited studies on the elimination of Eriochrome Black T dye using *Cannabis sativa* L. activated carbon as an adsorbent. All chemicals employed in this work were of analytical grade and were used without additional purification.

2.1. Preparation of Waste Hemp Activated Carbon (WHAC)

The method of preparation applied for the WHAC has two steps: carbonization and activation, as already described in our previous works [26,27]. After impregnation, to remove any excess of phosphoric acid, the solid was filtered under a vacuum. Then afterwards the waste hemp powder was pyrolyzed at 600 °C for 90 min in a muffle furnace (PR Series Hobersal). Furthermore, the carbon was completely washed with ultra-pure water to remove the remaining phosphoric acid until reaching a pH of (6.5). Lastly, the solids were dried in the oven at 105 °C for 24 h

2.2. Characterization of the Activated Carbon

In order to approximate the temperature of distribution at which waste hemp responds under a latent climate, a thermogravimetric analysis (TGA) was applied. Thermal analyses were conducted with STD 2960 TA and SDT Q600 instruments under a nitrogen flow of 100 mL/min. A temperature ramp of 10 °C/min from room temperature to 800 °C was employed during the analyses.

FTIR spectroscopy was used to examine the surface functionalities. A Thermo IS5 Nicolet (USA) spectrophotometer was used to obtain FTIR spectra, acquired from 400 to 4000 cm^{-1} at room temperature (16 scans and spectral resolution of 4 cm^{-1}); the peak positions were revealed using Origin software (Version 2021). Origin Lab Corporation, Northampton, MA, USA.

2.3. Functional Group Analysis by FTIR

To characterize the different functional groups at the surface of the precursor and the prepared activated carbon, FTIR spectra of the various materials (EBTA, WHAC, WHNAC, WH, WHAFC) were recorded between 4000 cm^{-1} to 400 cm^{-1}. Figure 1 depicts the obtained spectrum. From this figure, the precursor presents vibration bands around 607.46, 691.12, 862.02, 953.62; 1028.83, 1086.69, 1230.20, 1306.5, 1394.28, 1616.05, 1741.4, 2851.52, 2920.66 and 3291.89 cm^{-1}. The infrared spectrum of the mixture remaining after the adsorption of the EBTA colorant displays a total absence of the waves linked to the dye, obtaining two bungs which correspond to the water molecule, one bung at 3291.89 cm^{-1} and the other at 1616.05 cm^{-1}. On one hand, the WHAC carbonization and the WHAFC activation of the carbon present cyclic carbon compounds, and functional groups have disappeared such as alcohols, ketones, and aldehydes. On the other hand, the biomass is rich in witness groups and also present in addition to the OH groups linked to 3300 cm^{-1}. The table indicates the different leaves that contain cannabis. The other bonds are grouped in Table 1, where:

EBT-A: Eriochrome Black T after adsorption and filtration.
WHAC: waste hemp activated carbon.
WHNAC: waste hemp non-activated carbon.
WH: waste hemp (*Cannabis sativa* L.).
WHAFC: waste hemp activated carbon after adsorption.

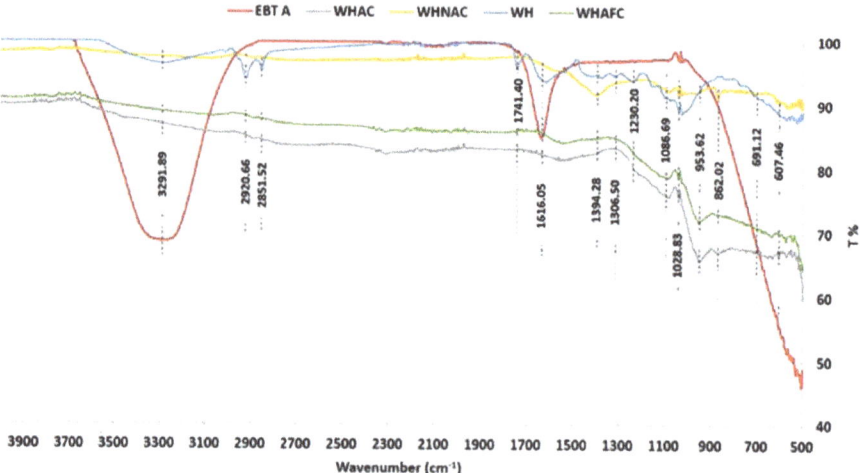

Figure 1. FTIR (Fourier transform infrared spectroscopy) spectra.

Table 1. FTIR analysis of WHAC.

Bond Type	Functional Group	Wave Numbers Range (cm^{-1})	
		σ_{th}	σ_{exp}
C-H	Alkane	2850–2925	2920.66
			2851.52
C=O	Aliphatic Ketone	1710–1735	1741.40
C-H	Aldehyde	1370–1390	1394.28
C-OH	Third Alcohol	1110–1250	1230.20
			1146.47
C-H	Cycloalkane	1012–1031	1028.83
=C-H (E)	Alkene	950–1010	953.62
Ar-C	Aromatic	850–890	862.02
=C-H (Z)	Alkene	650–750	691.12

2.4. SEM/EDX

SEM micrographs and elemental analysis spectra of various prepared materials shown in Figure 2 show that all the materials have cracks and pores on their surfaces. This may be due to the escape of gases released during the carbonization process [28,29]. As the rate of impregnation increases, the development of cracks and pores becomes more pronounced. The prepared materials consist mainly of carbon (47.85 to 54.70%), oxygen (28.72 to 36.57%), phosphorus (0.35 to 12.14%), calcium (0.88 to 6.41%), and silicon (0.27 to 1.09%). Other elements such as magnesium, aluminum, sulfur, potassium, and sodium are present in the form of traces, in Figure 3. The high carbon content coupled with the porous structure of all the materials prepared are important criteria for an adsorbent suitable for the elimination of colorants and heavy metals in an aqueous media [30].

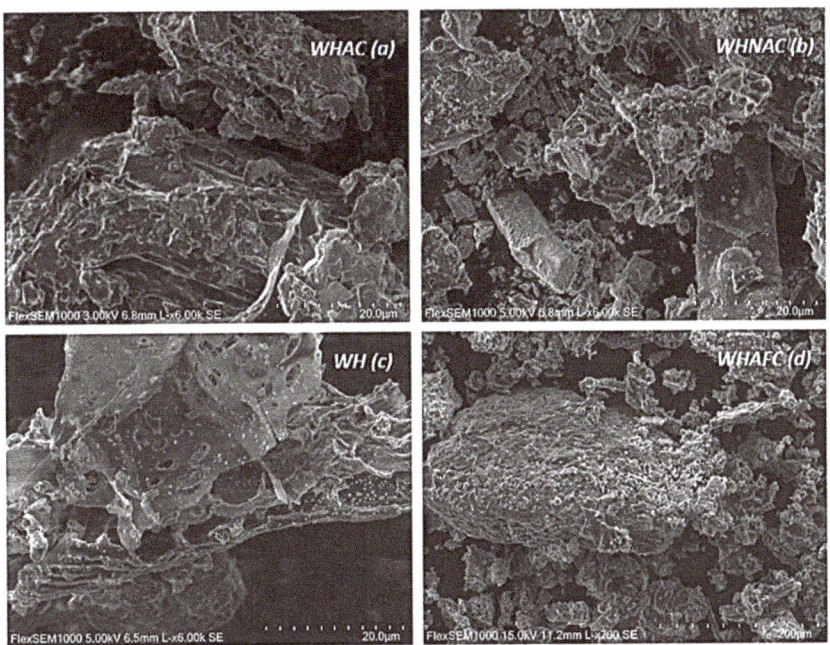

Figure 2. SEM (scanning electron microscopy) micrographs.

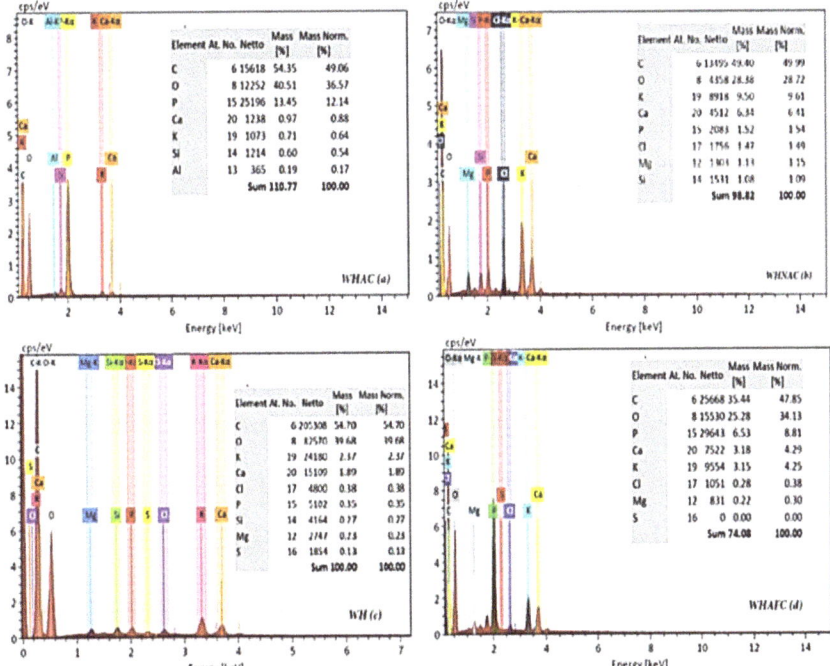

Figure 3. EDXA (energy dispersive X-ray analysis) diffractograms.

2.5. TGA/DTA Analysis

The waste hemp (*Cannabis sativa* L.) thermal performance was examined employing thermogravimetric analysis (TGA) and differential scanning calorimetry (DSC). Figure 4 depicts the TGA/DSC curve of WH for the heating rate of 50 °C/min. As a result, the thermal decomposition of WH was detected at three phases. The first phase occurs from room temperature to about 125 °C with a corresponding weight loss of 9.9%. The endothermic process that takes place at 81 °C could be assigned to the vaporization of water. The low value of weight loss at this stage is a result of the low moisture content of WH. In the second phase, which extends up to about 320 °C, the weight loss has considerably increased to a value of 56.33%. At this stage, the broad and intense exothermic peak detected at 304 °C can be attributed to the decomposition of celluloses, hemicelluloses, and part of lignin. According to Haykiri et al. [31], hemicellulose and part of lignin decomposes in the range 265–310 °C. During the third phase, there is a narrow peak centered at 405 °C which relates to the degradation of residual lignin. This phase corresponds to the combustion of released gases during the decomposition of lignin. In this phase, the mass loss was lower than in the previous phase corresponding to 31.07%. The shoulder at 373 °C corresponds to the transition from the combustion of celluloses to lignin [32]. Above 505 °C the weight loss becomes constant. This shows that all the lignocellulosic content has been decomposed. Therefore, T = 505 °C appears as a minimum temperature to produce WH-based activated carbon.

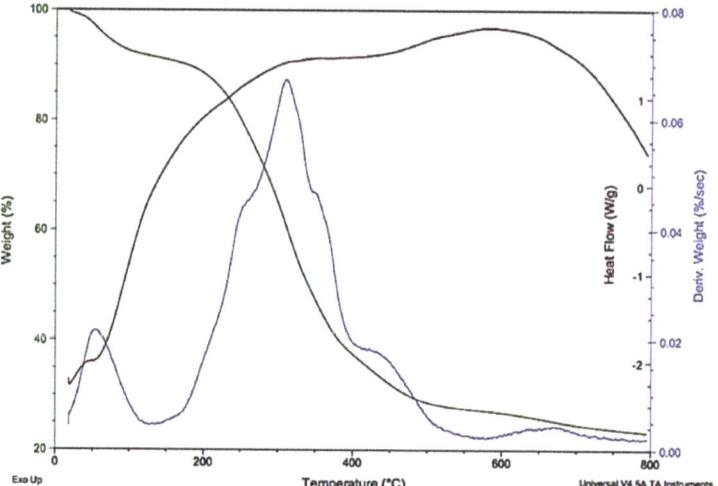

Figure 4. TGA/DTA Analysis.

3. Experimental Procedure

The adsorption tests were conducted, in triplicate, by adding 10 mg of activated carbon to 25 mL of the mixture, containing EBT dye. The stock concentration of the three mixtures was diluted to draw the calibration curve in a concentration range of EBT dye (from 10 to 70 mg.L^{-1}), and the absorbance measured using a spectrophotometer. The tests were disposed on a shaker with a stirring speed of 150 rpm. For adsorption kinetics, samples were taken at time intervals varying from 20 to 160 min, centrifuged for 2 min at 3000 rpm, and then the absorbance was measured. Regarding the isothermal tests, the initial concentrations used were 10; 20; 30; 40; 50; 60; and 70 mg.L^{-1}. Samples were taken after an equilibrium time of 90 min. The quantity of EBT adsorbed per gram of activated carbon q_e (mg.g^{-1}), was determined based on the following formula:

$$q_e = \frac{(C_i - C_e) \times V}{M} \tag{1}$$

$$R\% = \frac{(C_i - C_e)}{C_i} * 100 \qquad (2)$$

where C_i and C_e are the initial and final ion concentrations, respectively, expressed in (mg.L^{-1}). V is the volume in liters of the solution and M represents the mass of activated carbon in (g), and R%: removal.

4. Results and Discussion

4.1. pH Effect

Figure 5 shows the effect of pH on the elimination of the dye, it is observed that with the increase in pH the quantity adsorbed reduces this decrease due to the presence of ions (H$^+$) which causes the birth of protonation of the OH groups to dye in the acid medium by elimination of the water molecule and formation of a cycle of seven with two nitrogen atoms. In the basic medium, the existence of ions (HO$^-$) in the solution inhibits the adsorption of the dye on the surface of the cannabis and the adsorption becomes very hard with a minimum quantity of 1.7 mg.g^{-1} at pH = 12.

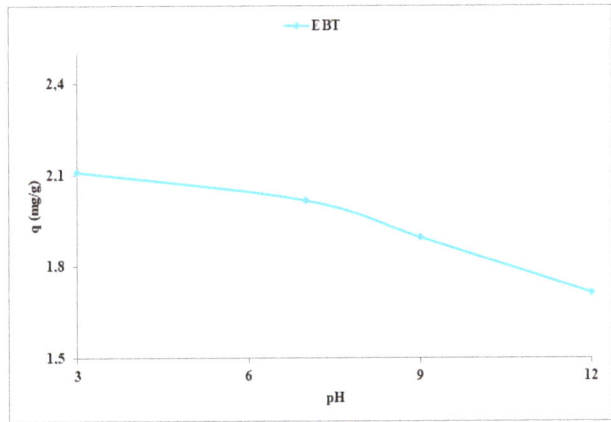

Figure 5. pH effect on the adsorption of EBT dye by activated carbon of cannabis (t = 90 min, T = 20 $\pm$ 1 °C, adsorbent dose 10 mg, (C_0 = 10 mg.L^{-1}), stirring speed = 150 rpm.

We present in (Equation (3)) the formula for predicting adsorption as a function of pH. This formula is obtained using polynomial interpolation. The interpolation error is given by the formula (Equation (4)).

$$Ad = 9.25926e - 5 \times pH^3 - 5.92593e - 3 \times pH^2 + 2.69444 \times pH + 2.07 \qquad (3)$$

where, Ad is the value of the adsorption

$$\forall x \in [pH_{min}, pH_{max}] \, we \, have, \; Er = \frac{Ad^{(n+1)}(x)}{(n+1)!} \prod_{i=0}^{n}(x - pH_i) \qquad (4)$$

where Er is the interpolation error, n is the polynomial degree. pH_{min} and pH_{max} are, respectively, the minimum and maximum pH values in the experiment. pH_i is the nth value of pH in the experiment. $Ad^{(n)}$ is the nth derivative of Ad, and $n! = n \times (n-1) \times \cdots \times 2 \times 1$. Figure 6 shows the comparison of the results of our model (Equation (3)) and the observed results.

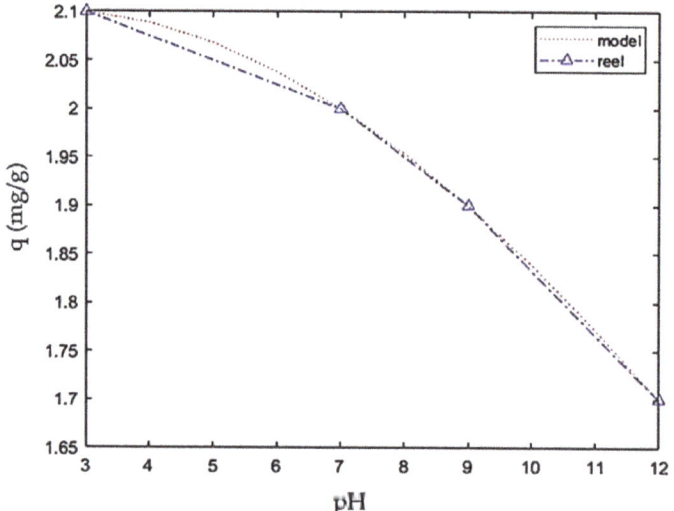

Figure 6. Comparison between the mathematical model (Equation (3)) and the observed results.

The coefficients in (Equation (3)) are calculated using the Lagrange interpolation formula given by:

$$Ad(pH) = \sum_{j=0}^{n} pH_i \left(\prod_{i=0, i \neq j}^{n} \frac{pH - pH_i}{pH_j - pH_i} \right)$$

4.2. Dose Effect

The histogram presented in Figure 7 gives the effect of the dose of cannabis on the elimination of the dye; it is observed that the yield increases with the increase in mass, this yield goes through 44.12% for m = 10 mg then continuously increases up to a yield of 60% when m = 40 mg, but for masses m > 50 mg the yield remains almost constant, fixed at 62% at this moment in equilibrium.

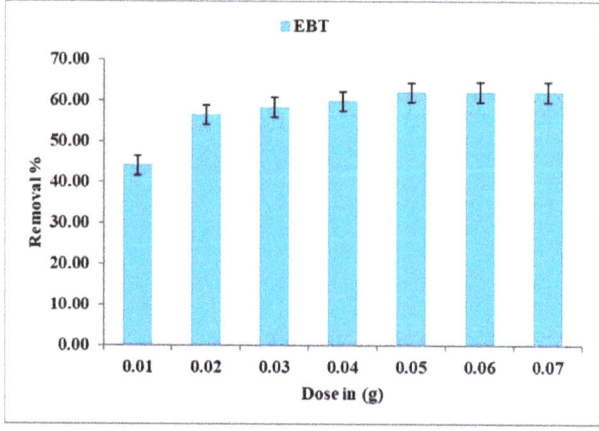

Figure 7. Influence of the mass of activated carbon of cannabis on adsorption of EBT dye (stirring speed = 150 rpm, t = 90 min, pH = 7 ± 0.2; C_0 = 10 mg.L^{-1} and temperature = 20 ± 1 °C).

The mathematical model describing the effect of the mass of the activated carbon on the adsorption of EBT is given by the formula (Equation (5)).

$$Re = 2.92222 \times 10^9 \times d^6 - 6.53083 \times 10^8 \times d^5 + 5.60264 \times 10^7 \times d^4$$
$$-2.31604 \times 10^6 \times d^3 + 47473.1 \times d^2 - 183.715 \times d + 0.673 \quad (5)$$

where Re is the removal and d is the dose in g. This formula is obtained by using the same technique used in (Equation (3)). We give in Figure 8 the comparison between our new mathematical model and the detected findings.

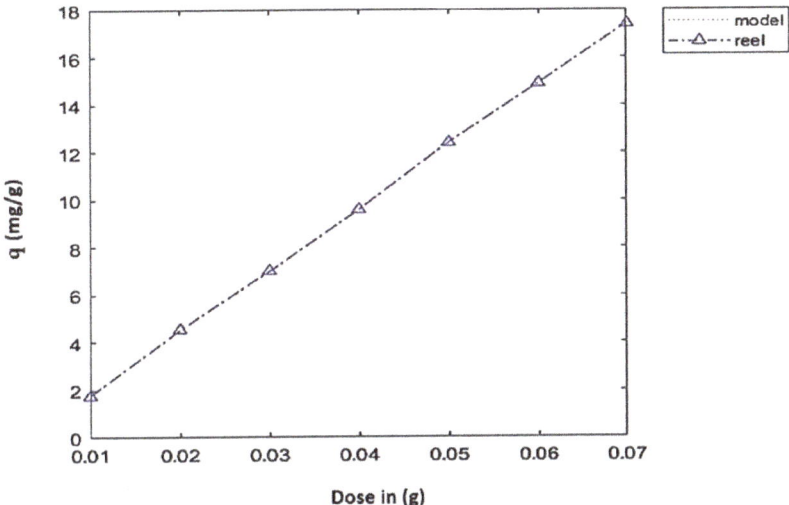

Figure 8. Comparison between the mathematical model and the observed results.

4.3. Effect of the Initial Concentration

With the aim to identify the impact of the preliminary concentration of EBT dye suggested for these studies on retention phenomena, solutions of 100 mL were prepared at different concentrations of metal ions between 10 to 70 mg.L^{-1}. The achieved results are presented in Figure 9 below. The illustrious results show that the adsorbed amount of EBT dye increases with increasing initial concentration. In fact, after an equilibrium time of 90 min, the adsorption capacity registers an increase from 2.21 to 10.17 mg.g^{-1}, for concentrations from 10 to 70 mg.L^{-1}. This action is explained by the fact that the more the concentration of EBT dye increases, the more the number of molecules in the solution increases, involving a higher absorption capacity [33–35].

The mathematical model describing the effect of the initial concentration of EBT dye adsorption by activated carbon of cannabis is given by the formula (Equation (6)).

$$q_e = -\frac{11 \times c^6}{7.2e8} + \frac{91 \times c^5}{2.4e7} - \frac{107 \times c^4}{2.88e4} + \frac{291 \times c^3}{1.6e4} - \frac{1.6657 \times c^2}{3.6e4} + \frac{1753 \times c}{300} - 25 \quad (6)$$

where q_e is the amount adsorbed at equilibrium and c is the initial concentration of EBT in mg/L. This formula is obtained by using the same technique used in (Equation (3)).

The comparison between our new mathematical model and the observed results is given in Figure 10.

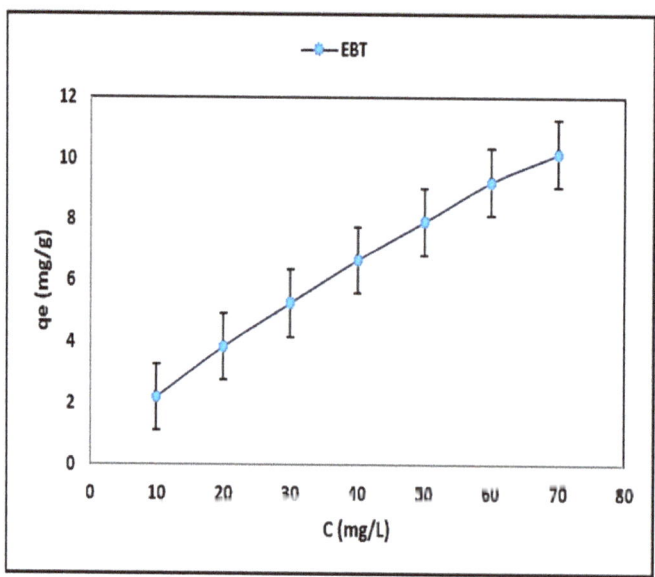

Figure 9. Effect of initial concentration of EBT dye adsorption by activated carbon of cannabis (t = 90 min, T = 20 ± 1 °C, adsorbent dose 10 mg, stirring= 150 rpm and pH = 7 ± 0.2).

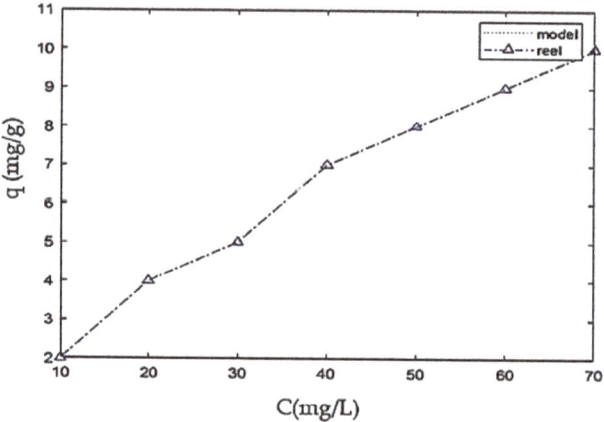

Figure 10. Comparison between the mathematical model and the observed results.

4.4. Effect of Contact Time

The adsorptions of Eriochrome Black T (EBT) by activated carbons obtained from hemp waste (*Cannabis sativa* L.) were studied at different time intervals (20 to 160 min) and a fixed amount of 10 mg.L^{-1}. Figure 11 shows that the absorption speed is fast during the first 20 to 60 min, and afterwards proceeds at a slower rate with a constant phenomenon of adsorption–desorption until the 100 min. After this period, the amount adsorbed did not change significantly. The initial rapid reaction is due to many vacant sites available at the initial stage; as a result, there is an increased concentration gradient between the adsorbate in the solution and the adsorbate in the adsorbent. Generally, the rapid initial adsorption results in a surface reaction. Slower adsorption ensues as available adsorption sites decrease with increasing occupancy and repulsive forces between favorable negatively charged dye (EBT) adsorption due to electrostatic attraction molecules on the phase's solid and bulk [36]. The maximum absorption of EBT after reaching pseudo-equilibrium was 1.9 mg/g.

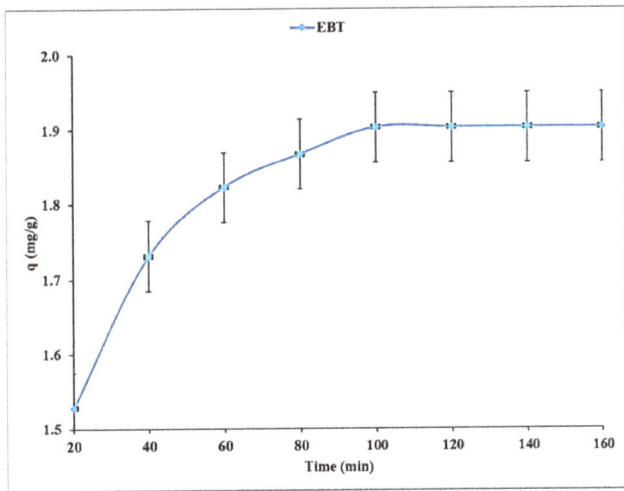

Figure 11. Effect of contact time of EBT dye adsorption by activated carbon of cannabis (T = 20 ± 1 °C, adsorbent dose 10 mg, C_0 = 10 mg.L^{-1}, stirring speed = 150 rpm and pH = 7 ± 0.2).

4.5. Effect of Temperature

The following figure represents the effect of temperature on the amount adsorbed by EBT on cannabis. From Figure 12, we observe that the temperature is a kinetic factor favoring the adsorption of the dye and also that the quantity adsorbed increases from 1.89 to 2 mg.g^{-1} when the temperature increases from 293°K to 313°K, then the continuous adsorbed amount increases up to 2.2 mg.g^{-1} when the temperature equals 333°K. This increase is owing to the effect of vibration of the dye molecules with the increase in shock numbers on the surface of the cannabis. Therefore, the adsorption of the examined ions seems to be an endothermic phenomenon. This could be also due to a relative increase in the mobility of ions in solution, which improves their exposure to active adsorption sites on the one hand and sends them to difficult-to-access sites on the other.

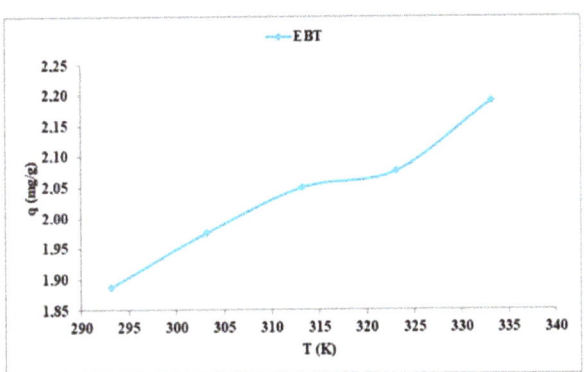

Figure 12. Effect of temperature of EBT dye adsorption by activated carbon of cannabis (adsorbent dose 10 mg, C_0 = 10 mg.L^{-1}, stirring speed = 150 rpm and pH = 7 ± 0.2).

4.6. Modeling of Adsorption Isotherms

To obtain the adsorption isotherm, a series of Erlenmeyer flasks were employed. In each Erlenmeyer were poured 25 mL of EBT solution dye of varying concentrations: 10; 20; 30; 40; 50; 60 and 70 mg.L^{-1}. The adsorption equilibrium study was carried out under the same optimum conditions mentioned above. After equilibration, the particles of the adsorbent were separated by centrifugation and the clarified mixture was analyzed by determination of the equilibrium concentration (C_e) of EBT using the same calibration curve used previously. The quantity of the adsorbed reagent at equilibrium (q_e, in mg.g^{-1}) was calculated by an equation (Equation (1)).

The following four conventional models, in their linear forms, are used to describe the adsorption isotherms:

The four models tested in this adsorption are presented by their nonlinear equation and also their linear form.

The Langmuir model (Equation (7)) is linearized according to the form given in (Equations (8) and (9)) [37,38] the linear form of the Freundlich model (Equation (9)) [39,40], the Temkin model (Equation (10)) [41], and finally the Dubinin–Radushkevich model (Equation (11)) [42], the potential of Polanyi (Equation (12)) energy (Equation (13)) [43]

$$q_e = \frac{q_m \, K_L C_e}{1 + K_L C_e} \tag{7}$$

$$\left(\frac{1}{q_e}\right) = \frac{1}{q_m K_L}\left(\frac{1}{C_e}\right) + \frac{1}{q_m} \tag{8}$$

$$R_L = \frac{1}{1 + K_L C_0} \tag{9}$$

$$Ln \, q_e = \frac{1}{n} Ln \, C_e + Ln \, K_F \tag{10}$$

$$q_e = \frac{RT}{b} Ln \, C_e + \frac{RT}{b} Ln \, K_T \tag{11}$$

$$Ln \, q_e = -K_D \, \varepsilon^2 + Ln \, q_m \tag{12}$$

$$\varepsilon = RTLn\left(1 + \frac{1}{C_e}\right) \tag{13}$$

$$E = \frac{1}{\sqrt{2K_D}} \tag{14}$$

Figure 13 represents the representation of the four linear forms of these isotherms and the choice of the model is subject to the correlation factor of the experimental points.

The linearization and the graphic representation of the four models tested in this study, and the obtained results synthesized in Table 2 above, indicate that the value of the linear correlation coefficient for the Freundlich model is closer to 1 for the EBT dye studied; these results also show the high value of the maximum adsorption capacity for the Langmuir model was 14.03 mg.g^{-1}. Similarly, some studies were written on the absorption phenomena of other such ions and dyes [44–52] (Table 3).

4.7. Modeling of Adsorption Kinetics

To evaluate the reaction parameters, a modeling of the adsorption kinetics is essential for the identification of the chemical or physical mechanisms that control the rate of adsorption. Four models are employed to link the experimental data of the absorption kinetics of the studied systems, namely pseudo-first order, pseudo-second order, and intraparticle diffusion models. Figure 14 and Table 4 show the adsorption Kinetics obtained in this study.

Table 2. Constant adsorption of four isotherms models of EBT dye on activated carbon of cannabis (T = 20 ± 1 °C, mass of adsorbent = 10 mg, stirring speed = 150 rpm and pH = 7 ± 0.2).

Isotherm Models	Constants	Activated Carbon of Cannabis
Langmuir	R^2	**0.9904**
	R_L	0.2636–0.7143
	K_L (L.mg^{-1})	0.0399
	q_m (mg.g^{-1})	14.025
Freundlich	R^2	**0.9996**
	K_F	0.8052
	n	1.4892
Temkin	R^2	**0.9545**
	K_T (L.g^{-1})	0.00012
	B_1 (J.mol^{-1})	3.4945
	b	697.096
Dubinin–Radushkevich	R^2	0.7805
	K_{ad} (mol^2.Kj^{-2}) × 10^{-5}	0.5
	E (Kj.mol^{-1})	316.2277
	q_m (mg.g^{-1})	7.5754

Table 3. The adsorption capacity of dyes and heavy metals in aqueous solutions by activated carbons of different biomass.

Adsorbate	Adsorbent Pollutants	Dose (mg)	C_0 (mg L^{-1})	pH	Kinetic	Isotherm	q_m (mg g^{-1})	Ref.
Zinc oxide-loaded activated char (ZnO-AC)	OG Rh-b	8–30	50	7	Pseudo-second-order	Langmuir	153.8 128.2	[46]
Rice straw (RS) biochar Wood chip (WC) biochar	CV-CR	01	500	7	Pseudo-second-order	Langmuir	620.3 195.6	[47]
Charcoal (tree branches) (BCA-TiO$_2$)	MB Cd^{2+}	** **	0.4 600	7 8	Pseudo-second-order	**	200 250	[48]
Sulfonated peanut shell (PNS-SO3H)	MB TC	20	900 ppm	10	Pseudo-second-order	Langmuir	1250 303	[49,50]
Shrimp shell (SS) Coal acid mine drainage (AMD)	Mn Fe	**	≤1 ≤15	6–9 5–9	Pseudo-second-order	Frendlich	17.43 3.87	[51]
Waste hemp activated carbon (WHAC)	EBT	10	10	7	Pseudo-second-order	Langmuir	14.025	This work

** Undetermined.

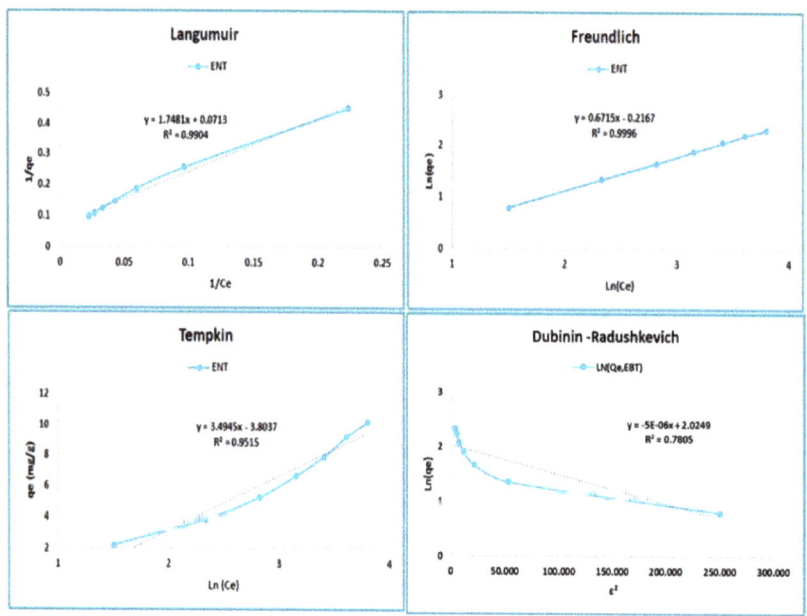

Figure 13. Langmuir, Freundlich, Temkin, and Dubinin–Radushkevich isotherm models curves of activated carbon of cannabis adsorption towards BET dye.

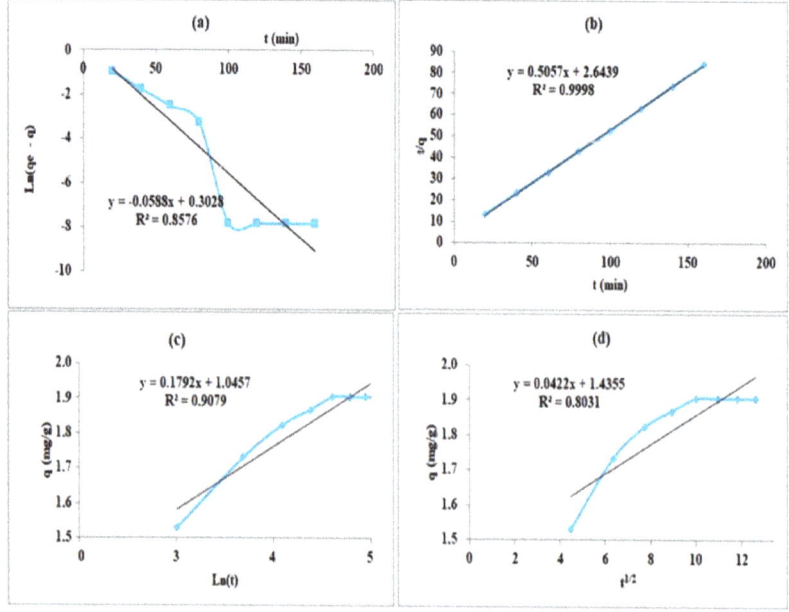

Figure 14. Adsorption kinetics models: (**a**) pseudo-first-order, (**b**) pseudo-second-order, (**c**) Elovich and (**d**) interparticle diffusion of BET dye on activated carbon of cannabis, (T = 20 ± 1 °C, adsorbent dose 10 mg, C_o = 10 mg.L^{-1}, stirring = 150 rpm and pH = 7 ± 0.2).

Table 4. Adsorption kinetics constants of BET dye on activated carbon cannabis (temperature = 20 ± 1 °C, mass of adsorbent = 10 mg, initial concentration of dye = 10 mg.L^{-1}; stirring speed = 150 rpm and pH = 7 ± 0.2).

Models	The Constants	Cannabis
Pseudo-first-order	R^2	0.8576
	K_1 (mL.min^{-1})	0.0588
	$q_{e,cal}$ (mg.g^{-1})	1.353
	$q_{e,exp}$ (mg.g^{-1})	1.903
Pseudo-second-order	R^2	0.9998
	K_2 (g.mg^{-1}.min^{-1})	0.0968
	$q_{e,cal}$ (mg.g^{-1})	1.9774
	$q_{e,exp}$ (mg.g^{-1})	1.903
Elovich	R^2	0.9079
	α (mg.g^{-1}.min^{-1})	45.4475
	β (g.mg^{-1})	5.5803
Intraparticle diffusion	R^2	0.8031
	K_i (mg.g^{-1}.min$^{0.5}$	0.0422
	C (mg.g^{-1})	1.4355

For a pseudo-first-order kinetics, Lagergen suggested in 1898 [53] the following equation:

$$\frac{dq}{dt} = K_1(q_e - q) \tag{15}$$

From the integration of (Equation (13)) and the application of the boundary conditions we find the following equation:

$$Ln(q_e - q_t) = Ln(q_e) - K_1 t \tag{16}$$

The pseudo-second-order model, or the Ho and Mckay model [54,55], turns out to be more appropriate for writing experimental data; this model is given by its following linear equation:

$$\frac{t}{q_t} = \frac{1}{K_2 q_e^2} + \left(\frac{1}{q_e}\right)t \tag{17}$$

The models established, respectively, by Morris and Weber and Urano Tachikawa [56] for internal diffusion were used with the aim of selecting the model or models best suited to the physical processes implicated in the adsorption of adsorbate on the activated carbon of cannabis used. This model is expressed in the following form:

$$q_t = K_i t^{\frac{1}{2}} + C \tag{18}$$

With: t the time in (min); q_e: the amount adsorbed at equilibrium (mg.g^{-1}); q_t: the quantity adsorbed at the instant t (mg.g^{-1}); K_1: the first-order rate constant (min^{-1}); K_2: the second-order rate constant (g.mg^{-1}.min^{-1}); C: the boundary layer thickness value (mg.g^{-1}); K_i: diffusion speed coefficient (min$^{-1/2}$).

4.8. Thermodynamic Study

The thermodynamic parameters were determined to qualify the phenomenon of absorption of EBT dye on activated carbon of cannabis. Thus, Gibbs free energy or free enthalpy of absorption; ΔG° (kJ.mol^{-1}), the enthalpy of adsorption; ΔH° (kJ.mol^{-1})

and adsorption entropy; $\Delta S°$ (KJ.mol^{-1}.K^{-1}) were calculated according to equations (Equations (18) and (19)) [52].

$$\Delta G^0 = -RT.Ln(K_d) \tag{19}$$

$$Ln(K_d) = -\frac{\Delta H^0}{RT} + \frac{\Delta S^0}{R} \tag{20}$$

$$K_d = \frac{q_e}{C_e} \tag{21}$$

where, K_d is the adsorption equilibrium constant, R is the gas constant perfect, and T is the temperature in (°K). From the results illustrated in Table 5 and Figure 15, the positive value of ($\Delta S°$) shows the good nature of the present adsorption phenomenon. Furthermore, positive values of ($\Delta G°$) show that the examined adsorption process is spontaneous up to a temperature of 60 °C. In addition, the positive value of ($\Delta H°$) demonstrates the endothermic nature of this phenomenon.

Table 5. Thermodynamics parameters data of EBT dye adsorption on activated carbon of cannabis.

Parameters		Cannabis
$\Delta H°$ (KJ.mol^{-1})		16.8467
$\Delta S°$ (J.mol^{-1}.K^{-1})		11.0808
$\Delta G°$ (kJ.mol^{-1})	T = 293°K	13.5999
	T = 303°K	13.48917
	T = 313°K	13.37838
	T = 323°K	13.26756
	T = 333°K	13.15675

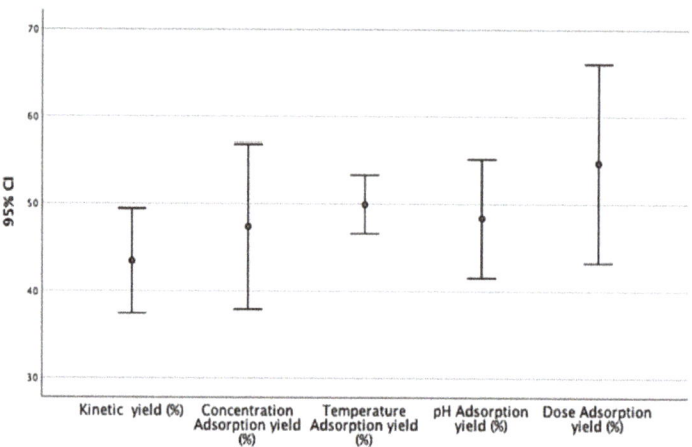

Figure 15. The 95% confidence intervals for the main analysis of influential adsorption parameters.

5. Conclusions

In this study, the performance of phosphoric acid-activated carbonaceous materials derived from waste hemp (*Cannabis sativa* L.) to remove Eriochrome Black T (EBT) from an aqueous mixture was investigated. The effects of the activator (liquid) to adsorbent (solid) on the textural, structural, and adsorption characteristics were investigated. The porosity of the adsorbents increased with increasing the activator: adsorbent ratios resulting in increased adsorption capacities. Equilibrium data were well explained by the Langmuir model with upper limit adsorption abilities of 14.03 mg.g^{-1} for WHAC corresponding to the activator: adsorbent ratios of 1:1. The second-order kinetic model was suitable with the experimental results. It was found that the prepared activated carbons worked as a potent adsorbent for the elimination of EBT from an aqueous medium. Since the *Cannabis sativa* L. plant is available in abundance in Morocco, it may be considered as an economically viable raw material.

Author Contributions: Conceptualization, F.E.M., A.M. and J.B.; methodology, F.E.M., H.T. and H.E.F.; validation, F.E.M., M.H.Z. and A.M.; investigation, F.E.M., H.T., G.P. and H.E.F.; resources, J.B.; writing—original draft preparation, F.E.M.; writing—review and editing, F.C., A.M., H.T. and J.C.G.E.D.S.; supervision, F.C., J.C.G.E.D.S. and J.B.; project administration, A.M., J.B. and J.C.G.E.D.S. All authors have read and agreed to the published version of the manuscript.

Funding: The Portuguese "Fundação para a Ciência e Tecnologia" (FCT, Lisbon) is acknowledged for funding the RD Units CIQUP (UIDB/000081/2020) and the Associated Laboratory IMS (LA/P/0056/2020).

Institutional Review Board Statement: Not applicable.

Informed Consent Statement: Not applicable.

Data Availability Statement: Not applicable.

Acknowledgments: The authors are thankful to Shimadzu and Merck Life Science Corporations for their continuous support.

Conflicts of Interest: The authors declare no conflict of interest.

References

1. Farinon, B.; Molinari, R.; Costantini, L.; Merendino, N. The seed of industrial hemp (*Cannabis sativa* L.): Nutritional quality and potential functionality for human health and nutrition. *Nutrients* **2020**, *12*, 1935. [CrossRef] [PubMed]
2. Russo, E.B.; Jiang, H.E.; Li, X.; Sutton, A.; Carboni, A.; del Bianco, F.; Mandolino, G.; Potter, D.J.; Zhao, Y.X.; Bera, S.; et al. Phytochemical and genetic analyses of ancient cannabis from Central Asia. *J. Exp. Bot.* **2008**, *59*, 4171–4182. [CrossRef] [PubMed]
3. Andre, C.M.; Hausman, J.-F.; Guerriero, G. Cannabis sativa: The plant of the thousand and one molecules. *Front. Plant Sci.* **2016**, *7*, 19. [CrossRef] [PubMed]
4. De Petrocellis, L.; Ligresti, A.; Moriello, A.S.; Allarà, M.; Bisogno, T.; Petrosino, S.; Stott, C.G.; Di Marzo, V. Effects of cannabinoids and cannabinoid-enriched Cannabis extracts on TRP channels and endocannabinoid metabolic enzymes. *Br. J. Pharmacol.* **2011**, *163*, 1479–1494. [CrossRef]
5. Zhang, J.; Mao, L.; Nithya, K.; Loh, K.C.; Dai, Y.; He, Y.; Tong, Y.W. Optimizing mixing strategy to improve the performance of an anaerobic digestion waste-to-energy system for energy recovery from food waste. *Appl. Energy* **2019**, *249*, 28–36. [CrossRef]
6. Wang, B.; Dong, F.; Chen, M.; Zhu, J.; Tan, J.; Fu, X.; Wang, Y.; Chen, S. Advances in recycling and utilization of agricultural wastes in China: Based on environmental risk, crucial pathways, influencing factors, Policy Mechanism. *Procedia Environ. Sci.* **2016**, *31*, 12–17. [CrossRef]
7. Sulyman, M.; Namiesnik, J.; Gierak, A. Low-cost Adsorbents Derived from Agricultural By-products/Wastes for Enhancing Contaminant Uptakes from wastewater: A Review. *Polish J. Environ. Stud.* **2017**, *26*, 479–510. [CrossRef]
8. Crini, G.; Badot, P.M. *Traitement et Epuration des Eaux Industrielles Polluées*; Presses Universitaires de Franche-Comté: Besançon, France, 2007; p. 353.
9. Sidi Zhu, Mingzhu Xia, Yuting Chu, Muhammad Asim Khan, Wu Lei, Fengyun Wang, Tahir Muhmood, Along Wang, Adsorption and Desorption of Pb(II) on l-Lysine Modified Montmorillonite and the simulation of Interlayer Structure. *Appl. Clay Sci.* **2019**, *169*, 40–47. [CrossRef]
10. Zhu, Sidi and Chen, Yexiang and Khan, Muhammad Asim and Xu, Haihua and Wang, Fengyun and Xia, Mingzhu, In-Depth Study of Heavy Metal Removal by an Etidronic Acid-Functionalized Layered Double Hydroxide. *ACS Appl. Mater. Interfaces* **2022**, *14*, 7450–7463. [CrossRef]
11. Chen, Y.; Zhu, Y.; Wang, Z.; Li, Y.; Wang, L.; Ding, L. Application of studies of activated carbon derived from rice husks produced by chemical–thermal process—A review. *Adv. Colloid Interface Sci.* **2011**, *163*, 39–52. [CrossRef]
12. Iqbal, M.J.; Ashiq, M.N. Adsorption of dyes from aqueous solutions on activated charcoal. *J. Hazard Mater.* **2007**, *139*, 57–66. [CrossRef] [PubMed]
13. Monvisade, P.; Siriphanon, P. Chitosan intercalated montmorillonite: Preparation, characterization and cationic dye adsorption. *Appl. Clay Sci.* **2009**, *42*, 427–431. [CrossRef]
14. Tan, I.A.; Ahmad, A.L.; Hameed, B.H. Adsorption of basic dye using activated carbon prepared from oil palm shell: Batch and fixed bed studies. *Desalin* **2008**, *225*, 13–28. [CrossRef]
15. Amin, N.K. Removal of direct blue-106 dye from aqueous solution using new activated carbons developed from pomegranate peel: Adsorption equilibrium and kinetics. *J. Hazard Mater.* **2009**, *165*, 52–62. [CrossRef]

16. da Silva, L.G.; Ruggiero, R.; Gontijo, P.M.; Pinto, R.B.; Royer, B.; Lima, E.C.; Fernandes, T.H.M.; Calvete, T.A. Adsorption of Brilliant Red 2BE dye from water solutions by a chemically modified sugarcane bagasse lignin. *Chem. Eng. J.* **2011**, *168*, 620–628. [CrossRef]

17. Mansouri, F.E.; Farissi, H.E.; Zerrouk, M.H.; Cacciola, F.; Bakkali, C.; Brigui, J.; Lovillo, M.P.; Esteves da Silva, J.C.G. Dye Removal from Colored Textile Wastewater Using Seeds and Biochar of Barley (*Hordeum vulgare* L.). *Appl. Sci.* **2021**, *11*, 5125. [CrossRef]

18. Rajeshwarisivaraj, C.; Namasivayam, K.; Kadirvelu, K. Orange peel as an adsorbent in the removal of Acid violet 17 (acid dye) from aqueous solutions. *Waste Manag.* **2001**, *21*, 105–110.

19. Sudaryanto, Y.; Hartono, S.; Irawata, W.; Hidarso, H.; Ismadji, S. High surface area activated carbons prepared from cassava peel by chemical activation. *Bioresour Technol.* **2006**, *97*, 734–739. [CrossRef]

20. Patnukao, P.; Pavasant, P. Activated carbon from eucalyptus camaldulensis dehn barkusing phosphoric acid activation. *Bioresour. Technol.* **2008**, *99*, 8540–8543. [CrossRef]

21. Gratuito, M.; Panyathanmaporn, T.; Chumnanklong, R.; Sirinuntawittaya, N.; Dutta, A. Production of activated carbon from coconut shell: Optimization using response surface methodology. *Bioresour Technol* **2008**, *99*, 4887–4895. [CrossRef]

22. Ozer, C.; Imamoglu, M.; Turhan, Y.; Boyan, F. Removal of methylene blue from aqueous solutions using phosphoric acid activated carbon produced from hazelnut husks. *Toxic Environ. Chem.* **2012**, *94*, 1283–1293. [CrossRef]

23. Li, W.; Zhang, L.; Peng, J.; Li, N.; Zhu, X. Preparation of high surface activated carbons from tobacco stems with K2CO3 activation using microwave irradiation. *Ind. Crop. Prod.* **2008**, *27*, 341–347. [CrossRef]

24. Rim, B.A.; Sarra, K.; Karine, M.; Achraf, G. Adsorptive removal of cationic and anionic dyes from aqueous solution by utilizing almond shell as bioadsorbent. *Euro-Mediterr. J. Environ. Integr.* **2017**, *2*, 20. [CrossRef]

25. Ghader, Z.; Mahsa, K.; Yusef, O.K.; Heshmatollah, N.; Shirin, E.; Mohammad, J.M.; Rajab, R. Eriochrme black-T removal from aqueous environment by surfactant modified clay: Equilibrium, kinetic, isotherm, and thermodynamic studies. *Toxin Rev.* **2018**, *38*, 307–317. [CrossRef]

26. el Farissi, H.; Lakhmiri, R.; Albourine, A.; Safi, M.; Cherkaoui, O. Adsorption study of charcoal of cistus ladaniferus shell modified by H3PO4 and NaOH used as a low-cost adsorbent for the removal of toxic reactive red 23 dye: Kinetics and thermodynamics. *Mater. Today Proc.* **2020**, *43*, 1740–1748. [CrossRef]

27. El Mansouri, F.; El Farissi, H.; Cacciola, F.; Talhaoui, A.; El Bachiri, A.; Tahani, A.; Esteves da Silva, J.C.G.; Brigui, J. Rapid elimination of copper (II), nickel (II) and chromium (VI) ions from aqueous solutions by charcoal modified with phosphoric acid used as a green biosorbent. *Polym. Adv. Technol.* **2022**, *33*, 2254–2264. [CrossRef]

28. Molina-Sabio, M.; Rodríguez-Reinoso, F. Role of chemical activation in the development of carbon porosity. *Colloids Surf. A Physicochem. Eng. Asp.* **2004**, *241*, 15–25. [CrossRef]

29. Foong, S.Y.; Liew, R.K.; Yang, Y.; Cheng, Y.W.; Yek, P.N.Y.; Mahari, W.A.W.; Lee, X.Y.; Han, C.S.; Vo, N.D.-V.; Le, Q.V.; et al. Valorization of biomass waste to engineered activated biochar by microwave pyrolysis: Progress, challenges, and future directions. *Chem. Eng. J.* **2020**, *389*, 124401. [CrossRef]

30. Zięzio, M.; Charmas, B.; Jedynak, K.; Hawryluk, M.; Kucio, K. Preparation and characterization of activated carbons obtained from the waste materials impregnated with phosphoric acid(V). *Appl. Nanosci.* **2020**, *10*, 4703–4716. [CrossRef]

31. Haykiri-Acma, H.; Yaman, S.; Alkan, M.; Kucukbayrak, S. Mineralogical characterization of chemically isolated ingredients from biomass. *Energy Convers. Manag.* **2014**, *77*, 221–226. [CrossRef]

32. Protásio, T.D.P.; Guimarães, M.; Mirmehdi, S.; Trugilho, P.F.; Napoli, A.; Knovack, K.M. Combustion of biomass and charcoal made from babassu nutshell. *Cerne* **2017**, *23*, 1–10. [CrossRef]

33. Park, D.; Yun, Y.S.; Park, J.M. Use of dead fungal biomass for the detoxification of hexavalent chromium: Screening and kinetics. *Process Biochem.* **2005**, *40*, 2559–2565. [CrossRef]

34. Begum, S.A.S.; Tharakeswar, Y.; Kalyan, Y.; Naidu, G.R. Biosorption of Cd (II), Cr (VI) Pb (II) from Aqueous Solution Using *Mirabilis jalapa* as Adsorbent. *J. Encapsulation Adsorpt. Sci.* **2015**, *5*, 93–104. [CrossRef]

35. Kondapalli, S.; Mohanty, K. Influence of Temperature on Equilibrium, Kinetic and Thermodynamic Parameters of Biosorption of Cr(VI) onto Fish Scales as Suitable Biosorbent. *J. Water Resour. Prot.* **2011**, *3*, 429–439. [CrossRef]

36. Dula, T.; Siraj, K.; Kitte, S.A. Adsorption of Hexavalent Chromium from Aqueous Solution Using Chemically Activated Carbon Prepared from Locally Available Waste of Bamboo (*Oxytenanthera abyssinica*). *ISRN Environ. Chem.* **2014**, *2014*, 4382452014. [CrossRef]

37. Langmuir, I. The Adsorption Of Gases On Plane Surfaces Of Glass, Mica And Platinum. *Verh. Deut. Phys. Ges.* **1918**, *40*, 1361–1403. [CrossRef]

38. Freundlich, H. *Colloid and Capilary Chemistry*, english translation of 3rd German ed.; Methuen: London, UK, 1926.

39. Freundlich, H.; Heller, W. The Adsorption of cis- and trans-Azobenzene. *J. Am. Chem. Soc.* **2002**, *61*, 2228–2230. [CrossRef]

40. Mahmoodi, N.M.; Salehi, R.; Arami, M.; Bahrami, H. Dye removal from colored textile wastewater using chitosan in binary systems. *Desalination* **2011**, *267*, 64–72. [CrossRef]

41. Ghasemi, M.; Javadian, H.; Ghasemi, N.; Agarwal, S.; Gupta, V.K. Microporous nanocrystalline NaA zeolite prepared by microwave assisted hydrothermal method and determination of kinetic, isotherm and thermodynamic parameters of the batch sorption of Ni (II). *J. Mol. Liq.* **2016**, *215*, 161–169. [CrossRef]

42. Wang, X.; Jiang, C.; Hou, B.; Wang, Y.; Hao, C.; Wu, J. Carbon composite lignin-based adsorbents for the adsorption of dyes. *Chemosphere* **2018**, *206*, 587–596. [CrossRef] [PubMed]

43. Shi, T.; Xie, Z.; Zhu, Z.; Shi, W.; Liu, Y.; Liu, M. Highly efficient and selective adsorption of heavy metal ions by hydrazide-modified sodium alginate. *Carbohydr. Polym.* **2022**, *276*, 118797. [CrossRef] [PubMed]
44. Maneechakr, P.; Mongkollertlop, S. Investigation on adsorption behaviors of heavy metal ions (Cd^{2+}, Cr^{3+}, Hg^{2+} and Pb^{2+}) through low-cost/active manganese dioxide-modified magnetic biochar derived from palm kernel cake residue. *J. Environ. Chem. Eng.* **2020**, *8*, 104467. [CrossRef]
45. Tao, Y.; Yang, B.; Wang, F.; Yan, Y.; Hong, X.; Xu, H.; Xia, M.; Wang, F. Green synthesis of MOF-808 with modulation of particle sizes and defects for efficient phosphate sequestration. *Sep. Purif. Technol.* **2022**, *300*, 121825. [CrossRef]
46. Saini, J.; Garg, V.K.; Gupta, R.K.; Kataria, N. Removal of Orange G and Rhodamine B dyes from aqueous system using hydrothermally synthesized zinc oxide loaded activated carbon (ZnO-AC). *J. Environ. Chem. Eng.* **2017**, *5*, 884–892. [CrossRef]
47. Sewu, D.D.; Boakye, P.; Woo, S.H. Highly efficient adsorption of cationic dye by biochar produced with Korean cabbage waste. *Bioresour. Technol.* **2017**, *224*, 206–213. [CrossRef]
48. Popa, N.; Visa, M. The synthesis, activation and characterization of charcoal powder for the removal of methylene blue and cadmium from wastewater. *Adv. Powder Technol.* **2017**, *28*, 1866–1876. [CrossRef]
49. Islam, M.T.; Hyder, A.G.; Saenz-Arana, R.; Hernandez, C.; Guinto, T.; Ahsan, M.A.; Alvarado-Tenorio, B.; Noveron, J.C. Removal of methylene blue and tetracycline from water using peanut shell derived adsorbent prepared by sulfuric acid reflux. *J. Environ.Chem. Eng.* **2019**, *7*, 102816. [CrossRef]
50. Isa, K.M.; Daud, S.; Hamidin, N.; Ismail, K.; Saad, S.A.; Kasim, F.H. Thermogravimetric analysis and the optimisation of bio-oil yield from fixed-bed pyrolysis of rice husk using response surface methodology (RSM). *Ind. Crops Prod.* **2011**, *33*, 481–487. [CrossRef]
51. Núñez-gómez, D.; Rodrigues, C.; Rubens, F. Adsorption of heavy metals from coal acid mine drainage by shrimp shell waste: Isotherm and continuous-flow studies. *J. Environ. Chem. Eng.* **2019**, *7*, 102787. [CrossRef]
52. Ho, Y.S.; McKay, G. Pseudo-second order model for sorption processes. *Process Biochem.* **1999**, *34*, 451–465. [CrossRef]
53. Urano, K.; Hirotaka, T. Process development for removal and recovery of phosphorus from wastewater by a new adsorbent. II. Adsorption rates and breakthrough curves. *Ind. Eng. Chem. Res.* **1991**, *30*, 1897–1899. [CrossRef]
54. Venkat, P.V.V.B.; Mane, S. Studies on the adsorption of Brilliant Green dye from aqueous solution onto low-cost NaOH treated saw dust. *Desalination* **2011**, *273*, 321–329. [CrossRef]
55. Jin, G.P.; Wang, X.L.; Fu, Y.; Do, Y. Preparation of tetraoxalyl ethylenediamine melamine resin grafted-carbon fibers for nano-nickel recovery from spent electroless nickel plating baths. *Chem. Eng. J.* **2012**, *203*, 440–446. [CrossRef]
56. Mahjoub, B.; Ncibi, M.C.; Seffen, M. Adsorption d'un Colorant Textile Réactif sur un Biosorbant Non-Conventionnel: Les Fibres de *Posidonia oceanica* (L.) Delile. *Can. J. Chem. Eng.* **2008**, *86*, 23–29. [CrossRef]

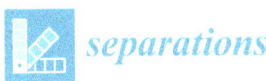

MDPI

Article

Wound Healing Potential of *Commiphora gileadensis* Stems Essential Oil and Chloroform Extract

Hassan N. Althurwi [1], Mohammad Ayman A. Salkini [2], Gamal A. Soliman [1,3], Mohd Nazam Ansari [1], Elmutasim O. Ibnouf [4,5] and Maged S. Abdel-Kader [2,6,*]

[1] Department of Pharmacology, College of Pharmacy, Prince Sattam Bin Abdulaziz University, P.O. Box 173, Al-Kharj 11942, Saudi Arabia
[2] Department of Pharmacognosy, College of Pharmacy, Prince Sattam Bin Abdulaziz University, P.O. Box 173, Al-Kharj 11942, Saudi Arabia
[3] Department of Pharmacology, College of Veterinary Medicine, Cairo University, Giza 12211, Egypt
[4] Department of Pharmaceutics, College of Pharmacy, Prince Sattam Bin Abdulaziz University, P.O. Box 173, Al-Kharj 11942, Saudi Arabia
[5] Department of Medical Microbiology, Faculty of Medical Laboratory Sciences, Omdurman Islamic University, Omdurman P.O. Box 382, Sudan
[6] Department of Pharmacognosy, Faculty of Pharmacy, Alexandria University, Alexandria 21215, Egypt
* Correspondence: m.youssef@psau.edu.sa; Tel.: +966-545539145

Citation: Althurwi, H.N.; Salkini, M.A.A.; Soliman, G.A.; Ansari, M.N.; Ibnouf, E.O.; Abdel-Kader, M.S. Wound Healing Potential of *Commiphora gileadensis* Stems Essential Oil and Chloroform Extract. *Separations* 2022, 9, 254. https://doi.org/10.3390/separations9090254

Academic Editor: Ernesto Reverchon

Received: 19 August 2022
Accepted: 6 September 2022
Published: 8 September 2022

Publisher's Note: MDPI stays neutral with regard to jurisdictional claims in published maps and institutional affiliations.

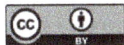
Abstract: Essential oils (EOs) prepared from the fresh and dried stems of *Commiphora gileadensis* were compared qualitatively and quantitatively. Although the components were closely similar, the amount of oil decreased from 2.23 to 1.77% upon drying. Both samples showed equal potencies in the antimicrobial testing. The chloroform extract (CE) of the fresh stems with reported antimicrobial activity was compared with the EO sample of the fresh stems for wound healing potential. For the wound healing assay, 11 mm-diameter full-thickness skin excision wounds were made on the backs of four groups of rats (n = 6). The negative control group I was treated with the cream base. Group II was treated with 2% Fucidin cream, which served as a reference, and groups III and IV were treated with 1% EO- and 3% CE-containing creams, respectively. Treatments were applied topically one time daily. The wound healing potential was evaluated by recording the wound contraction percentages, epithelialization period, and histopathological changes of wounds. The topical application of CE significantly promoted the healing of wounds in rats. The effectiveness was demonstrated through the speed of wound contraction and the shortening of the epithelialization period in an animal treated with CE cream when compared to the NC group. Histopathological studies of the CE cream-treated group also expressed the effectiveness of CE in improving the wound healing process. These findings suggested that CE cream can enhance the process of wound healing in rats.

Keywords: *Commiphora gileadensi*; essential oil; GC-MS; wound healing; antimicrobial; rats

1. Introduction

The resins obtained from members of the genus *Commiphora* are used for the management of microbial infections, wounds, tumors, obesity, pain, inflammation, arthritis, gastrointestinal diseases, and fractures [1]. Plants of *Commiphora gileadensis* (synonymous with *Commiphora opobalsamum*) have many applications in traditional medicine [2]. The bark of the plant is used to treat infected wounds [3], a fact supported by the broad-spectrum antimicrobial activity against both Gram-negative, Gram-positive bacteria, and fungi [4,5]. *C. gileadensis* can disturb the bacterial lectin-dependent adhesion process essential for the survival of *Pseudomonas aeruginosa*. The traditional claims of the ability of balsam obtained from the plant to control infections were also supported by their ability to interfere with bacterial lectin-dependent adhesion [6]. The leaves' methanol extract expressed antiviral activity against two enveloped viruses: HSV-2 and RSV B [7].

We recently reported on the isolation of four *ent*-verticillane-type diterpenes, namely *ent*-Verticillol, *(13S,14S)-ent*-13,14-epoxyverticillol, *(9S,10S)-ent*-9,10-epoxyverticillol, *(1S,3E, 7E,11R)*-(+)-verticilla-3,7,12(18)-triene, as well as gileadenol with novel diterpene skeleton from the fresh *C. gileadensis* stems' $CHCl_3$ extract. Four triterepenes were also isolated, and the antimicrobial potential of the isolated compounds was demonstrated [8].

The main goal of the current study was the evaluation of the wound healing potential of the different *C. gileadensis* extracts and the essential oil and the correlation of this effect with the antimicrobial activity.

2. Materials and Methods

2.1. Plant Material

The plants of *Commiphora gileadensis* (L.) C.Chr were described earlier [8].

2.2. Chemicals

Hematoxylin, eosin, Masson trichrome, petrolatum, and sorbitan monolaurate were purchased from Merck, KGaA, Darmstadt, Germany. Mueller–Hinton agar, Sabouraud dextrose agar, M_H broth, S-D broth, M_H agar, and S-D agar were obtained from Scharlau, Barcelona, Spain. Tween 80 was obtained from Chem Sino, China. All solvents used were of analytical grades.

2.3. Preparation of the Oils

Samples of 300 g of the fresh stems and 200 g of shade dried stems (obtained from drying 300 gm of fresh stems) of *C. gileadensis* were used to prepare the essential oil by hydrodistillation for 5 h using Clevenger apparatus. Fresh stems were cut into pieces about 2 cm long and were utilized for oil isolation, while the intact stems were dried in in the shade under a controlled temperature for two weeks, then ground and used for oil preparation. The resulting oil layers were separated, and the condensates were extracted with ether. The ether extract was added to the separated oil and dehydrated using anhydrous sodium sulfate. The ether was then evaporated under the reduced pressure of 350 m bar leaving the essential oil (EO). Each experiment was repeated three times.

2.4. GC/MS Analysis

Diluted EO samples (5 ppm) in methanol (1 uL of 5 ppm concentration) were injected (1 uL) into GC/MS apparatus (Agilent Model 7890 MSD) fitted with capillary column (30 m × 0.25 mm i.d., 0.25 µm coating) HP-5MS using the Autosampler and applying the splitless mode. The starting temperature was set at 60 °C for 10 min and raised at the rate of 4 °C/min until it reached 220 °C where it was held for 5 min. The temperature was raised again at a rate of 10 °C/min to 290 °C and was kept isothermally for 5 min. The carrier gas was Helium (99.999% purity) with a flow rate of 1.0 mL/min. Quadrupole MS analysis conditions were set to an electronic impact ionization mode at 70 eV with a mass range of 30 to 600 m/z. The components of the EO were identified by comparing the obtained mass spectra with that stored in the library of the National Institute of Standards and Technology (NIST 2017) (Figure 1). The results were analyzed and controlled by MASSHUNTER software (Agilent MassHunter Workstation Software-Quantitative Analysis program version B.04.xx, Agilent Technologies, Inc., Santa Clara, CA USA).

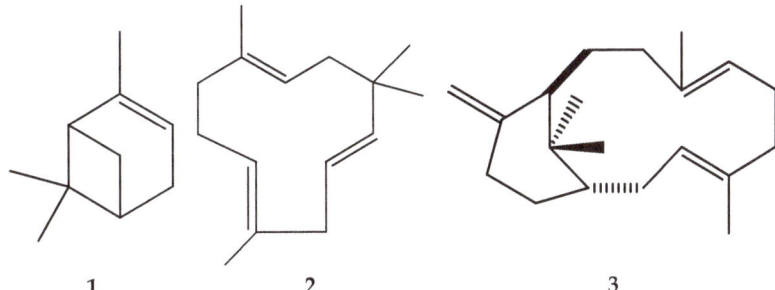

Figure 1. Chemical structure of β-Pinene (**1**), humulene (**2**) and (1*S*,3*E*,7*E*,11*R*)-(+)-verticilla-3,7,12(18)-triene (**3**). (**3**) from the essential oils of *C. gileadensis*.

2.5. GC Analysis

The GC chromatograms were recorded on GC Agilent 7890B, fitted with an HP-5 19091J-413 capillary column (30 m × 0.25 mm) and FID detector using the same conditions of GC/MS analysis. The relative retention index (RRI) to *n*-alkanes series was applied for the identification of peaks. Computerized peak areas were used for the quantitative determination of each compound.

2.6. Extraction

Fresh stems (5.8 kg) were macerated in $CHCl_3$ at room temperature (10 L × 5) to yield 117.5 g of the $CHCl_3$ soluble extract (CE) after the solvent was evaporated using a rotary vacuum under it to reduce pressure. The fresh stems were then similarly extracted with MeOH (10 L × 5) to yield 226.7 g of the MeOH soluble extract (ME). Extraction of the fresh leaves (2.3 kg) was performed in the same fashion and provided 32.2 g of the $CHCl_3$ soluble extract and 90.25 g of the MeOH soluble extract.

2.7. Antimicrobial Activity

2.7.1. Bacterial Strains

American Type Culture Collection (ATCC) strains and National Collection of Type Culture (NCTC) maintained in the Microbiology Laboratory at the College of Pharmacy/Prince Sattam University (Al-Kharj- Saudi Arabia), *Bacillus subtilis* and *Staphylococcus aureus*, *Escherichia coli*, and *Klebsiella pneumonia*, as well as the fungus *Candida albicans*, were used in the study. The strains were grown aerobically at 37 °C. The suspension of organisms equivalent to a 0.5 McFarland standard was utilized.

2.7.2. Antimicrobial Assay

The MIC of the tested materials was measured following the broth dilution method adopted by the Clinical and Laboratory Standards Institute guidelines [9]. Both EO and CE were prepared in 10 mg/mL, where serial dilutions were prepared. The testing was performed in the range of 50–3.125 μg/mL. From each tested organism, 10 μL of the culture was inoculated with the used concentrations. Sterility was assured by the incubation of Mueller–Hinton broth (MHB, Scharlau) alone. Negative control results were obtained by the incubation of MHB with different concentrations of DMSO. After the incubation period of 24 h at 37 °C, the lowest concentration that inhibited visible microbial growth was designated as the MIC [9,10].

2.8. Evaluation of Wound Healing Activity

2.8.1. Experimental Animals

In this study, 24 healthy male Wistar rats weighing 180–200 g were experimented on. Rats were bred and housed in the lab animal unit, College of Pharmacy; University of Prince Sattam bin Abdulaziz in ventilated cages (Rat IVC Blue Line, Techniplast, Buguggiate VA,

Italy). The animals were maintained in controlled environmental conditions ($25 \pm 1\,^\circ$C and 12 h/12 h light/dark cycle) with food and water *ad libitum*. The care and handling complied with the internationally accepted guidelines for use of animals 33. Furthermore, the animal experiments were approved by the Bioethical Research Committee (BERC) at Prince Sattam bin Abdulaziz University (ref No. BERC-008-04-21).

2.8.2. Preparation of Creams

The topical creams were prepared by melting petrolatum (21.16 g) in a water bath at $70\,^\circ$C. Tween 80 (2 g) was dispersed in the oil phases, respectively, and 0.5 g of EO or 1.5 g of EC were added. Quantities of glycerol (4.67 g) were mixed together accordingly with the aqueous phase composed of water (17.17 mL) and sorbitan monolaurate (5 g). The oily phase was added to the aqueous phase slowly with continuous stirring at 500 rpm using a Kenwood kitchen mixer. After the addition of the oil phase was completed, further mixing for another 5 min was applied before the cream was allowed to set [11].

2.8.3. Experimental Design

Creams of essential oil (EO) and fresh stems (CE) of *C. gileadensis* were evaluated for their wound healing potential in rats using the excision wound model [12]. Twenty-four rats were anesthetized using ketamine hydrochloride (5 mg/kg i.p.) and xylazine (2 mg/kg i.p.). In the dorsal area of each rat, the skin was shaved by an electrical clipper and disinfected with 70% alcohol. A uniform wound of 11 mm in diameter was excised from the shaved region of each rat with the aid of sterile toothed forceps and sharp pointed scissors (Figure 2). Rats were randomly grouped into four groups, with 6 rats/group.

Group 1: Negative control group (NC); treated with the plain cream base topically.
Group 2: Reference group (REF); topically with 2% Fucidin cream.
Group 3 and 4 were treated with either 1% EO or with 3% CE creams, respectively.

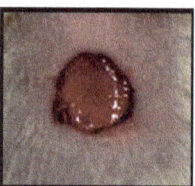

Figure 2. Photographic representation of wound area on 0th day.

Different treatments were distributed topically over the wound area once a day starting from the day of wounding (day 0) until the complete healing of wounds was achieved. The wound area was assessed every 4 days by drawing its borders with the help of a transparent sheet. These wound drawings were retraced on a sheet of 1 mm^2 graph paper. The wound areas were obtained by counting the squares [13].

The percentage reduction of wound contraction was calculated based on the initial wound area [14].

$$\% \text{ Wound Contraction} = \frac{\text{wound area on day 0} - \text{wound area on day n}}{\text{wound area on day 0}} \times 100$$

where n = number of days (4th, 8th, 12th, 16th, and 20th day).

The epithelialization period was calculated as the period of days required for the scab to fall off and leave no raw wounds behind [15].

2.9. Histopathological Examination

At the end of the study, tissues from the wounded area were collected in 10% buffered formalin and prepared in an automatic tissue processing machine (ASP300s, Leica Biosystems, Deer Park, IL, USA). After that, tissue samples were soaked in paraffin wax blocks, and sections of 5 μ thickness were prepared using a rotary microtome (SHUR/Cut 4500, TBS, Durham, NC, USA) [16]. Two sections of each block were stained either by hematoxylin and eosin (H&E) or Masson trichrome (MT) [17]. For hematoxylin and eosin, stain sections were dewaxed and rehydrated with descending grades of alcohol to water. The sections were stained in hematoxylin (HX082464, MERK, Darmstadl, Germany) for 10 min, washed with running tap water until the sections were 'blue' for 5–10 min, then stained in 1% eosin Y for 1–3 min and washed with running tap water for 1–3 min. Sections were then dehydrated with alcohol and mounted in DPX [18]. Masson trichrome techniques were used according to Hamad et al., (2016) [17].

2.10. Data Analysis

The data are presented as mean ± SEM. Analysis of the results was performed by SPSS version 19 to apply a one-way analysis of variance (ANOVA), followed by Dunnett's multiple comparison tests. Graphical representation was carried out using Microsoft Excel 2010. The differences between mean values were considered significant at $p < 0.05$.

3. Results and Discussion

3.1. Preparation of the Oil and GC-MS Study

The average yield of EO from the fresh and dried stems of *C. gileadensis* showed a 0.46% loss in the dried sample (Table 1). Regarding the oil composition revealed by GC-MS analysis, little difference was found in the number of compounds (Table 2). However, great changes were observed in the percentage of the components. It was noticed that the lighter monoterpene components, such as β-Pinene (**1**) (Figure 1), dramatically declined from 62.974% in the oil obtained from the fresh plant samples to 4.462% in the oil derived from the dried samples. Components with higher molecular weights were expected to be less volatile, and consequently, their relative percentages increased in the oil obtained from the dried samples. For example, Eugenol percentage increased from 5.834% in the fresh oil samples to 35.366% in the essential oil samples prepared from the dried plants (Table 2). The diterpene hydrocarbon 1S,3E,7E,11R)-(+)-verticilla-3,7,12(18)-triene (**3**) was identified via direct comparison with the isolated compound [8], and its percentage increased to 20.638 in the essential oil of the dried samples.

Table 1. Yield of essential oil from fresh and dried stem samples of *C. gileadensis*.

Condition	Weight (g)	Weight of Oil (g)	% *w/w*
Fresh	300.00	6.69	2.23
Dried	200.00	3.55	1.77

Table 2. Components of fresh and dried stem samples essential oil of *C. gileadensis*.

Components	RT	RRI	Area % Fresh	Area % Dry
β-Pinene (**1**)	9.7833	978	62.974	4.462
Eugenol	26.7184	1365	5.834	35.366
Caryophyllene	28.7625	1444	4.543	34.469
Humulene (**2**)	29.8557	1460	-	1.718
cis-Calamenene	32.0615	1533	12.29	0.687
Isoeugenol acetate	32.2167	1618	1.926	0.483
1S,3E,7E,11R)-(+)-verticilla-3,7,12(18)-triene (**3**)	63.1821	2040	11.374	20.638
Total			**98.941**	**97.823**

3.2. Antimicrobial Activity

Two Gram-positive bacteria (*Bacillus subtilis* and *Staphylococcus aureus*), two Gram-negative bacteria (*Escherichia coli* and *Klebsiella pneumonia*), and the fungus (*Candida albicans*) were utilized to study the antimicrobial effect of the EO obtained from the fresh and dried stems. The activity of the CE and methanol extract (ME) of the fresh stems of *C. gileadensis* was previously reported [8]. The MIC was determined for all of the tested materials (Table 3). The two essential oil samples were active against all of the tested organisms with equal potencies, although the yield of the oil was less in the cases of dried samples, and the relative percentages of the components were different. This indicated that the effect is due to combined action of all the components [19,20]. The CE expressed stronger activity against *k. pneumonia* and *C. albicans* than the EO.

Table 3. MIC (mg/mL) of different essential oil and different extracts.

	Staph. aureus	B. subtilis	E. coli	k. pneumonia	C. albicans
Fresh Stem Oil	0.75	0.75	0.5	0.5	0.25
Dried stem Oil	0.75	0.75	0.5	0.5	0.25
Fresh stem CHCl$_3$ Ext.	0.75	0.75	0.75	0.25	0.125
Fresh stem MeOH Ext.	75	25	75	50	25
Fresh Leaves CHCl$_3$ Ext.	0.75	0.5	0.75	0.25	0.125
Fresh Leaves MeOH Ext.	75	25	75	25	75

3.3. Wound Healing Activity

The wound healing properties of *C. guidottii* and *C. myrrha* have been reported, while *C. gileadensis* was mentioned in the early Islamic era to be used by the Prophet and his companions for the treatment of wounds [21,22]. As the wound healing effect can be correlated to the antimicrobial activity, both EO and CE of the fresh stem sample were selected for the wound healing study. Both products were formulated as creams [11] containing 1% EO and 3% CE.

In the experiment for the evaluation of the wound healing activity of EO and CE, all animals survived, and no complications related to the procedure were observed. The sizes of wounded areas, percentages of wound contraction, and the periods of epithelialization are represented in Figures 3–6. On day 0, the wound areas in all groups were almost similar, and there was no significant difference between different groups. The topical application of EO and CE creams on the wounds of rats reduced their areas in comparison to the NC group. The group treated with Fucidin cream had a smaller wound size than that of the other tested creams (Figure 3).

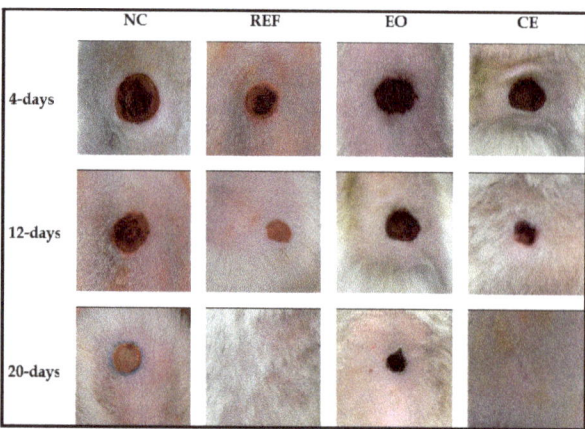

Figure 3. Photograph of wound area after topical application of Fucidin cream (REF) and essential oil (EO) and chloroform extract (CE) creams of *Commiphora gileadensis* in rats.

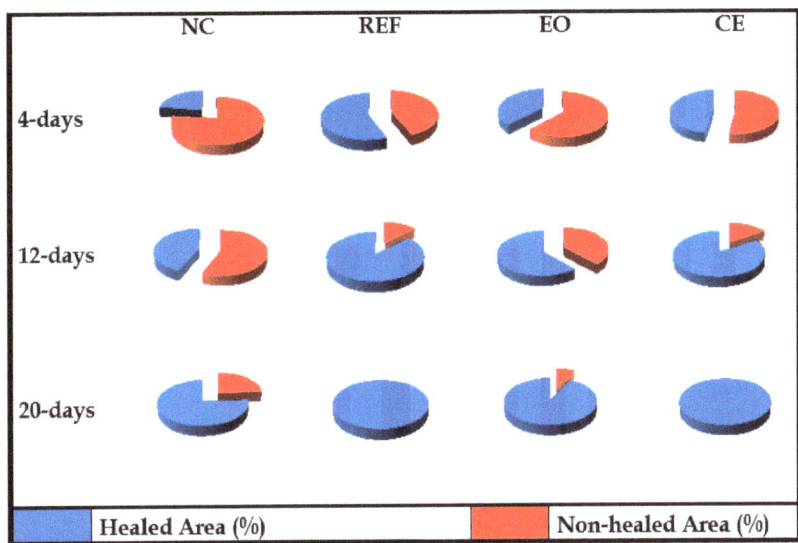

Figure 4. Effect of Fucidin cream (REF), essential oil (EO), and chloroform extract (CE) creams of *Commiphora gileadensis* on the percentages of wound contractions in rats.

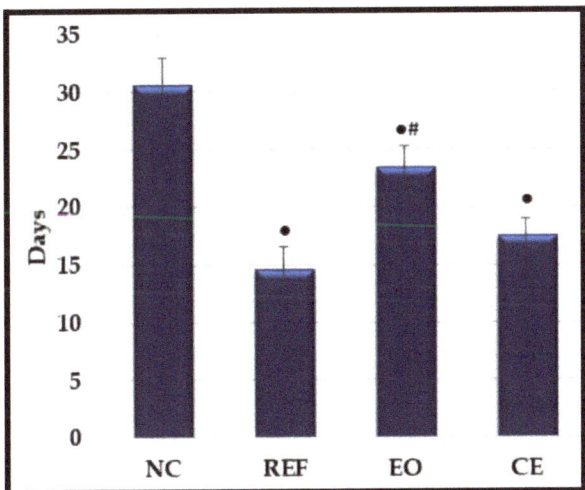

Figure 5. Effect of Fucidin cream (REF), essential oil (EO), and chloroform extract (CE) creams of *Commiphora gileadensis* on the epithelialization periods in rats. Values are expressed as mean ± S.E.M., n = 6 animals/group. • Significant compared to NC group at $p < 0.05$. # Significant compared to REF group at $p < 0.05$.

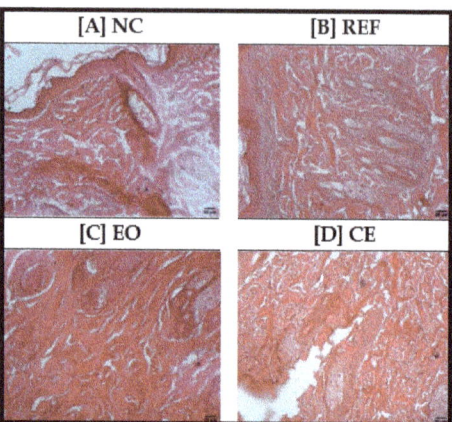

Figure 6. Histological sections of the wound tissue of rats after topical application of cream base (**A**), Fucidin cream (**B**), EO cream (**C**), and CE cream (**D**). H&E stain, magnification: ×100.

In this study, the percentages of wound contraction were calculated on the 4, 8, 12, 16, and 20 post-wounding days, as shown in Figure 4. Wound contraction facilitates the re-epithelialization of the wounded skin and helps in restoring the function of skin as a physical barrier. The topical application of the reference Fucidin cream on the wounds resulted in a significant increase in the wound contraction rate when compared to the NC group. Significant effects were also observed for the groups treated with EO and CE creams compared to the NC group (Figure 4). Interestingly, the percentages of wound contraction were significantly higher in CE-treated rats, reaching 96.49 ± 1.71 and $100.0 \pm 0.00\%$ after 16 and 20 days, respectively (Figure 4). In EO-treated rats, 77.37 ± 2.43 and $92.63 \pm 1.51\%$ of wound contractions were recorded after 16 and 20 days of topical application, respectively.

The rates of epithelialization (in days) were also evaluated in wounded rats, with epithelialization being the proliferation and migration of epithelial cells across the wound. The time for compelling this process is an important parameter to evaluate the wound healing potential. The group treated with the cream base took a longer time (30.67 ± 2.36 days) to achieve epithelialization (Figure 5). The mean time taken for complete epithelialization in groups treated with EO and CE creams was reduced. Moreover, the mean healing time in CE-treated rats (17.50 ± 1.50 days) was comparable to that of the reference Fucidin cream-treated group (14.67 ± 1.86 days).

3.4. Histopathological Study

Histopathological examination using Mayer's hematoxylin stain and Masson trichrome technique was used as a general parameter for the evaluation of wound healing potential. Masson trichrome develops a blue color with collagen, giving an indication about fibrosis of the examined tissues [23]. The histological examination of skin samples of the NC group showed multiple areas of tissue damage, degeneration, and a wide area of necrosis (Figure 6A). Furthermore, the skin of NC rats showed multiple areas of lost collagen fibers (Figure 7A). Skin samples of the REF group showed normal skin tissue samples (Figure 6B) with normal contents and distribution of collagen fibers (Figure 7B). Skin samples of the EO-treated rats showed moderate improvement (Figure 6C) with areas of lost collagen (Figure 7C). The skin of the CE-treated rats showed much improvement (Figure 6D) and an almost normal content of collagen fibers (Figure 7D).

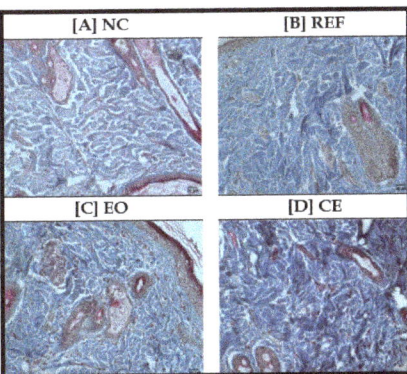

Figure 7. Histological sections of the wound tissue of rats after topical application of cream base (**A**), Fucidin cream (**B**), EO cream (**C**), and CE cream (**D**). Masson Trichrome stain, Magnification: ×400.

Our recent phytochemical study on the CE of the fresh stems resulted in the isolation of diterpenes and triterpenes, all with significant antimicrobial activity [8]. EO lacks these components due to their higher molecular weight. This can explain the stronger effects of the CE in the antimicrobial testing and as a wound healing promoter compared with the EO.

4. Conclusions

The process of drying had a great impact on the yield and percentage of components of the EO prepared from the fresh and dried stems of *C. gileadensis*. Antimicrobial testing using Gram-positive and Gram-negative bacteria in addition to pathogenic fungus (*Candida albicans*) indicated that the EOs of the fresh and dry stems were equally active. The CE of the fresh stems was more active than the EO, while the ME was almost inactive.

The present study results suggest that CE and EO creams enhance wound healing in rats. The CE cream was more effective and comparable with that of Fucidin cream, as shown by the reduction in the percentage of wound contraction, reduction in the period of epithelization, and the improvement in the skin histopathological parameters. Further, the wound healing efficacy of CE seems to be correlated with its antimicrobial effect. Our findings suggest that CE cream is valuable for the treatment and management of wounds.

Author Contributions: Conceptualization, M.S.A.-K., G.A.S. and H.N.A.; methodology, M.N.A., M.A.A.S., M.S.A.-K. and E.O.I.; software, M.A.A.S., M.N.A. and H.N.A.; validation, G.A.S., H.N.A. and M.N.A.; formal analysis, M.N.A. and H.N.A.; investigation, M.N.A., M.A.A.S., H.N.A. and E.O.I.; resources, M.S.A.-K.; data curation, G.A.S., H.N.A. and E.O.I.; writing—original draft preparation, M.N.A., M.A.A.S. and E.O.I.; writing—review and editing, M.S.A.-K., G.A.S. and H.N.A.; visualization, M.N.A., M.A.A.S. and E.O.I.; supervision, M.S.A.-K. and G.A.S.; project administration, M.S.A.-K.; funding acquisition, M.S.A.-K. All authors have read and agreed to the published version of the manuscript.

Funding: The project was funded by the Deputyship for Research & Innovation, Ministry of Education in Saudi Arabia via project number (IF-PSAU-2021/03/18755).

Institutional Review Board Statement: The study was conducted in accordance with the Declaration of Helsinki, and approved by the Bioethical Research Committee (BERC) at Prince Sattam bin Abdulaziz University (ref No. BERC-008-04-21).

Informed Consent Statement: Not applicable.

Data Availability Statement: Not applicable.

Acknowledgments: The authors would like to thank A. Hamad, College of Applied Medical Science at Prince Sattam University for the histopathological study.

Conflicts of Interest: The authors declare no conflict of interest.

References

1. Marcotullio, M.C.; Rosati, O.; Lanari, D. Phytochemistry of *Commiphora erythraea*: A review. *Nat. Prod. Comm.* **2018**, *13*, 1209–1212. [CrossRef]
2. El Rabey, H.A.; Al-sieni, A.I.; Al-seeni, M.N.; Alsieni, M.A.; Alalawy, A.I.; Almutairi, F.M. The antioxidant and antidiabetic activity of the Arabian balsam tree "*Commiphora gileadensis*" in hyperlipidaemic male rats. *J. Taibah Univ. Sci.* **2020**, *14*, 831–841. [CrossRef]
3. Miller, A.G.; Morris, M.; Stuart-Smith, S. *Plants of Dhofar, the Southern Region of Oman: Traditional, Economic, and Medicinal Uses*; Office of the Adviser for Conservation of the Environment, Diwan of Royal Court: Muscat, Oman, 1988.
4. Al-mahbashi, H.M.; El-shaibany, A.; Saad, F.A. Evaluation of acute toxicity and antimicrobial effects of the bark extract of Bisham (*Commiphora gileadensis* L.). *J. Chem. Pharm. Res.* **2015**, *7*, 810–814.
5. Al Zoubi, O.M. Evaluation of anti-microbial activity of ex vitro and callus extracts from *Commiphora gileadensis*. *Pak. J. Biol. Sci.* **2019**, *22*, 73–82.
6. Iluz, D.; Hoffman, M.; Gilboa-Garber, N.; Amar, Z. Medicinal properties of *Commiphora gileadensis*. *Afr. J. Pharm. Pharmacol.* **2010**, *4*, 516–520.
7. Bouslama, L.; Kouidhi, B.; Alqurashi, Y.M.; Chaieb, K.; Papetti, A. Virucidal Effect of Guggulsterone Isolated from *Commiphora gileadensis*. *Planta Med.* **2019**, *85*, 1225–1232. [CrossRef]
8. Abdel-Kader, M.S.; Ibnouf, E.O.; Alqarni, M.H.; AlQutaym, A.S.; Salkini, M.A.; Foudah, A.I. Terpenes from the Fresh Stems of *Commiphora gileadensis* with Antimicrobial Activity. *Rec. Nat. Prod.* **2022**, *16*, 605–613. [CrossRef]
9. Alkahtani, J.; Elshikh, S.M.; Almaary, K.S.; Ali, S.; Imtiyaz, Z.; Ahmad, B.S. Anti-bacterial, anti-scavenging and cytotoxic activity of garden cress polysaccharides. *Saudi J. Biol. Sci.* **2020**, *27*, 2929–2935. [CrossRef]
10. Gonelimali, F.D.; Lin, J.; Miao, W.; Xuan, J.; Charles, F.; Chen, M.; Hatab, S.R. Antimicrobial Properties and Mechanism of Action of Some Plant Extracts Against Food Pathogens and Spoilage Microorganisms. *Front. Microbiol.* **2018**, *9*, 1639. [CrossRef]
11. Chauhan, L.; Gupta, S. Creams: A Review on Classification, Preparation Methods, Evaluation and its Applications. *J. Drug Deliv. Ther.* **2020**, *10*, 281–289. [CrossRef]
12. Mukherjee, P.K.; Verpoorte, R.; Suresh, B. Evaluation of in-vivo wound healing activity of *Hypericum patulum* (Family: Hypericaceae) leaf extract on different wound model in rats. *J. Ethnopharmacol.* **2000**, *70*, 315–321. [CrossRef]
13. Ponrasu, T.; Suguna, L. Efficacy of *Annona squamosa* on wound healing in streptozotocin-induced diabetic rats. *Int. Wound J.* **2012**, *9*, 613–623. [CrossRef] [PubMed]
14. Sadaf, F.; Saleem, R.; Ahmed, M.; Ahmad, S.I.; Navaid-ul-Zafar. Healing potential of cream containing extract of *Sphaeranthus indicus* on dermal wounds in Guinea pigs. *J. Ethnopharmacol.* **2006**, *107*, 161–163. [CrossRef] [PubMed]
15. Manjunatha, B.K.; Vidya, S.M.; Rashmi, K.V.; Mankani, K.L.; Shilpa, H.J.; Singh, S.D. Evaluation of wound-healing potency of *Vernonia arborea* Hk. *Ind. J. Pharmacol.* **2005**, *37*, 223–226. [CrossRef]
16. Hamad, A.M.; Ahmed, H.G. Association of some carbohydrates with estrogen expression in breast lesions among Sudanese females. *J. Histotechnol.* **2018**, *41*, 2–9. [CrossRef]
17. Hamad, A.M.; Ahmed, H.G. Association of connective tissue fibers with estrogen expression in breast lesions among Sudanese females. *Int. Clin. Pathol. J.* **2016**, *2*, 97–102. [CrossRef]
18. Suvarna, S.K.; Christopher, L.; Bancroft, J.D. *The Hematoxyline and Eosin. Bancroft's Theory and Practice of Histological Techniques*, 8th ed.; Elsevier: Amsterdam, The Netherlands, 2018.
19. Alqarni, M.H.; Salkini, M.A.; Abujheisha, K.Y.; Daghar, M.F.; Al-khuraif, F.A.; Abdel-Kader, M.S. Qualitative, Quantitative and Antimicrobial Activity Variations of the Essential Oils Isolated from *Thymus Vulgaris* and *Micromeria Fruticosa* Samples Subjected to Different Drying Conditions. *Arab. J. Sci. Eng.* **2022**, *47*, 6861–6867. [CrossRef]
20. Bassolé, I.H.; Juliani, H.R. Essential oils in combination and their antimicrobial properties. *Molecules* **2012**, *17*, 3989–4006. [CrossRef]
21. Gebrehiwot, M.; Asres, K.; Bisrat, D.; Mazumder, A.; Lindemann, P.; Bucar, F. Evaluation of the wound healing property of *Commiphora guidottii* Chiov. ex. Guid. *BMC Complement. Altern. Med.* **2015**, *15*, 282. [CrossRef]
22. Bisrat, D.; Mazumder, A.; Lindemann, P. Effects of Resin and Essential Oil from *Commiphora myrrha* Engl. on Wound Healing. *Ethiop. Pharm. J.* **2016**, *32*, 85–100.
23. Krishna, M. Role of special stains in diagnostic liver pathology. *Clin. Liver Dis.* **2013**, *2*, 8–10. [CrossRef] [PubMed]

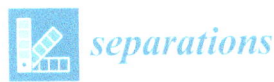 *separations*

MDPI

Article

Ecofriendly Validated RP-HPTLC Method for Simultaneous Determination of the Bioactive Sesquiterpene Coumarins Feselol and Samarcandin in Five *Ferula* Species Using Green Solvents

Maged S. Abdel-Kader [1,2,*], Mohammed H. Alqarni [1], Sura Baykan [3], Bintug Oztürk [3],
Mohammad Ayman A. Salkini [1], Hasan S. Yusufoglu [4], Prawez Alam [1] and Ahmed I. Foudah [1]

1   Department of Pharmacognosy, College of Pharmacy, Prince Sattam Bin Abdulaziz University,
     Al-Kharj 11942, Saudi Arabia
2   Department of Pharmacognosy, Faculty of Pharmacy, Alexandria University, Alexandria 21215, Egypt
3   Department of Pharmaceutical Botany, Faculty of Pharmacy, Ege University, 172/98, Izmir 35040, Turkey
4   Department of Pharmacognosy & Pharmaceutical Chemistry, College of Dentistry & Pharmacy,
     Buraydah Private College, Buraydah 52385, Saudi Arabia
*   Correspondence: m.youssef@psau.edu.sa; Tel.: +966-545-539-145

Citation: Abdel-Kader, M.S.; Alqarni, M.H.; Baykan, S.; Oztürk, B.; Salkini, M.A.A.; Yusufoglu, H.S.; Alam, P.; Foudah, A.I. Ecofriendly Validated RP-HPTLC Method for Simultaneous Determination of the Bioactive Sesquiterpene Coumarins Feselol and Samarcandin in Five *Ferula* Species Using Green Solvents. *Separations* 2022, 9, 206. https://doi.org/ 10.3390/separations9080206

Academic Editor: Ernesto Reverchon

Received: 16 July 2022
Accepted: 5 August 2022
Published: 8 August 2022

Publisher's Note: MDPI stays neutral with regard to jurisdictional claims in published maps and institutional affiliations.

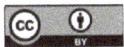
Abstract: An environmentally friendly unreported rapid and simple reverse-phase high-performance thin-layer chromatography (RP-HPTLC) has been designed for the simultaneous determination of bioactive sesquiterpene coumarins feselol and samarcandin in the methanol extract of five *Ferula* species. The method was developed using glass plates coated with RP-18 silica gel 60 F254S and a green solvent system of ethanol–water mixture (8:2 v/v) as mobile phase. After development, the plates were quantified densitometrically at 254 for feselol and samarcandin. Feselol and samarcandin peaks from methanol extract of five *Ferula* species were identified by comparing their single band at Rf = 0.43 ± 0.02 and Rf = 0.60 ± 0.01, respectively. Valid linear relationships between the peak areas and concentrations of feselol and samarcandin in the range of 1000–7000 ng/band respectively were obtained. The method was subjected to the validation criteria of the international conference on harmonization (ICH) for precision, accuracy, and robustness. The new method provides an analytical tool to enumerate the therapeutic doses of feselol and samarcandin in herbal formulations and/or crude drugs. The obtained results indicated that *F. drudeana* was the richest species in the more active samarcandin, with 0.573% w/w, while *F. duranii* had the largest quantity of the less active feselol, 0.813% w/w. *F. drudeana* was superior to the other species in the sum of the two active compounds, 1.4552% w/w, and was consequently expected to be the most active aphrodisiac among the five studied species.

Keywords: feselol; samarcandin; *Ferula*; HPTLC; ICH guidelines; quantitative

1. Introduction

The family Apiaceae is one of the largest families of flowering plants, with approximately 450 genera and 3700 species, growing in the northern temperate regions [1]. The family members are economically important as food, flavoring agents, and ornamental plants [2]. One of the important genera in the family is *Ferula* L., which contains 180–185 species found in Central and Southwest Asia [1]. In Turkey, more than 130 species were recognized. About 100 of these species are endemic [3]. *Ferula* species members are generally tall perennials or biennials characterized by stout stems and finely divided leaves with inflated sheaths [4]. Plants belonging to the *Ferula* genus are well-documented for their therapeutic value in the Middle East area's traditional medicine. Among the reported traditional medicinal uses of *Ferula* species are for treating rheumatism, inflammation, pain, convulsion, neurological disorders, and diabetes [5]. Many members of the genus have been used in Chinese traditional medicine for stomach disorders and rheumatoid arthritis. Recent pharmacological investigations have proved the antibacterial, antioxidant, antiulcerative, immunopharmacological, and hypotensive activities of the genus [6–8]. The antihyperlipidemic and antihyperglycemic effects of *F. assa-foetida, F. tenuissima, F. drudeana,* and *F. huber-morathii* were demonstrated [9,10].

The most common traditional use of *Ferula* species members is as an aphrodisiac [11]; for example, *F. hermonis* is commonly used in Syria and Lebanon [12]. *F. narthex* is used for its aphrodisiac properties in Ayurvedic medicine [13]. In the USA [14] and Brazil [15] *F. assa-foetida* extracts have been applied for the treatment of erectile dysfunction. Other *Ferula* members such as *F. elaeochytris* and *F. communis* are listed as aphrodisiacs in the Turkish traditional medicine [16].

Ferula species are the source of important biologically active secondary metabolites as sesquiterpene coumarin derivatives and sulphur compounds [17]. The biological activities of the plants' genus are partially attributed to the volatile oil contents [18].

Our investigation of the aphrodisiac effect of *F. drudeana* listed in Turkish traditional medicine and phytochemical study resulted in the isolation of two active sesquiterpene coumarins, feselol and samarcandin [19]. In this investigation, we designed a validated RP-HPTLC method for the analyses of feselol and samarcandin biomarker in five *Ferula* spices, utilizing RP18 silica gel plates. The proposed method was proved to be precise, accurate, and compliant with all the ICH guidelines [20].

2. Materials and Methods

2.1. Standard and Chemicals

Standard feselol and samarcandin (Figure 1) were previously purified and characterized from of *F. drudeana* [19]. All the used solvents were of HPLC grade and other chemicals were of analytical reagent (AR) grade.

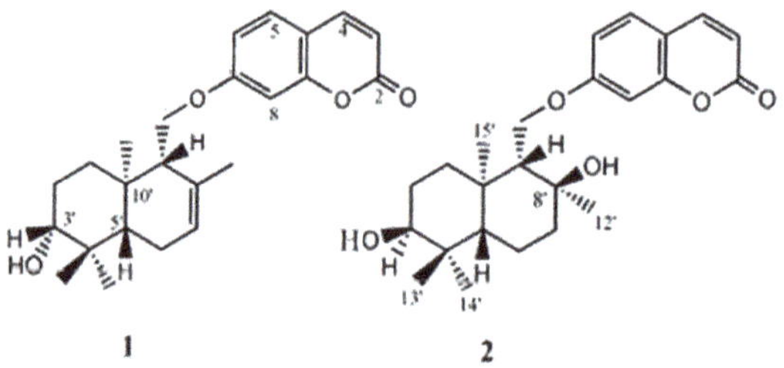

Figure 1. Structures of feselol (**1**) and samarcandin (**2**).

2.2. Preparation of Standard Solutions

Accurately weighed 10 mg of the standard feselol and samarcandin were separately dissolved in the green solvent ethanol and the volume was completed to 10 mL volumetric flasks to obtain 1000 μg/mL concentration. From this working standard, 1, 2, 3, 4, 5, 6 and 7 μL equivalent to 1000, 2000, 3000, 4000, 5000, 6000, and 7000 ng, respectively, were applied as bands on the RP 18-TLC. Two calibration curves for feselol and samarcandin were plotted in the range of 1000–7000 ng/band, correlating peak areas with the corresponding concentrations of the analytes per band. This solution was used as a reference solution.

2.3. Plant Material

The plants of *F. drudeana, F. tenuissima, F. Huber-morathii, F. duranii,* and *F. assa-foetida* were collected from the Turkey and were previously described in [9,10,19].

2.4. Extractions Procedure

The dried powdered parts of different plant species (10 g) were extracted by percolation at room temperature with ethanol (4 × 70 mL) until exhaustion. The combined solvents were evaporated using rotary vacuum evaporator and the left extracts were dissolved in

50 mL volumetric flask with ethanol. These test solutions were used in the TLC (Thin Layer Chromatography)densitometric analysis.

2.5. Chromatographic Conditions

Glass-backed plates 10 × 20 cm coated with 0.2 mm layers of RP18 silica gel 60 F254S (E-Merck, Darmstadt, Germany) were used for densitometric analysis. Samples were applied as 6 mm bands using a Camag Automatic TLC Sampler 4 (ATS4) sample applicator (Muttenz, Switzerland) integrated with a Camag microlitre syringe. The application rate was adjusted to 150 nL/s. The plates were developed to 80 mm distance using ethanol/water 8:2 (%, *v/v*) as mobile phase in a Camag Automatic Developing Chamber 2 (ADC2). Saturation of the camber with mobile phase was allowed for 30 min at 22 °C.

2.6. Method Validation

The designed HPTLC method was subjected to validation according to the ICH guidelines [20]. Linearity of the method for feselol and samarcandin were checked between 1000–7000 and peak area was plotted against concentration.

2.6.1. Accuracy

Accuracy was determined using the standard addition method. Preanalyzed samples of feselol and samarcandin (2000 ng/band) were spiked with extra amounts of the analytes (0, 50, 100, and 150%) and the mixtures were reanalyzed. Both percentage recovery and relative standard deviation (RSD, %) were obtained for each concentration level as indication for accuracy.

2.6.2. Precision

Precision was determined as repeatability and intermediate precision. Repeatability of sample was determined as intraday variation, while intermediate precision was proved from the interday variation for analysis of feselol and samarcandin at three different dilutions (300, 400, and 500 ng/band) in six replicates.

2.6.3. Robustness

Robustness was used to evaluate the influence of small deliberate changes in the chromatographic conditions on the new designed method. Small changes to duration of mobile-phase saturation, mobile-phase composition, mobile-phase volume, and activation of HPTLC plates during the analyses of feselol and samarcandin could be applied.

2.6.4. Limit of Detection (LOD) and Limit of Quantification (LOQ)

The two values known as limit of detection (LOD) and limit of quantification (LOQ) were obtained, applying the standard deviation (SD) method. The two were calculated using the slope of the calibration (S) curve, SD of the blank sample, and applying the following formulas:

$$LOD = 3.3 \times SD/S$$

$$LOQ = 10 \times SD/S$$

The standard deviation of the response was determined using the y-intercepts of regression lines' standard deviation.

2.6.5. Quantification of Feselol and Samarcandin in Ethanol Extract of *Ferula* Species

Different *Ferula* species samples were applied on the RP18-TLC plates, and same conditions for analysis of standard feselol and samarcandin were used to obtain test samples' chromatograms. The area of the peak corresponding to the Rf value of feselol and samarcandin standard were observed and the amounts present were obtained using the regression equation obtained from the calibration plot.

3. Results

3.1. Method Development

The densitometric HPTLC method for analysis of feselol and samarcandin was achieved by optimizing the mobile-phase composition. The mobile phase composed of ethanol–water 8:2 (%, v/v) resulted in a compact, symmetrical, and well-resolved peak at Rf value of 0.43 ± 0.02 and 0.60 ± 0.01 for feselol and samarcandin, respectively (Figure 2). UV spectra showed λ_{max} absorbance at 254 nm for both feselol and samarcandin bands.

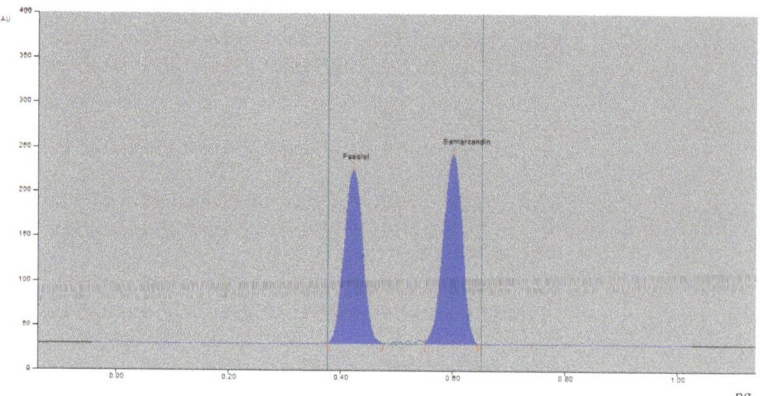

Figure 2. HPTLC densitogram of standard feselol and samarcandin.

3.2. Method Validation

The calibration plot of the peak area against the concentrations of feselol (Figure 3A) and samarcandin (Figure 3B) showed linearity in the range of 1000–7000 ng/band. Linear regression data obtained from the plot indicated a good linear relationship (Table 1).

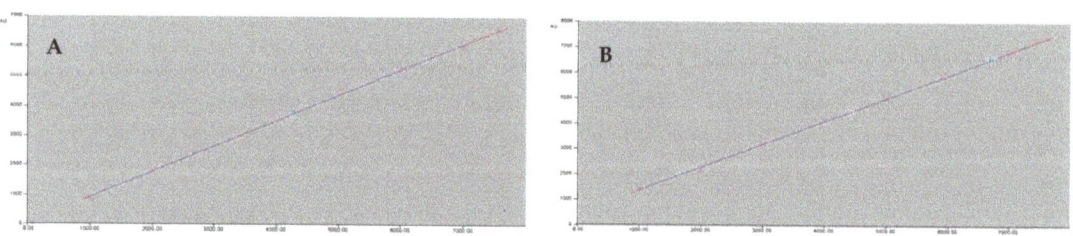

Figure 3. The linearity graph of feselol (**A**) and samarcandin (**B**).

Table 1. Linear regression data for the calibration curve of feselol and samarcandin (n = 6).

Parameters	Feselol	Samarcandin
Linearity range (ng/band)	1000–7000	1000–7000
Regression equation	Y = 0.8399x + 115.43	Y = 0.9507x + 42.314
Correlation coefficient	0.9996	0.9995
Slope ± SD	0.8399 ± 0.2321	0.9507x ± 0.1250
Intercept ± SD	115.43 ± 71.45	42.314 ± 78.08
Standard error of slope	0.0520	0.0456
Standard error of intercept	44.31	54.03
95% confidence interval of slope	10.316–9.841	13.54–12.11
95% confidence interval of intercept	5343–5671	3120–3270
p value	<0.0001	<0.0001

The accuracy of the method expressed as recovery is shown in Table 2. In Table 3, the results of repeatability and intermediate precision, expressed as SD (%), are presented. Robustness of the presented new HPTLC method explored by introducing a small deliberate change into the densitometric TLC procedure. Results of robustness are presented in Table 4. LOD and LOQ of the proposed method were found to be 12.34 and 38.45 as well as 14.03 and 56.12 ng/band for feselol and samarcandin, respectively.

Table 2. Accuracy of the proposed method (n = 6).

Excess Analyte (%)	Theoretical Content (ng)	Conc. Found (ng) ± SD	% Recovery	% RSD
		Feselol		
0	2000	1986.33 ± 8.52	99.32	0.43
50	3000	2953.67 ± 40.71	98.42	1.38
100	4000	3990.83 ± 10.07	99.77	0.25
150	5000	4959.00 ± 43.98	99.18	0.89
		Samarcandin		
0	2000	1981.33 ± 19.46	99.07	0.98
50	3000	2963.33 ± 27.90	98.78	0.94
100	4000	3994.83 ± 3.87	99.87	0.10
150	5000	4974.35 ± 40.35	99.50	0.81

Table 3. Precision of the proposed method of feselol and samarcandin.

Conc. (ng/band)	Repeatability (Intraday Precision)			Intermediate Precision (Interday)		
	Avg Conc. ± SD (n = 6)	Standard Error	% RSD	Avg Conc. ± SD (n = 6)	Standard Error	% RSD
			Feselol			
3000	2603.60 ± 28.15	11.49	1.08	2569.60 ± 32.68	13.35	1.27
4000	3545.00 ± 23.45	9.58	0.66	3533.00 ± 34.50	14.09	0.98
5000	4385.00 ± 8.94	3.65	0.20	4393.00 ± 18.62	7.60	0.42
			Samarcandin			
3000	2889.00 ± 7.55	3.08	0.26	2865.00 ± 32.94	13.45	1.15
4000	3821.00 ± 21.16	8.64	0.55	3837.00 ± 34.10	13.92	0.89
5000	4648.00 ± 15.06	6.15	0.32	4664.00 ± 30.11	12.29	0.65

Table 4. Robustness of the proposed HPTLC method of feselol and samarcandin.

Conc. (ng/band)	Mobile-Phase Composition (Ethanol: Water)					
	Original	Used		Area ± SD (n = 3)	% RSD	Rf
			Feselol			
4000	8:2	6.9:3.1	−0.1, +0.1	3513 ± 20.41	0.58	0.44
		8:2	0.0	3533 ± 26.65	0.75	0.43
		7.1:2.9	+0.1, −0.1	3523 ± 16.33	0.46	0.42
			Samarcandin			
4000	8:2	8.9:2.1	−0.1, +0.1	3776 ± 38	1.02	0.62
		8:2	0.0	3788 ± 32	0.83	0.60
		8.1:1.9	+0.1, −0.1	3780 ± 30	0.79	0.58

4. Discussion

Sesquiterepene coumarins are unique secondary metabolites of limited distribution in the plant kingdom. They were reported from the genera *Ferula*, *Daucus*, *Heptaptera* and *Dorema* (Apiaceae); *Achillea, Artemisia, Anthemis, Brocchia,* and *Tanacetum* (Asteraceae), *Euphorbia* and *Jatropha* (Euphorbiaceae) and *Aegle* (Rutaceae). However, most of the isolated sesquiterpene coumarins came from herbs from the *Ferula* genus. According to Li et al. [21], 181 sesquiterpene coumarins have been reported, among which 135 were identified from *Ferula* species. For example, the study of *F. samarkandica* led to the isolation of 22 sesquiterpene coumarins [22]. Sesquiterpene coumarins can be considered as biomarkers for the genus *Ferula*. Most of the genus bioactivities were attributed to sesquiterpene coumarins. The aphrodisiac effect of *F. drudeana* was traced to feselol and samarcandin [19]. Quantification of these two compounds in the genus member can give an indication to their aphrodisiac potential.

The developed method was challenged against all parameters required by the ICH [20] for validation. The linearity of both feselol and samarcandin were observed in the range of 1000–7000 ng (Figure 3A,B). The correlation coefficient (R2) was highly significant ($p < 0.0001$), and values were 0.9996 and 0.9995 for feselol and samarcandin, respectively (Table 1). The obtained R2 values gave indication about the strength of the correlations between the two variables. The % recoveries of 98.42–99.77 and 98.78–99.87 for feselol and samarcandin (Table 2) after standard addition of 0, 50, 100, and 150% to preanalyzed sample with 2000 ng/band of both feselol and samarcandin indicated that the method is accurate for the determination of the two standards.

Repeatability and intermediate precision were determined as intraday precision and interday variation (n = 6) (Table 3). The obtained % RSD for feselol at 0.2–1.08; 0.42–1.27 in the intraday precision and interday variation as well as those for samarcandin at 0.26–0.55; 0.65–1.15 gave a firm indication regarding the method's precision. The robustness is an important parameter for the method's validation, as minute experimental-condition variations are expected to happen very frequently. We proved the developed method robustness by small changes in the mobile-phase composition (Table 4). The obtained % RSD for feselol at 0.46–0.75 and at 0.79–1.02 for samarcandin were within the acceptable range, with small change in the Rf values indicating that the developed method was robust.

The LOD and LOQ of the proposed method were found to be 12.34; 38.45 and 14.03, 56.12 ng/band for feselol and samarcandin, respectively, indicating the sensitivity of the method and ability to analyze ng quantities. The method was specific for the quantification of feselol and samarcandin as indicated from their corresponding Rf values at 0.43 ± 0.02 and 0.60 ± 0.01, respectively. The UV absorption curves of the corresponding bands at λ_{max} 254 nm in the different extract were completely identical.

The amounts of feselol and samarcandin were estimated, applying the developed, validated green HPTLC method in five *Ferula* species (Table 5). The highest amount of festetol were found in *F. duranii* (0.813% w/w), while samarcandin was higher in *F. drudeana* (0.573% w/w). Our previous investigation indicated that samarcandin was more active than feselol [19]. Considering the sum of the two compounds in each of the studied species, *F. drudeana* was superior, with 1.375% w/w, followed by *F. duranii*, with 1.034% w/w. *F. tenuissima* showed the lowest concentration of both compounds (0.217% w/w). Based on available data, *F. drudeana* was expected to be the most active species as an aphrodisiac among the five studied species. However, further phytochemical and biological studies are need for this genus.

Table 5. Contents of feselol and samarcandin in methanol extract of different species of *Ferula*.

Samples	Feselol (%*w/w*)	Samarcandin (%*w/w*)	Sum (%*w/w*)
F. drudeana	0.802	0.573	1.375
F. tenuissima	0.107	0.047	0.217
F. Huber-morathii	0.089	0.549	0.638
F. duranii	0.813	0.221	1.034
F. assa-foetida	0.652	0.285	0.937

5. Conclusions

The developed green HPTLC method designed for the simultaneous quantification of feselol and samarcandin was simple, accurate, reproducible, sensitive, and is applicable to the analysis of plant species or products containing these compounds. This proposed method was developed using green solvent (ethanol and water) and RP-HPTLC plates. Statistical data indicated that the new method is selective for the analysis of feselol and samarcandin with added advantages of short time, being environmentally friendly, and requiring minimal sample preparation, in addition to the low cost. Based on the analysis of the individual biologically active feselol and samarcandin, as well as the sum total of their concentration, the relative potency of the species as aphrodisiacs can be expected.

Author Contributions: Conceptualization, M.S.A.-K., M.H.A. and A.I.F.; methodology, P.A., M.A.A.S. and H.S.Y.; software, M.H.A., A.I.F. and P.A.; validation, M.H.A., A.I.F. and H.S.Y.; formal analysis, M.S.A.-K. and M.A.A.S.; investigation, M.A.A.S., M.H.A. and P.A.; resources, B.O., S.B. and H.S.Y.; data curation, M.H.A. and A.I.F.; writing—original draft preparation, M.H.A., P.A. and A.I.F.; writing—review and editing, M.S.A.-K.; visualization, M.S.A.-K. and M.H.A.; supervision, M.S.A.-K. All authors have read and agreed to the published version of the manuscript.

Funding: This research received no external funding.

Institutional Review Board Statement: Not applicable.

Informed Consent Statement: Not applicable.

Data Availability Statement: Not applicable.

Acknowledgments: This work was supported by Deanship of Scientific Research at Prince Sattam Bin Abdulaziz University.

Conflicts of Interest: The authors declare no conflict of interest.

References

1. Pimenov, M.G.; Leonov, M.V. The Asian Umbelliferae Biodiversity Database (ASIUM) with particular reference to South-West Asian Taxa. *Turk. J. Bot.* **2004**, *78*, 139–145.
2. Baser, B.; Sagıroglu, M.; Dogan, G.; Duman, H. Morphology of pollen in *Ferula* genus (Apiaceae). *PhytoKeys* **2021**, *179*, 111–128. [CrossRef]
3. Chamberlain, D.F.; Rechinger, K.H. *Ferula* L. In *Flora Iranica*; Umbelliferae; Rechinger, K.H., Ed.; Akademische Druck und Verlagsanstalt: Graz, Austria, 1987; Volume 162, pp. 387–425.
4. Kurzyna-Mlynik, R.; Oskolski, A.A.; Downie, S.R.; Kopacz, R.; Wojewódzka, A.; Spalik, K. Phylogenetic position of the genus *Ferula* (Apiaceae) and its placement in tribe Scandiceae as inferred from nr DNA ITS sequence variation. *Plant Syst. Evol.* **2008**, *274*, 47–66. [CrossRef]
5. Asili, J.; Sahebkar, A.; Bazzaz, B.S.F.; Sharifi, S.; Iranshahi, M. Identification of essential oil components of *Ferula badrakema* fruits by GC-MS and 13C-NMR methods and evaluation of its antimicrobial activity. *J. Essent. Oil Bear. Plants* **2009**, *12*, 7–15. [CrossRef]
6. Sahebkar, A.; Iranshahi, M. Volatile constituents of the Genus *ferula* (Apiaceae): A review. *J. Essent. Oil Bear. Plants* **2011**, *14*, 504–531. [CrossRef]
7. Li, G.; Li, X.; Cao, L.; Shen, L.; Zhu, J.; Zhang, J.; Wang, J.; Zhang, L.; Si, J. Steroidal esters from *Ferula sinkiangensis*. *Fitoterapia* **2014**, *97*, 247–252. [CrossRef] [PubMed]
8. Yang, J.; An, Z.; Li, Z.; Jing, S.; Qina, H. Sesquiterpene coumarins from the roots of *Ferula sinkiangensis* and *Ferula teterrima*. *Chem. Pharm. Bull.* **2006**, *54*, 1595–1598. [CrossRef] [PubMed]
9. Yusufoglu, H.S.; Soliman, G.A.; Abdel-Rahman, R.F.; Abdel-Kader, M.S.; Genaie, M.A.; Bedir, E.; Baykan, S.; Oztürk, B. Antioxidant and Antihyperglycemic Effects of *Ferula drudeana* and *Ferula huber-morathii* in Experimental Diabetic Rats. *Int. J. Pharmacol.* **2015**, *11*, 738–748. [CrossRef]
10. Yusufoglu, H.S.; Soliman, G.A.; Abdel-Rahman, R.F.; Abdel-Kader, M.S.; Ganaie, M.A.; Bedir, E.; Baykan, S.; Oztürk, B. Antihyperglycemic and Antihyperlipidemic Effects of *Ferula assa-foetida* and *Ferula tenuissima* Extracts in Diabetic Rats. *Pak. J. Biol. Sci.* **2015**, *18*, 314–323. [CrossRef]
11. Mohammadhosseini, M.; Venditti, A.; Sarker, S.D.; Nahar, L.; Akbarzadeh, A. The genus *Ferula*: Ethnobotany, phytochemistry and bioactivities—A review. *Ind. Crops Prod.* **2019**, *129*, 350–394. [CrossRef]
12. Al-Ja'fari, A.; Vila, R.; Freixa, B.; Tomi, F.; Casanova, J.; Costa, J.; Cañigueral, S. Composition and antifungal activity of the essential oil from the rhizome and roots of *Ferula hermonis*. *Phytochemistry* **2011**, *72*, 1406–1413. [CrossRef] [PubMed]
13. Achliya, G.S.; Wadodkar, S.G.; Dorle, A.K. Evaluation of sedative and anticonvulsant activities of Unmadnashak Ghrita. *J. Ethnopharmacol.* **2004**, *94*, 77–83. [CrossRef] [PubMed]

14. Eli Lilly and Company. *Lilly's Handbook of Pharmacy and Therapeutics*; Eli Lilly and Co.: Indianapolis, IN, USA, 1898.
15. Elisabetsky, E.; Figueiredo, W.; Oliveria, G. Traditional Amazonian Nerve Tonics as Antidepressant Agent. *J. Herbs Spices Med. Plants* **1992**, *1*, 125–162. [CrossRef]
16. Tufan, S.; Toplan, G.G.; Mat, A. Ethnobotanical usage of plants as aphrodisiac agents in Anatolian folk medicine. *Marmara Pharm. J.* **2018**, *22*, 142–151. [CrossRef]
17. Iranshahy, M.; Iranshahi, M. Traditional uses, phytochemistry and pharmacology of asafetida (Ferula assa-foetida oleo-gum-resin): A review. *J. Ethnopharmacol.* **2011**, *134*, 1–10. [CrossRef]
18. Maggi, F.; Cecchini, C.; Cresci, A.; Coman, M.M.; Tirillini, B.; Sagratini, G.; Papa, F. Chemical composition and antimicrobial activity of the essential oil from *Ferula glauca* L. (*F. communis* L. subsp. Glauca) growing in Marche (central Italy). *Fitoterapia* **2009**, *80*, 68–72. [CrossRef] [PubMed]
19. Alqarni, M.H.; Soliman, G.A.; Salkini, M.A.; Alam, P.; Yusufoglu, H.S.; Baykan, S.; Oztürk, B.; Abdel-Kader, M.S. The potential aphrodisiac effect of *Ferula drudeana* korovin extracts and isolated sesquiterpene coumarins in male rats. *Phcog. Mag.* **2020**, *16*, 404–409.
20. ICH. Q2 (R2): Validation of Analytical Procedures–Text and Methodology. In Proceedings of the International Conference on Harmonization (ICH), Geneva, Switzerland, 31 March 2022.
21. Li, N.; Guo, T.; Zhou, D. Bioactive sesquiterpene coumarins from plants. In *Studies in Natural Products Chemistry*; ur-Rahman, A., Ed.; Elsevier: Amsterdam, The Netherlands, 2018; Volume 59, pp. 251–282.
22. Kamoldinov, K.; Li, J.; Eshbakova, K.; Sagdullaev, S.; Xu, G.; Zhou, Y.; Li, J.; Aisa, H.A. Sesquiterpene coumarins from Ferula samarkandica Korovin and their bioactivity. *Phytochemistry* **2021**, *187*, 112705. [CrossRef] [PubMed]

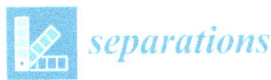 *separations*

Article

A High-Performance Thin-Layer Chromatographic Method for the Simultaneous Determination of Curcumin I, Curcumin II and Curcumin III in *Curcuma longa* and Herbal Formulation

Maged S. Abdel-Kader [1,2,*], Ayman A. Salkini [1], Prawez Alam [1], Khaled A. Alshahrani [1], Ahmed I. Foudah [1] and Mohammed H. Alqarni [1]

[1] Department of Pharmacognosy, College of Pharmacy, Prince Sattam Bin Abdulaziz University, Al-Kharj 11942, Saudi Arabia; m.salkini@psau.edu.sa (A.A.S.); p.alam@psau.edu.sa (P.A.); ph.khaled1997@gmail.com (K.A.A.); a.foudah@psau.edu.sa (A.I.F.); m.alqarni@psau.edu.sa (M.H.A.)
[2] Department of Pharmacognosy, Faculty of Pharmacy, Alexandria University, Alexandria 21215, Egypt
* Correspondence: m.youssef@psau.edu.sa or mpharm101@hotmail.com; Tel.: +966-545-539-145

Citation: Abdel-Kader, M.S.; Salkini, A.A.; Alam, P.; Alshahrani, K.A.; Foudah, A.I.; Alqarni, M.H. A High-Performance Thin-Layer Chromatographic Method for the Simultaneous Determination of Curcumin I, Curcumin II and Curcumin III in *Curcuma longa* and Herbal Formulation. *Separations* 2022, 9, 94. https://doi.org/10.3390/separations9040094

Academic Editor: Ernesto Reverchon

Received: 16 March 2022
Accepted: 8 April 2022
Published: 10 April 2022

Publisher's Note: MDPI stays neutral with regard to jurisdictional claims in published maps and institutional affiliations.

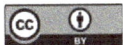

Abstract: *Curcuma longa* (turmeric) has traditionally been used in Ayurvedic, Unani and herbal drugs to cure numerous ailments. Due to the high demand, the quantitative standardization of herbal products is challenging to maintain their quality. We aim to develop a rapid, sensitive and validated high-performance thin-layer chromatography (HPTLC) method for the simultaneous determination and quantification of curcumin I, curcumin II and curcumin III in *C. longa* and herbal formulation. The three standards were separated using centrifugal preparative thin-layer chromatography (CPTLC) silica gel and identified by different spectroscopic methods. The developed HPTLC method was validated by following ICH guidelines (linearity; limit of detection, LOD; limit of quantitation; accuracy; precision; and robustness). The calibration curves of both the compounds were linear (50–500 ng/spot), with a correlation coefficient (r^2) of >999. The developed HPTLC method was effectively applied to the concurrent detection and quantification of curcumins I–III in fresh, dry rhizomes and the herbal formulation of *C. longa* extracts was obtained by hot and cold extraction methods.

Keywords: CPTLC; spectroscopic identification; HPTLC; method development; curcumins; *Curcuma longa*

1. Introduction

The genus *Curcuma* is a rhizomatous annual or perennial herb in the Zingiberaceae family comprising about 120 species [1]. Most of the species of *Curcuma* are naturally present in tropical evergreen areas [2,3]. Many members of the genus are well known in traditional medicine. *C. amada* rhizomes are used as an appetizer, carminative, digestive, stomachic, demulcent, vulnerary, aphrodisiac, laxative, diuretic, expectorant, anti-inflammatory and antipyretic [4]. The rhizomes of *C. angustifolia* are used as a demulcent and antipyretic, are effective against gravel Stomatitis and aid in blood coagulation [5]. In combination with astringents and aromatics, the rhizomes of *C. aromatic* are used for bruises, sprains, hiccough, bronchitis, cough, leukoderma and skin eruptions [6]. The rhizome of *C. zedoaria* are used as an appetizer and tonic, and are particularly prescribed to ladies after childbirth. In Ayurveda, it is an ingredient of "Braticityādi kwatha", used in high fever [7].

Ayurvedic systems have widely used *Curcuma longa* (turmeric) for centuries in the treatment of many inflammatory conditions and diseases such as biliary disorders, anorexia, cough, diabetic wounds, hepatic disorders, rheumatism and sinusitis [8]. Turmeric has been used as a remedy for all kinds of poisonous conditions, ulcers and wounds [9]. It gives a good complexion to the skin and is applied to face as a depilatory and facial tonic. The drug is also useful in cold, cough, bronchitis, conjunctivitis and liver affections [10,11]. Several pharmacological studies were conducted to support the use of *C. longa*. Water-

and fat-soluble extracts of turmeric and its main active component, curcumin, exhibited strong antioxidant activity, comparable to vitamins C and E. Curcumin was found to be eight times more powerful than vitamin E in preventing lipid peroxidation [12]. Turmeric's hepatoprotective effects have been proven in a number of animal studies. Curcumin has choleretic activity that increases bile output and solubility, which may be helpful in treating gallstones [13]. An open, phase II trial was performed on 25 patients with endoscopically diagnosed gastric ulcer treated with 600 mg of powdered turmeric five times daily. After four weeks, the ulcers had completely healed in 48 percent of patients and the percentage reached 76 after 12 weeks of treatment. No significant adverse reactions or blood abnormalities were noted [14].

The active constituents of *C. longa* are the curcumins [15]. Turmeric contains up to 5% curcumin and up to 5% of essential oils. Other constituents include sugars, proteins and resins [16]. The main oil components were identified as ar-turmerone (31.7%), α-turmerone (12.9%), β-turmerone (12.0%) and (Z) β-ocimene (5.5%), α-bisabolene (13.9%), *trans*-ocimene (9.8%), myrcene (7.6%), 1,8-cineole (6.9%), thujene (6.7%) and thymol (6.4%) [17].

Curcumin has anti-inflammatory properties [18] mediated via downregulation of the nuclear factor (NF)-κB [19] and cyclooxygenase 2 (Cox-2) [20]. Animal studies have indicated that oral curcumin possess antinociceptive [21] and indicated the involvement of ATP-sensitive potassium channels [22]. Pilot human studies of curcumin have demonstrated promise for improving the symptoms of rheumatoid arthritis and inflammatory bowel disease [23,24]. Curcumin also demonstrated antiviral, anti-inflammatory, antibacterial, antifungal, antidiabetic, antifertility and cardiovascular protective and immunostimulant activity [11]. Curcumin, one of the most studied chemopreventive agents, allows suppression, retardation or inversion of carcinogenesis. Curcumin is also described as an antitumoral, anti-oxidant and anti-inflammatory agent capable of inducing apoptosis in numerous cellular systems [25]. Both in vitro studies utilizing human cell lines and in vivo studies have demonstrated curcumin's ability to inhibit carcinogenesis at three stages: tumor promotion, angiogenesis and tumor growth [26]. Curcumin exhibits anticoagulant activity by inhibiting collagen and adrenaline-induced platelet aggregation in vitro as well as in vivo in rat thoracic aorta [27].

The aim of the current study is to develop and validate the high-performance thin-layer chromatography (HPTLC) method for the quantification of curcumins I–III in different extracts of *C. longa* and formulation. There are several advantages of using HPTLC for the analysis, such as the ability to analyze crude samples containing multi-components. Several samples can be separated parallel to each other on the same plate, resulting in a high output and a rapid low-cost analysis. The choice of solvents for the HPTLC development is wide, as the mobile phases evaporated before the spot detection. Spray reagents can be used to detect separated spots [28]. The HPTLC method uses much less amounts of the mobile phase, minimizing exposure to organic solvents and reducing environment pollution [29,30].

2. Materials and Methods

2.1. Chemicals and Plant Materials

A standard curcumin mixture was procured from Sigma-Aldrich, St. Louis, MO, USA. All other reagents utilized for the extraction and method development were of analytical grade. The rhizomes of *Curcuma longa* and its herbal formulation containing 500 mg of curcuma extract per capsule were obtained randomly from the hypermarket in Al-Kharj, Saudi Arabia. Chromatographic and analytical grade reagent (AR) were used for the extraction and method development. Centrifugal preparative TLC (CPTLC) was preformed using a chromatotron (Harrison Research Inc. model 7924, Harrison Research, Palo Alto, CA, USA): a 4 mm silica gel P254 disc. Pre-coated, glass-baked TLC plates obtained from E. Merck (silica gel-60F254; thickness: 0.2 mm; area: 20 × 10 cm) were used for quantification.

2.2. Purification of Individual Curcumins

The standardly composed mixture of the three major curcumins was purified to obtain the individual compounds for the quantification. From the standard mixture, 100 mg were separated using CPTLC on 4 mm silica gel GF254 disks (solvents: 0.5% MeOH in CHCl$_3$). Three zones were collected from the chromatotron and corresponded to curcumins I–III (Figure 1).

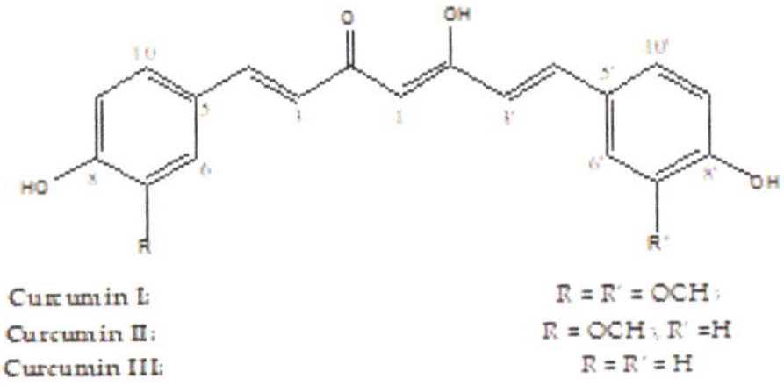

Curcumin I: R = R' = OCH$_3$
Curcumin II: R = OCH$_3$, R' =H
Curcumin III: R = R' = H

Figure 1. Structures of Curcumins I–III.

2.3. Charaterization of Curcumins

NMR data (Figures S1 and S2) were measured using a Bruker UltraShield Plus 500 MHz spectrometer (Bruker, Fällanden, Switzerland) at the NMR Unite, College of Pharmacy, Prince Sattam Bin Abdulaziz, and was operated at 500 MHz for protons and 125 MHz for carbon atoms, respectively. Chemical shift values were reported in δ (ppm) relative to the residual solvent peaks. HRESIMS (Figures S3–S5) were determined by direct injection using a Thermo Scientific UPLC RS Ultimate 3000-Q Exactive hybrid quadrupole-Orbitrap mass spectrometer (Thermo Scientific, Waltham, MA, United States) combined with the high-performance quadrupole precursor selection with high resolution and accurate-mass (HR/AM) Orbitrap™ detection.

2.4. Extraction Procedure

Fresh and dried curcuma purchased from the local market and a formulation containing 500 mg of curcuma extract per capsule were extracted with MeOH by maceration (×3) at room temperature, using the soxhlet apparatus for 6 h to obtain the corresponding six extracts, two for each sample. All extracts were filtered and dried using the rotary vacuum evaporator to obtain the corresponding dry extracts.

2.5. HPTLC Conditions

HPTLC (Camag, Muttenz, Switzerland) was performed on glass-backed TLC silica-gel plates (20 cm × 10 cm). Purified curcumin I, curcumin II and curcumin III and sample solutions were separately spotted with nitrogen flow on a plate with a 6-mm-wide band at 8-mm from the bottom by using the automatic Camag-TLC (Linomat V, Camag, Muttenz, Switzerland) applicator. The (linear ascending) development of TLC plates was performed in a twin glass Camag chamber (automatic ADC2, Camag). The chamber was filled with 20 mL of mobile phase for a fixed time of 15 min.

2.6. Method Validation

Different validation parameters for the simultaneous determination of curcumin I, curcumin II and curcumin III were determined as per the ICH-Q2 (R1) guidelines [31].

2.6.1. Accuracy

Accuracy was determined by the standard addition method. The preanalyzed samples of curcumin I, curcumin II and curcumin III were spiked with the extra 0, 50, 100 and 150% of the standard curcumin I, curcumin II and curcumin III, and the solutions were reanalyzed in six replicates by the proposed method. The accuracy of the HPTLC technique for the simultaneous determination of curcumin I, curcumin II and curcumin III was estimated as % recovery.

2.6.2. Precision

Precision of the proposed method was determined at two levels i.e., repeatability and intermediate precision. Repeatability was determined as the intraday precision, whereas the intermediate precision was determined by carrying out an inter-day variation for the determination of curcumin I, curcumin II and curcumin III. The precision of the HPTLC technique for the simultaneous estimation of curcumin I, curcumin II and curcumin III was expressed as the percent relative standard deviation (% RSD).

2.6.3. Robustness

The robustness of the proposed HPTLC method was determined to evaluate the influence of small deliberate changes in the chromatographic conditions during the determination of curcumin I, curcumin II and curcumin III. The robustness of the HPTLC technique for the simultaneous determination of curcumin I, curcumin II and curcumin III was evaluated by introducing small deliberate changes in the composition of mobile phase components, total run length, saturation time and detection wavelength.

2.6.4. Limit of Detection and Quantification (Sensitivity)

The sensitivity of the HPTLC technique for the simultaneous determination of curcumin I, curcumin II and curcumin III was determined in terms of detection (LOD) and quantification (LOQ) limits. The limit of detection (LOD) and limit of quantification (LOQ) were determined by the standard deviation (SD) method. They were determined from the slope of the calibration (S) curve and SD of the blank sample using the following equations:

$$LOD = 3.3 \times SD/S$$

$$LOQ = 10 \times SD/S$$

2.6.5. Specificity

The specificity of the proposed TLC densitometric method was confirmed by the R_f and spectra of the spot with that of the standards of curcumin I, curcumin II and curcumin III.

2.7. Quantification of Curcumins I–III in C. longa and Herbal Formulation

Curcumin I, curcumin II and curcumin III peaks in *C. longa* and herbal formulation were identified by comparing their spots at that of the standard curcumin I, curcumin II and curcumin III. The amount of curcumin I, curcumin II and curcumin III present in the *C. longa* and herbal formulation was quantified from the regression equation obtained from the calibration plot of HPTLC.

3. Results
3.1. Method Validation
3.1.1. Linearity

Calibration curves for curcumins I–III are presented in Figures S6–S8. The results for the least square regression analysis of the calibration curves (CCs) of curcumins I–III are included in Table 1.

Table 1. Linear regression data for the calibration curve of curcumins I–III (*n* = 6).

Parameters	Curcumin I	Curcumin II	Curcumin III
Linearity range (ng/spot)	50–500	50–500	50–500
Regression equation	Y = 4.3931x + 424.66	Y = 8.1074x + 254.62	Y = 13.66x + 2.858
Correlation coefficient	0.998	0.999	0.997
Slope ± SD	4.3931 ± 0.1123	8.1074 ± 0.1342	13.66 ± 0.1391
Intercept ± SD	424.66 ± 56.12	254.62 ± 53.23	2.858 ± 62.90
Standard error of slope	0.0310	0.0538	0.0457
Standard error of intercept	28.15	33.07	30.18
95% confidence interval of slope	12.456–13.032	11.89–12.12	13.34–15.02
95% confidence interval of intercept	6540–6712	4651–5478	5231–5365
p value	<0.0001	<0.0001	<0.0001

3.1.2. Accuracy

The accuracy of the HPTLC technique for the simultaneous determination of curcumins I–III was estimated as % recovery, and the results are included in Table 2.

Table 2. Accuracy of the proposed method of curcumins I–III (*n* = 6).

Excess Drug Added to Analyte (%)	Theoretical Content (ng)	Conc. Found (ng) ± SD	% Recovery	% RSD
		Curcumin I		
0	100	98.67 ± 0.52	98.67	0.52
50	150	145.83 ± 2.23	97.22	1.53
100	200	194.50 ± 2.88	97.25	1.48
150	300	293.67 ± 3.14	97.89	1.07
		Curcumin II		
0	100	97.83 ± 1.17	97.83	1.19
50	150	147.33 ± 1.37	98.22	0.93
100	200	195.83 ± 2.04	97.92	1.04
150	300	295.67 ± 6.12	98.56	0.63
		Curcumin III		
0	100	97.17 ± 0.98	97.17	1.01
50	150	145.83 ± 2.48	97.22	1.70
100	200	295.17 ± 1.72	98.39	0.58

3.1.3. Precision

The precision of the HPTLC technique for the simultaneous estimation of curcumin I, curcumin II and curcumin III was estimated in terms of instrumental and intra/inter-assay precision and expressed as the percent relative standard deviation (% RSD). The results of intra/inter-assay precisions for the simultaneous determination of curcumins I–III using the HPTLC technique are included in Table 3.

Table 3. Precision of the proposed method of curcumins I–III.

Conc. (ng/spot)	Repeatability (Intraday Precision)			Intermediate Precision (Interday)		
	Avg Conc. ± SD (*n* = 6)	Standard Error	% RSD	Avg Conc. ± SD (*n* = 6)	Standard Error	% RSD
			Curcumin I			
200	1360.00 ± 21.24	8.67	1.56	1354.50 ± 23.24	9.49	1.72
300	1747.50 ± 13.58	5.54	0.78	1750.17 ± 18.99	7.75	1.08
400	2149.83 ± 24.27	9.91	1.13	2156.33 ± 28.14	11.49	1.30

Table 3. *Cont.*

Conc. (ng/spot)	Repeatability (Intraday Precision)			Intermediate Precision (Interday)		
	Avg Conc. ± SD (n = 6)	Standard Error	% RSD	Avg Conc. ± SD (n = 6)	Standard Error	% RSD
			Curcumin II			
200	1842.50 ± 16.53	6.75	0.90	1873.00 ± 22.72	9.28	1.21
300	2694.83 ± 28.53	11.65	1.06	2674.00 ± 32.43	13.24	1.21
400	3574.17 ± 17.36	7.09	0.49	3572.33 ± 26.52	10.83	0.74
			Curcumin III			
200	2617.83 ± 27.23	11.12	1.04	1589.49 ± 22.75	9.29	1.43
300	4217.00 ± 32.12	13.12	0.76	4214.17 ± 25.44	10.39	0.60
400	5627.33 ± 20.45	8.35	0.36	5631.17 ± 24.91	10.17	0.44

3.1.4. Robustness

The robustness of the HPTLC technique for the simultaneous determination of curcumins I–III was evaluated by introducing small deliberate changes in the composition of mobile phase components, total run length, saturation time, and detection wavelength. The results of the robustness analysis after changing the mobile phase components are included in Table 4.

Table 4. Robustness of the proposed HPTLC method of curcumins I–III.

Conc. (ng/spot)	Original	Used		Area ± SD (n = 3)	% RSD	R_f
				Curcumin I		
		8.9:1.1	−0.1, +0.1	2148 ± 28	1.33	0.43
400	9:1	9:1	0.0	2149 ± 23	1.09	0.45
		9.1:0.9	+0.1, −0.1	2158 ± 22	1.01	0.46
				Curcumin II		
		8.9:1.1	−0.1, +0.1	3573 ± 27	0.75	0.51
400	9:1	9:1	0.0	3574 ± 26	0.73	0.52
		9.1:0.9	+0.1, −0.1	3574 ± 13	0.36	0.49
				Curcumin III		
		8.9:1.1	−0.1, +0.1	5645 ± 31	0.55	0.60
400	9:1	9:1	0.0	5650 ± 22	0.39	0.61
		9.1:0.9	+0.1, −0.1	5641 ± 25	0.45	0.63

3.1.5. Sensitivity

The sensitivity of the HPTLC technique for the simultaneous determination of curcumin I, curcumin II and curcumin III was determined in terms of detection (LOD) and quantification (LOQ) limits.

3.1.6. Specificity

The specificity of the proposed TLC densitometric method was confirmed by the R_f at 0.45 ± 0.02, 0.52 ± 0.02 and 0.61 ± 0.04 and the spectra of the spot with that of the standards curcumins I–III (Figure 2). The proposed method was found to be specific by comparing the R_f of *C. longa* rhizomes, herbal formulation and standard, as well as the overlaid spectra at peak start, peak apex and peak end position of the spot, showing λ_{max} 423 nm for curcumin I, curcumin II and curcumin III (Figure S9).

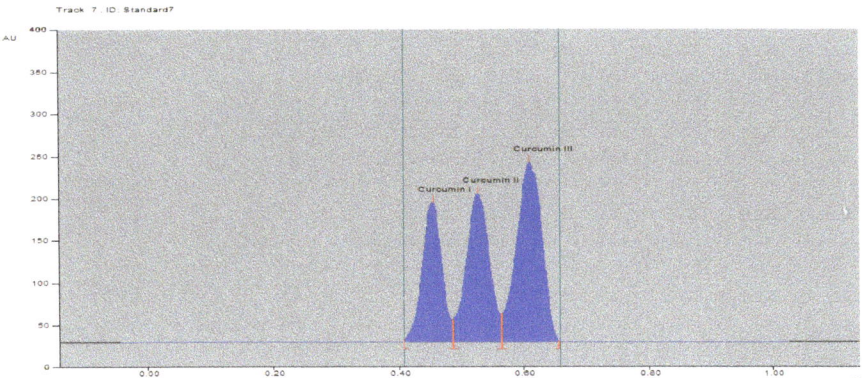

Figure 2. HPTLC densitogram of standard curcumins I–III.

3.2. Quantification of Curcumins I–III in C. longa and Herbal Formulation

The curcumins I–III peaks in the *C. longa* and herbal formulation were identified by comparing their spots at R_f = 0.45, 0.52 and 0.61 with that of purified curcumins I–III (Figure 2) as well as the overlay UV spectra of the spots with the same R_f value (Figure S9). The amount of curcumins I–III present in the *C. longa* (Figures 3–5) and herbal formulation was quantified from the regression equation obtained from the calibration plot of HPTLC. The amounts of curcumins I–III in *C. longa* and herbal formulation are presented in Table 5.

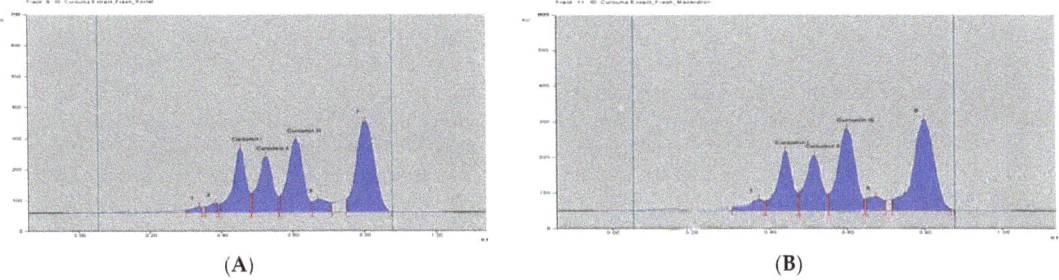

(A)   (B)

Figure 3. HPTLC densitogram of fresh *C. longa* extract by (**A**) soxhlet and (**B**) maceration.

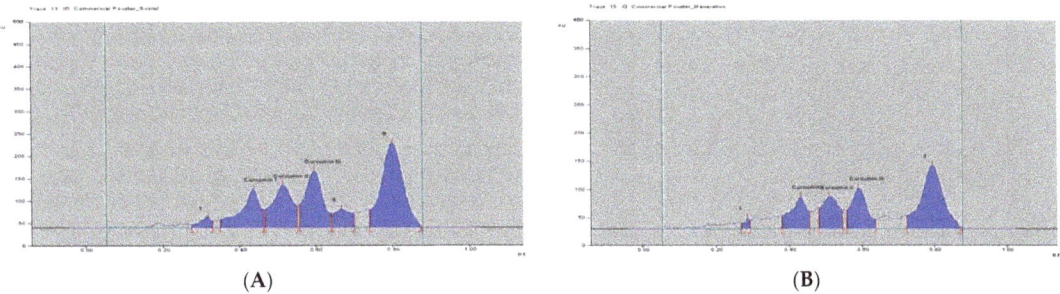

(A)   (B)

Figure 4. HPTLC densitogram of dry *C. longa* extract by (**A**) soxhlet and (**B**) maceration.

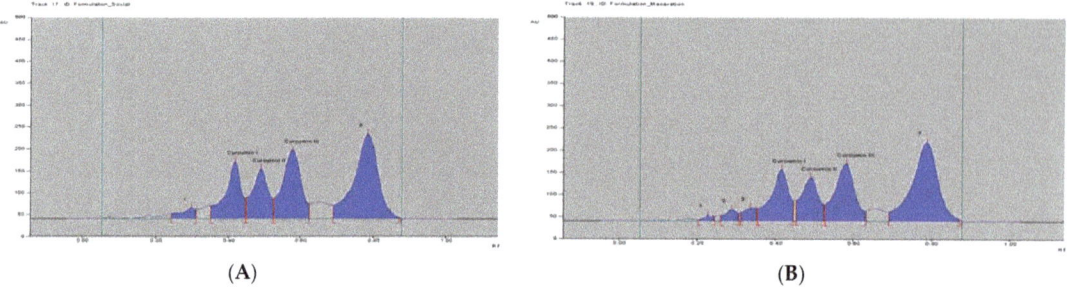

(A)   (B)

Figure 5. HPTLC densitogram of *C. longa* formulation extract by (**A**) soxhlet and (**B**) maceration.

Table 5. Contents (% *w/w*) of curcumins I–III in different samples of *C. longa*.

Samples	Cur. I	Cur. II	Cur. III
1. Curcuma Ext_Fresh (Maceration)	0.44	0.28	0.65
2. Curcuma Ext_Fresh (Soxhlet)	0.53	0.37	0.76
3. Commercial Powder (Maceration)	0.23	0.15	0.33
4. Commercial Powder (Soxhlet)	0.34	0.25	0.47
5. Formulation (Maceration)	0.26	0.19	0.41
6. Formulation (Soxhlet)	0.28	0.22	0.46

4. Discussion

4.1. Characterization of Curcumins

The three purified curcumins I–III shared the same carbon chain composed of C-1, C-2, C-2′, C-3, C-3′, C-4 and C-4′ with two trans-oriented methine carbons assigned for C-3, 3′ and C-4, 4′, which have trans orientation based on the *J* value of 16.0 Hz between H-3, 3′ and H-4, 4′ (Supplementary Materials). Curcumin I ^{1}H, ^{13}C NMR spectrum, showed ABX spin system in a 1, 3, 4 trisubstituted aromatic ring (Figures S1A and S2A). Two overlapped OCH$_3$ appeared at δ_H 3.98 and δ_C 55.84 ppm. High resolution electrospray ionization mass spectroscopy (HRESIMS) (Figure S3) showed an M$^+$−1 at *m/z* 367.1188, M$^+$+1 at 369.1328 and M$^+$+Na 391.1147. The data were identical with those reported for curcumin I [32–34]. ^{1}H NMR of curcumin II (Figure S1B) showed one system ABX system assigned for 6, 9 and 10 at δ_H 7.19 (s), 6.80 (bd, *J* = 7.5 Hz) and 7.08 (d, *J* = 7.0 Hz) in a tri-substituted benzene ring and an AX system assigned for a para-substituted benzene ring at δ_H 6.80 (bd, *J* = 7.5 Hz) and 7.46 (d, *J* = 7.5 Hz). Signals for one OCH$_3$ at δ_H 3.83 and δ_C 56.04 ppm were also observed. HRESIMS (Figure S4) showed an M$^+$−1 at *m/z* 337.1084, M$^+$+1 at 339.1226 and M$^+$+Na at 361.1043. The data were identical with those reported for curcumin II [32–34]. The ^{1}H NMR of curcumin III (Figure S1C) showed only two aromatic proton signals at δ_H 6.80 (d, *J* = 8.2) and 7.47 (d, *J* = 8.2) each integrated for four protons diagnostic for two identical para-substituted benzene rings. HRESIMS showed (Figure S5) an M$^+$−1 at *m/z* 307.0977, M$^+$+1 at 309.1120 and M$^+$+Na at 331.0938. The data were identical with those reported for curcumin III [32–34].

4.2. HPTLC Analysis

Standard curcumins are available as a mixture of the three main curcumins. For the purpose of quantification, the mixture was purified on chromatoron using normal silica gel and the resulted compounds were used as a standard after their identification spectroscopically. The calibration curve for curcumins I–III was observed as linear in the range of 50–500 ng band-1. The results demonstrated a good linear relationship between the concentration and spot area of curcumins I–III. The determination coefficient (R2) value for curcumins I–III was obtained as 0.998, 0.999 and 0.997, respectively, which were highly significant (*p* < 0.05) (Table 1). The R2 values represents the strength of the correlations between the two variables. All these observations and results suggested that the sustainable HPTLC technique was linear and acceptable for the simultaneous estimation of curcumin I, curcumin II and curcumin III.

The preanalyzed sample of curcumins I–III were spiked with the extra 0, 50, 100 and 150% of the standard curcumins I–III, and the solutions were reanalyzed in six replicates by the proposed method. The % of recoveries of curcumins I–III were estimated as 97.22–98.67, 97.83–98.22 and 99.32–100.84%, respectively, using the HPTLC technique (Table 2). The estimated % recoveries within the limit that exhibited the HPTLC technique was accurate for the simultaneous determination of curcumins I–III.

The precision of the proposed method was determined at two levels, i.e., repeatability and intermediate precision. The repeatability was determined as an intra-day precision, whereas the intermediate precision was determined by carrying out inter-day variation for the determination of curcumins I–III. Intra-day and inter-day precisions ($n = 6$) for curcumin I, curcumin II and curcumin III were found to be 0.78–1.56% and 1.08–1.72%, 0.49–1.06 and 0.74–1.21 and 0.36–1.04 and 0.44–1.43, respectively (Table 3), which demonstrated the good precision of the proposed method.

The robustness of the HPTLC technique for the simultaneous determination of curcumins I–III was evaluated by introducing small deliberate changes in the composition of mobile phase components. The % RSD for curcumins I–III after this change were determined as 1.01–1.33, 0.36–0.75 and 0.45–0.55%, respectively. In addition, the R_f values for curcumins I–III were recorded as 0.43–0.46, 0.49–0.52 and 0.61–0.63, respectively (Table 4). The small differences in the R_f values and lower % RSD demonstrated the robustness of the HPTLC technique for the simultaneous determination of curcumins I–III.

The LOD and LOQ values for curcumin I were determined as 4.36 and 12.79 ng band-1, respectively. The LOD and LOQ values for curcumin II, were determined as 4.59 and 12.67 ng band−1, respectively. However, the LOD and LOQ values for curcumin III, were determined as 4.66 and 12.84 ng band-1, respectively. The recorded values of LOD and LOQ suggested that the HPTLC technique was highly sensitive for the simultaneous estimation and quantification of curcumins I–III.

The specificity was proven by comparing the R_f at 0.45 ± 0.02, 0.52 ± 0.02 and 0.61 ± 0.04 and spectra of the spots in the *C. longa* extract and formulation with that of the purified curcumins I–III. The proposed method was found to be specific by comparing the R_f of rhizomes of *C. longa* and herbal formulation and standard as well as the overlaid spectra at peak start, peak apex and peak end position of the spot showing λ_{max} 423 nm for curcumins I–III (Figure S9). The specificity or peak purity for the proposed analytical method was suggested by the similar UV-absorption spectra, Rf values and detection wavelength of curcumins I–III.

4.3. Quantification of Curcumins I–III in C. longa and Herbal Formulation

Extraction methods selection is mainly based on the nature of the components to be obtained. Solvent extraction is the most widely used method. Solvent extraction includes maceration, percolation and reflux extraction. It usually requires a large volume of the organic solvents and long extraction time. Some modern extraction methods, such as the super critical fluid extraction, pressurized liquid extraction and microwave-assisted extraction, have been used in extraction. These methods lower organic solvent consumption, shorten extraction time and are more selective. However, they require more sophisticated and expensive instrumentation [35]. Maceration is a very simple extraction method with the disadvantage of long extraction time and low extraction efficiency. It could be used for the extraction of thermolabile components. On the other hand, the soxhlet extraction method integrates the advantages of the reflux extraction and percolation, which utilizes the principle of reflux and siphoning to continuously extract the plant materials with fresh solvent. The soxhlet extraction is an automatic continuous extraction method with high extraction efficiency that requires less time and solvent consumption than maceration or percolation. However, soxhlet extraction is not suitable for plant materials with thermolabile or volatile components [35]. In the current study, for comparison, both the maceration and soxhlet extraction were applied for the extraction of curcumins from *C. longa* fresh rhizomes, dry powdered rhizomes and the formulation, using methanol as an extraction solvent. The amounts of the three main curcumins were estimated by applying the proposed and validated HPTLC method. The results of the analysis are presented in Figures 3–5 and Table 5. The content of curcumin I–III in fresh rhizome and dry powdered by maceration and soxlet extraction was determined as 0.44, 0.28, 0.65 and 0.53, 0.37, 0.76 and 0.23, 0.15, 0.33 and 0.34, 0.25, 0.47% *w/w*, respectively, using the proposed analytical method. The content of curcumin I–III in formulation by maceration and soxhlet extraction was determined as 0.26, 0.19, 0.41 and 0.28, 0.22, 0.46% *w/w*, respectively, using the proposed analytical method.

As expected in all cases, the soxhlet extraction was more efficient than the maceration and gives better yield of the extracted compounds. Moreover, the soxhlet saves much time and solvent consumption. The results also indicated that the fresh plant materials were superior to the dry powdered plants in term of the percentage *w/w* of the three curcumins. This fact may be explained by the loss of some contents during the drying and processing of the plant material by oxidation or other factors. The amount of curcumin III was the highest in all estimations followed by curcumin I, while curcumin II was present in a lower concentration.

5. Conclusions

In conclusion, curcumins I–III were purified and characterized by various spectro scopic methods from the standard curcumin mixture available on the market. An HPTLC method was developed, validated and applied to estimate the amount of curcumins in the fresh, dry plant materials and formulation containing *C. longa*. Two extraction methods were applied to obtain the target curcumins from the raw plant materials. The soxhlet extraction gives better yields of the three curcumins than maceration, indicating the thermal stability of the compounds under used conditions. The fresh plant materials contained more amounts of curcumins than the dry plant materials.

Supplementary Materials: The following supporting information can be downloaded at: https://www.mdpi.com/article/10.3390/separations9040094/s1. Figure S1. 1HNMR of the aromatic protons of curcumins I–III (A–C). Figure S2. 13CNMR of the aromatic carbons of curcumins I–III (A–C). Figure S3. Mass spectra of curcumin I (A: Negative Mode B: Positive Mode). Figure S4. Mass spectra of curcumin II (A: Negative Mode B: Positive Mode). Figure S5. Mass spectra of Curcumin III (A: Negative Mode B: Positive Mode). Figure S6. Calibration curve of curcumin I. Figure S7. Calibration curve of curcumin II. Figure S8. Calibration curve of curcumin III. Figure S9: Overlay UV absorption spectra of curcumins I–III and corresponding spots in *C. longa* extracts and formulations.

Author Contributions: Conceptualization, M.S.A.-K. and P.A.; methodology, P.A., A.A.S., K.A.A. and M.H.A.; software, A.I.F. and M.H.A.; validation, A.I.F. and M.H.A.; formal analysis, M.S.A.-K., A.I.F. and M.H.A.; investigation, P.A., A.A.S. and K.A.A.; resources, M.S.A.-K.; data curation, P.A., A.A.S. and K.A.A.; writing—original draft preparation, P.A., A.A.S. and K.A.A.; writing—review and editing, M.S.A.-K., M.H.A. and A.I.F.; visualization, M.S.A.-K.; supervision, M.S.A.-K.; project administration, M.S.A.-K. All authors have read and agreed to the published version of the manuscript.

Funding: This research received no external funding.

Institutional Review Board Statement: Not applicable.

Informed Consent Statement: Not applicable.

Data Availability Statement: Not applicable.

Acknowledgments: The authors would like to thank the Deanship of Scientific Research at Prince Sattam Bin Abdulaziz University, Al-Kharj, Saudi Arabia for supporting this research.

Conflicts of Interest: The authors declare no conflict of interest.

References

1. Kress, W.J.; Prince, L.M.; Williams, K.J. The phylogeny and a new classification of the gingers (Zingiberaceae): Evidence from molecular data. *Am. J. Bot.* **2002**, *89*, 1682–1696. [CrossRef] [PubMed]
2. Larsen, K. A preliminary checklist of the Zingiberaceae of Thailand. *Thai For. Bull.* **1996**, *24*, 35–49.
3. Xia, Q.; Zhao, K.J.; Huang, Z.G.; Zhang, P.; Dong, T.T.; Li, S.P.; Tsim, K.W. Molecular genetic and chemical assessment of Rhizoma Curcumae in China. *J. Agric. Food Chem.* **2005**, *53*, 6019–6026. [CrossRef] [PubMed]
4. Gupta, M.; Shaw, B.P.; Mukherjee, A. A new glycosidic flavonoid from *Jwarhar mahakashay* (antipyretic) Ayurvedic preparation. *Int. J. Ayurveda Res.* **2010**, *1*, 106–111. [CrossRef] [PubMed]
5. Banerjee, A.; Nigam, S.S. Antifungal activity of the essential oil of Curcuma angustifolia. *Indian J. Pharmacol.* **1977**, *39*, 143–145.
6. Warrier, P.K.; Nambiar, V.P.; Ramankutty, C. *Indian Medicinal Plants*; Orient Longman Ltd.: Madras, India, 1994; pp. 1–5.
7. Thakur, R.S.; Puri, H.S.; Husain, A. *Major Medicinal Plants of India*; CIMAP: Lucknow, India, 1989; pp. 50–52.
8. Hanif, R.; Qiao, L.; Shiff, S.J. Curcumin., a natural plant phenolic food additive, inhibits cell proliferation and induces cell cycle changes in colon adenocarcinoma cell lines by a prostaglandin-independent pathway. *J. Laborat. Clin. Med.* **1997**, *130*, 576–584. [CrossRef]
9. Kolammal, M. *Pharmacognosy of Ayurvedic Drugs*; Ayurveda College: Trivandrum, India, 1979.
10. Kurup, P.N.; Ramdas, V.N.; Joshi, P. *Handbook of Medicinal Plants*; New Delhi, Oxford and IBH Publishing Co pvt Ltd.: Delhi, India, 1979.
11. Nadkarni, A.K. *Indian Materia Medica*; Popular Prakashay: Bombay, India, 1954; Volume 408, p. 1476.
12. Toda, S.; Miyase, T.; Arich, H. Natural antioxidants. Antioxidative compounds isolated from rhizome of Curcuma longa. *Laborat Chem. Pharmacol. Bullet.* **1985**, *33*, 1725–1728. [CrossRef]
13. Park, E.J.; Jeon, C.H.; Ko, G. Protective effect of curcumin in rat liver injury induced by carbon tetrachloride. *J. Pharm. Pharmacol.* **2000**, *52*, 437–440. [CrossRef]
14. Ammon, H.P.T.; Wahl, M.A. Pharmacology of Curcuma longa. *Planta Med.* **1991**, *57*, 1–7. [CrossRef]
15. Tayyem, R.F.; Heath, D.D.; Al-Delaimy, W.K.; Rock, C.L. Curcumin content of turmeric and curry powders. *Nutr. Cancer* **2006**, *55*, 126–131. [CrossRef]
16. Goh, C.L.; Ng, S.K. Allergic contact dermatitis to Curcuma longa (turmeric). *Cont. Dermat.* **1987**, *17*, 186.
17. Chempakam, B.; Parthasarathy, V.A.; Zachariah, T.J. *Chemistry of Spices*; Chempakam, B., Parthasarathy, V.A., Eds.; Turmeric; CABI Publishing: Oxford, UK, 2008.
18. Asher, G.N.; Spelman, K. Clinical utility of curcumin extract. *Altern. Ther. Health Med.* **2013**, *19*, 20–22.
19. Sandur, S.K.; Pandey, M.K.; Sung, B.; Ahn, K.S.; Murakami, A.; Sethi, G. Curcumin, demethoxycurcumin, bisdemethoxycurcumin, tetrahydrocurcumin and turmerones differentially regulate anti-inflammatory and anti-proliferative responses through a ROS-independent mechanism. *Carcinogenesis* **2007**, *28*, 1765–1773. [CrossRef] [PubMed]
20. Samad, T.; Abdi, S. Cyclooxygenase-2 and antagonists in pain management. *Curr. Opin. Anaesthesiol.* **2001**, *14*, 527–532. [CrossRef]
21. Tajik, H.; Tamaddonfard, E.; Hamzeh-Gooshchi, N. The effect of curcumin (active substance of turmeric) on the acetic acidinduced visceral nociception in rats. *Pak. J. Biol. Sci.* **2008**, *11*, 312–314. [CrossRef]
22. De Paz-Campos, M.A.; Chavez-Pina, A.E.; Ortiz, M.I.; Castaneda-Hernandez, G. Evidence for the participation of ATP sensitive potassium channels in the antinociceptive effect of curcumin. *Korean J. Pain.* **2012**, *25*, 221–227. [CrossRef]
23. Chandran, B.; Goel, A. A randomized, pilot study to assess the efficacy and safety of curcumin in patients with active rheumatoid arthritis. *Phytother. Res.* **2012**, *26*, 1719–1725. [CrossRef]
24. Holt, P.R.; Katz, S.; Kirshoff, R. Curcumin therapy in inflammatory bowel disease: A pilot study. *Digest Dis. Sci.* **2005**, *50*, 2191–2193. [CrossRef]
25. Duvoix, A.; Blasius, R.; Delhalle, S.; Schnekenburger, M.; Morceau, F.; Henry, E.; Dicato, M.; Diederich, M. Chemopreventive and therapeutic effects of curcumin. *Cancer Lett.* **2005**, *223*, 181–190. [CrossRef]
26. Srivastava, R.; Puri, V.; Srimal, R.C.; Dhawan, B.N. Effect of curcumin on platelet aggregation and vascular prostacyclin synthesis. *Arzneimittelforschung* **1986**, *36*, 715–717.
27. Limtrakul, P.; Lipigorngoson, S.; Namwong, O. Inhibitory effect of dietary curcumin on skin carcinogenesis in mice. *Cancer Lett.* **1997**, *116*, 197203. [CrossRef]
28. Wagner, H. *Plant Drug Analysis: A Thin Layer Chromatography Atlas*, 2nd ed.; Springer: Berlin/Heidelberg, Germany, 1996.
29. Shewiyo, D.H.; Kaaleb, E.; Rishab, P.G.; Dejaegherc, B.; Verbekec, J.S.; Heydenc, Y.V. HPTLC methods to assay active ingredients in pharmaceutical formulations: A review of the method development and validation steps. *J. Pharm. Biomed. Anal.* **2012**, *66*, 11–23. [CrossRef] [PubMed]
30. Shuijun, L.; Gangyi, L.; Jingying, J.; Xiaochuan, L.; Chen, Y. Liquid chromatography-negative ion electrospray tandem mass spectrometry method for the quantification of ezetimibe in human. *Plasma J. Pharm. Biomed. Anal.* **2006**, *40*, 987–992.
31. ICH. Q2 (R2): Validation of Analytical Procedures–Text and Methodology. In Proceedings of the International Conference on Harmonization (ICH), Geneva, Switzerland, 31 March 2022.
32. Chearwae, W.; Wu, C.P.; Chu, H.Y.; Lee, T.R.; Ambudkar, S.V.; Limtrakul, P. Curcuminoids purified from turmeric powder modulate the function of human multidrug resistance protein 1 (ABCC1). *Cancer Chemother. Pharmacol.* **2006**, *57*, 376–388. [CrossRef]

33. Ahmed, M.; Abdul, Q.M.; Imtiaz, S.M.; Muddassar, M.; Hameed, A.; Nadeem, A.M.; Asiri, A.M. Curcumin: Synthesis optimization and in silico interaction with cyclin dependent kinase. *Acta Pharm.* **2017**, *67*, 385–395. [CrossRef] [PubMed]
34. Naidu, M.M.; Shyamala, B.N.; Manjunatha, J.R.; Sulochanamma, G.; Srinivas, P. Simple HPLC method for resolution of curcuminoids with antioxidant potential. *J. Food Sci.* **2009**, *74*, C312–C318. [CrossRef] [PubMed]
35. Zhang, Q.W.; Lin, L.G.; Ye, W.C. Techniques for extraction and isolation of natural products: A comprehensive review. *Chin. Med.* **2018**, *13*, 20. [CrossRef] [PubMed]

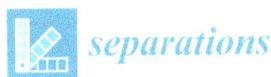 *separations*

Communication

Fractional Separation and Characterization of Cuticular Waxes Extracted from Vegetable Matter Using Supercritical CO$_2$

Mariarosa Scognamiglio, Lucia Baldino * and Ernesto Reverchon

Department of Industrial Engineering, University of Salerno, Via Giovanni Paolo II, 132, 84084 Fisciano, Italy;
mrscogna@unisa.it (M.S.); ereverchon@unisa.it (E.R.)
* Correspondence: lbaldino@unisa.it

Abstract: Cuticular waxes can be used in high-value applications, including cosmetics, foods and nutraceuticals, among the others. The extraction process determines their quality and purity that are of particular interest when biocompatibility, biodegradability, flavor and fragrance are the main features required for the final formulations. This study demonstrated that supercritical fluid extraction coupled with fractional separation can represent a suitable alternative to isolate cuticular waxes from vegetable matter that preserve their natural properties and composition, without contamination of organic solvent residues. Operating in this way, cuticular waxes can be considered as a fingerprint of the vegetable matter, where C$_{27}$, C$_{29}$ and C$_{31}$ are the most abundant compounds that characterize the material; the differences are mainly due to their relative proportions and the presence of hydrocarbon compounds possessing other functional groups, such as alcohols, aldehydes or acids. Therefore, selectivity of supercritical fluid extraction towards non-polar or slightly polar compounds opens the way for a possible industrial approach to produce extracts that do not require further purification steps.

Keywords: cuticular waxes; extraction; fractional separation; supercritical CO$_2$; gas chromatography-mass spectroscopy

Citation: Scognamiglio, M.; Baldino, L.; Reverchon, E. Fractional Separation and Characterization of Cuticular Waxes Extracted from Vegetable Matter Using Supercritical CO$_2$. *Separations* **2022**, *9*, 80. https://doi.org/10.3390/separations9030080

Academic Editor: Hailei Zhao

Received: 15 February 2022
Accepted: 16 March 2022
Published: 20 March 2022

Publisher's Note: MDPI stays neutral with regard to jurisdictional claims in published maps and institutional affiliations.

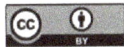
1. Introduction

Cuticular waxes are compounds ubiquitously present on the surface of all kinds of vegetable matter. They cover leaves, flowers, seeds and other vegetable structures, exerting the main functions of (i) controlling the perspiration, (ii) insulating the plant from external water and (iii) protecting it from pathogens [1,2], biotic and abiotic stresses and plant-insect interaction [3–5]. A cuticular wax is a complex mixture of long-chain alkanes, alkenes, alcohols, aldehydes, alkyl esters, fatty acids and other compound families [2,4,5]; although the large majority is represented by long-chain hydrocarbons [2]. Depending on the plant species, the total amount and composition of cuticular waxes can vary widely [4,6]: i.e., every vegetable species (and even organs from the same vegetable) can exhibit a unique composition. Cuticular waxes are not only interesting from an analytical point of view; they can have industrial applications in the field of cosmetic formulations and healthcare products [7,8], since they show a very large affinity with human skin thanks to the prevalence of odd long-chain hydrocarbons with respect to the analogous products coming from fossil feedstocks [8,9].

The current methods for extracting natural waxes from vegetable matter use large quantities of toxic organic solvents [10]. Guo and Jetter [11] studied cuticular waxes coming from potato leaves and other potato organs, after extraction using chloroform; the samples were extracted twice for 30 s. The same procedure was adopted by Jetter et al. [12] to process *Prunus laurocerasus* L. leaves. Cheng et al. [1] extracted cuticular waxes from rose petals and leaves using chloroform as the extraction solvent, in which the samples were immersed three times for 30 s. Trivedi et al. [2] used the same organic solvent to extract cuticular waxes from bilberry fruits; the immersion was 1 min long. Pimentel et al. [13]

processed *Croton* leaves using three consecutive immersions of 30, 20 and 10 s duration in dichloromethane. They systematically identified C_{19} to C_{33} alkanes and C_{18} to C_{34} alcohols.

Therefore, the extraction of cuticular waxes is carried out, as a rule, by liquid solvent extraction and chloroform is the most frequently used solvent. Moreover, the process is performed in a very fast manner to minimize the co-extraction of other undesired compounds [14]. However, when other extraction techniques are used, as in the case of Soxhlet method that can last some hours, other compounds and intracuticular waxes can be also extracted and the authors generally do not give indications about these co-extracts. In particular, cuticular waxes represent interfering compounds that are extracted together with the desired ones, since the target compounds generally have a biological/industrial interest, such as essential oil, coloring matter, antioxidants and active principles for pharmaceutical applications [8]. However, they are systematically co-extracted during solvent extraction, as previously discussed [15], and during alternative processes [16], like ultrasound assisted extraction (UAE), microwave assisted extraction (MAE), pressurized liquid extraction (PLE) and supercritical fluid extraction (SFE). Therefore, they have to be eliminated by post-processing procedures, such as the so-called winterization [17], in which the extract, dissolved in the organic solvent, is cooled at very low temperatures (e.g., from $-10\,°C$ to $-40\,°C$) for several hours to precipitate cuticular waxes that are subsequently separated by filtration [10].

CO_2 at supercritical conditions (SC-CO_2) is largely used to extract the compounds of interest from vegetable matter. In particular, above its critical point (P_c = 73.8 bar and T_c = 31 °C), CO_2 shows a liquid-like density and a gas-like diffusivity that favor the extraction of chemically affine compounds from solid matrices. Several studies [19–24] reported in the scientific literature describe the main advantages of using this green technique instead of the traditional ones, such as lower operative temperatures and higher selectivity. Moreover, post-processing steps, adopted to purify the extracts from cuticular waxes, are not required when winterization is performed in series to the extraction process in the same operative plant. In particular, Reverchon and co-workers demonstrated in several papers [25–27] that, by using SC-CO_2 extraction coupled with high-pressure fractional separation, it is possible to separate cuticular waxes during the extraction process by the selective precipitation from the overall extract [28]. Specifically speaking, the compounds of interest for extraction are generally located well inside the vegetable structure; whereas cuticular waxes are located on the surface of the vegetable material and show a non-negligible solubility in SC-CO_2 [28]. For this reason, they are inevitably co-extracted at all SC-CO_2 processing conditions due to the overlap of mass transfer limitations and thermodynamic (solubility) limits [28]. However, since they are generally considered as an interfering matter that reduces the quality (purity) of the extracts, a procedure has been developed that allows the selective separation of cuticular waxes from the extract by cooling the mixture CO_2 plus overall extract at the exit of the extractor down to temperatures lower than 0 °C [25–27,29,30]. Operating at these process conditions, the solubility of cuticular waxes reduces to near zero in SC-CO_2 and, therefore, they can be precipitated in a separator before the final collection of the extract of interest.

Therefore, according to the previous discussion of the literature, the scope of this work is to attempt, for the first time, a systematic analysis of cuticular waxes extracted by SC-CO_2 plus fractional separation from several vegetables. After performing the specific SC-CO_2 extraction processes, several high-resolution gas chromatography-mass spectroscopy (GC-MS) identifications are carried out on cuticular waxes obtained from more than ten different vegetable species, to analyze their composition and dependence on the vegetable tested, and to show that their composition can be specific for the different vegetable species and tissue analyzed.

2. Materials and Methods

2.1. Materials

Basil leaves (*Ocimum basilicum* L.), cannabis inflorescence (*Cannabis sativa* L.), chamomile flower heads (*Chamomilla recutita* L. Rausch.), clove buds (*Eugenia caryophyllata* Thun.), ginger rhizomes (*Zingiber officinale* Roscoe), lavender inflorence, marjoram leaf (*Origanum Majorana* L.), rosemary leaf (*Rosmarinus officinalis* L.), tangerine peels and tobacco leaves were supplied by Planta Medica srl (Pistrino di Citerna (PG), Italy). Jasmine concrete (*Jasminum grandiflorum* L.) was supplied by Chauvet (Seillans, France). Vegetable materials (except for jasmine concrete) were dried and ground using an electric stainless-steel grinder (KYG, mod. 304, China); mean particle size was determined by mechanical sieving. Carbon dioxide (CO_2, 99.9% purity, Morlando Group srl, Naples, Italy) was used to carry out SFE processing.

2.2. SFE Plant Description

SC-CO_2 extraction experiments were carried out in a homemade laboratory apparatus equipped with a 490 cm^3 internal volume extractor. One hundred grams of vegetable matter, with a mean particle size of 600 μm, were used in all the experiments. In the case of jasmine concrete, since it was a semi-solid material and can produce undesired caking/channeling phenomena during extraction, it was mixed with glass beads (3 mm diameter) to create an inert core surrounded by a thin shell of jasmine concrete. Extracts were recovered using two separation vessels with an internal volume of 200 cm^3 each, operated in series. The first separator was cooled down to −10 °C using a thermostated bath (Julabo, mod. F38-EH, Milan, Italy); the second one allowed the continuous discharge of the extract using a valve located at the bottom of the vessel. It was operated at 25 bar and 15 °C. A high-pressure pump (Lewa, mod. LDB1 M210S, Leonberg, Germany) pumped liquid CO_2 at the desired flow rate. CO_2 was then heated to the extraction temperature in a thermostated bath (Julabo, mod. CORIO C-B27, Milan, Italy). CO_2 flow rate was monitored by a calibrated rotameter (ASA, mod. d6, Sesto San Giovanni (MI), Italy), located after the last separator, coupled with a volumetric meter (Sacofgas 1927 SpA, mod. G.4, Milan, Italy). Temperature and pressure along the plant were measured by thermocouples and test gauges, respectively. More details about the apparatus and the experimental procedure are published elsewhere [25,27,30,31].

The operative conditions selected for the experiments carried out in this work were 90 bar and 50 °C ($\rho_{CO2} \approx 0.280$ g/cm^3) in the extractor, 90 bar and −10 °C in the first separator and 25 bar and 15 °C in the second one. CO_2 flow rate was fixed at 0.8 kg/h for all the experiments. The first separator, used for cuticular waxes precipitation, was operated at the same extraction pressure and at a temperature lower than 0 °C since, operating in this way, the solubility of cuticular waxes in CO_2 drastically reduced [25,27,28,30,31].

2.3. Characterization of Cuticular Waxes

Gas chromatography-mass spectroscopy (GC-MS) analysis was carried out using a Varian 3900 apparatus (Varian, Inc., San Fernando, CA, USA), equipped with a fused-silica capillary column (mod. DB-5, J & W, Folsom, CA, USA) of 30 m length, 0.25 mm internal diameter and 0.25 μm film thickness, and connected to a Varian Saturn Detector 2100T (Varian, Inc., San Fernando, CA, USA). Helium was used as the carrier gas, at a flow rate of 1 mL/min. Column temperature was set at 120 °C and held for 5 min; then, it was ramped up to 320 °C, at 2 °C/min, where it was held for 10 min. An injection step was performed using 1 μL of a 1:10 *n*-hexane solution in split mode; the injector temperature was set at 320 °C. The mass spectrometer operated at an ionization voltage of 70 eV in the 40–650 a.m.u. range, at a scanning speed of 5 scans/s. The retention indices (RI) were determined considering the retention time (Rt) values of homologous series of *n*-alkanes (C_{21}-C_{40}) obtained at the same operating conditions. The various components were also identified by a comparison of their RI with published data in the scientific literature. Further identifications were performed, by comparison, of the mass spectra with those stored in the

NIST 02 (National Institute of Standards and Technology, Gaithersburg, MD, USA) library. The relative amounts of the components were evaluated as a percentage of normalized peak area.

3. Results and Discussion

As reported in the literature, the major constituents of cuticular waxes extracted by SFE processing plus high-pressure fractionation of the vegetable matter were paraffinic compounds and, among them, heptacosane, nonacosane, hentriacontane and tritriacontane showed the larger percentages [32–38]. Moreover, odd-carbon-atom hydrocarbons were largely more represented than the homologous, even-carbon atoms. This is an interesting characteristic from an applicative point of view; indeed, differently from paraffins coming from fossil fractions, odd-carbon-atom hydrocarbons are largely more compatible with the human skin and can be applied in cosmetics and health care products [9,39–42].

A photograph of the cuticular waxes extracted during SFE processing of cannabis inflorescence is reported in Figure 1. In all cases, the precipitated material looks like a white powder, sometimes with a light smell, similar to that of the starting vegetable species.

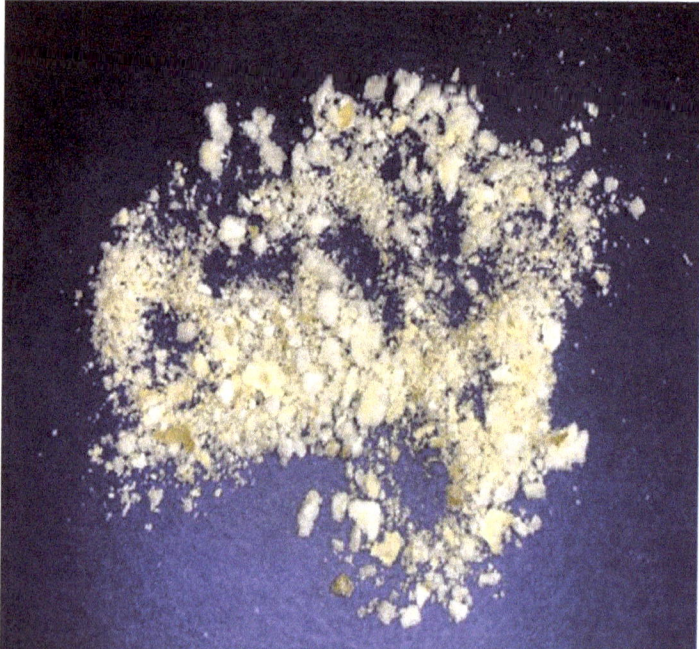

Figure 1. Macroscopic and qualitative example of cuticular waxes extracted by SFE processing of cannabis inflorescence.

Eleven GC-MS traces of the produced cuticular waxes are summarized in Figure 2, for overall comparison purposes. These traces can give a qualitative perspective of the compounds present in the various plants tested and their relative abundance.

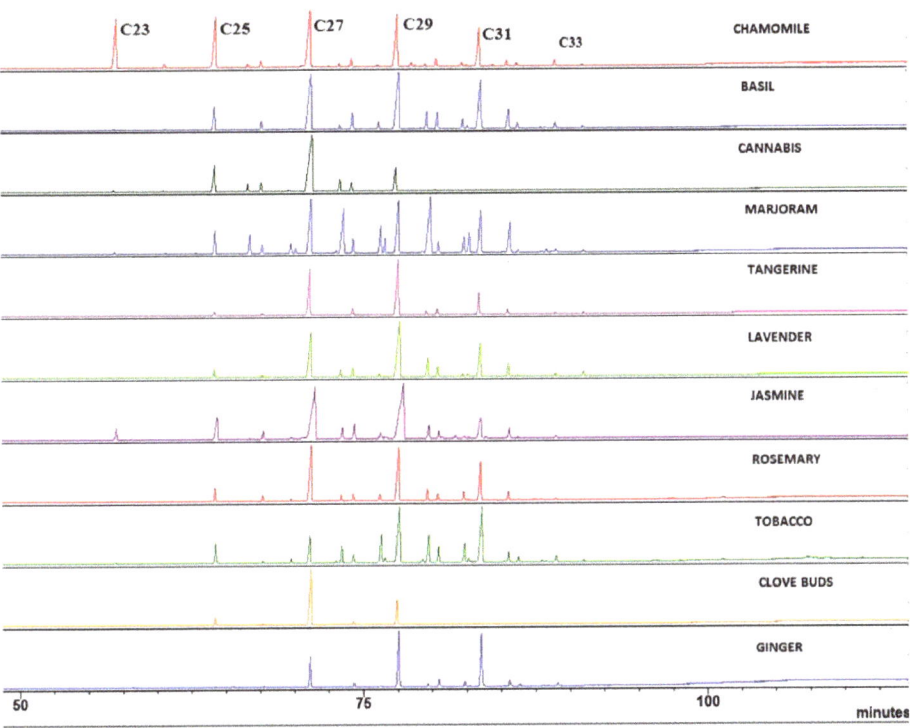

Figure 2. Comparison of GC−MS traces of cuticular waxes extracted by SC−CO₂ plus fractional separation from different vegetable matter, studied in this work.

Extensive identification of the cuticular waxes extracted and analyzed in this work is reported in Table 1. In particular, Figure 2 and Table 1 confirm that the most abundant compounds present in the cuticular waxes extracted by SC-CO$_2$ are C$_{27}$, C$_{29}$ and C$_{31}$ for all the vegetable species studied. These results are in agreement with the previous literature related to the same vegetable matter [32–39]. However, data in the literature are referred only to straight paraffins. Analysis performed in this work demonstrates, instead, the presence of some high-molecular-weight paraffinic alcohols (namely, C$_{24}$, C$_{26}$, C$_{28}$ and C$_{30}$). The largest percentages of these compounds are found in marjoram (16.22%), tobacco (5.94%) and lavender (5.48%). Additionally, aldehydes and traces of a paraffinic acid, namely octacosanoic acid, are detected in jasmine and tobacco. More specifically, C$_{28}$ and C$_{30}$ aldehydes are the most widespread compounds and the largest percentage of C$_{28}$ aldehyde is found in tobacco (6.57%) and marjoram (6.40%).

The prevalence of long-chain alkanes is confirmed, and they range from C$_{23}$ to C$_{33}$, with a prevalence of odd paraffins, as C$_{27}$, C$_{29}$ and C$_{31}$, that largely confirm as the major components, though their relative proportions vary from one vegetable species to another [43,44]. Some small quantities of paraffinic alcohols, aldehydes and fatty acids are also identified, as expected. They all show the same carbon atoms' skeleton of the identified paraffins, with the further presence of a functional group: i.e., alcoholic, aldehydic or acid group.

Table 1. Percentage (area %) of the compounds identified by GC−MS of cuticular waxes extracted by SC−CO$_2$ plus fractional separation from different vegetable matter, studied in this work.

Compound Identified	Chamomile	Basil	Ginger	Jasmine	Lavender	Tobacco	Marjoram	Tangerine	Cannabis	Rosemary	Clove Buds
Tricosane, C$_{21}$H$_{48}$	10.69	0.10	-	1.25	-	-	0.05	-	0.04	0.07	-
Tetracosane, C$_{24}$H$_{50}$	0.99	0.15	-	0.18	-	0.08	0.12	-	0.51	0.07	-
Pentacosane, C$_{25}$H$_{52}$	15.12	5.38	-	6.88	2.32	3.97	3.53	2.17	12.04	3.41	5.80
1-Tetracosanol, C$_{24}$H$_{50}$O	0.65	-	-	-	0.69	-	2.81	-	2.36	0.09	-
Hexacosane, C$_{26}$H$_{54}$	1.26	1.76	-	1.75	-	0.39	1.41	0.73	3.08	1.45	1.50
Methylhexacosane, C$_{27}$H$_{56}$	-	-	-	-	-	-	1.38	-	0.44	0.62	-
Heptacosane, C$_{27}$H$_{56}$	20.94	22.52	8.33	28.70	20.40	3.69	2.93	28.45	61.85	23.01	65.80
1-Hexacosanol, C$_{26}$H$_{54}$O	0.65	-	-	2.52	2.32	1.69	9.78	0.41	4.06	1.41	-
Octacosane, C$_{28}$H$_{58}$	1.63	3.33	1.07	3.19	2.74	-	1.85	3.56	2.88	1.87	3.90
Octacosanal, C$_{28}$H$_{56}$O	-	1.51	0.38	1.42	-	6.57	5.40	0.23	0.14	1.74	-
Nonacosane, C$_{29}$H$_{60}$	16.47	21.53	19.01	33.24	31.60	18.34	1.54	41.09	15.73	22.25	22.30
Methylhexacosanoate, C$_{17}$H$_{34}$O$_2$	0.78	-	0.73	-	-	-	-	-	-	-	-
1-Octacosanol, C$_{28}$H$_{58}$O	0.33	3.46	-	2.94	5.48	5.94	6.22	1.65	-	2.46	-
Triacontane, C$_{30}$H$_{62}$	1.36	3.34	2.09	1.61	2.54	3.11	1.40	2.93	0.35	1.67	-
Octacosanoic acid, C$_{28}$H$_{56}$O$_2$	-	-	-	0.85	-	0.09	-	-	-	-	-
Methylheptacosanoate, C$_{29}$H$_{58}$O$_2$	0.69	2.40	1.74	0.51	-	4.02	2.36	0.34	-	2.14	-
Triacontanal, C$_{30}$H$_{60}$O	-	0.57	-	0.19	-	1.14	2.84	0.12	-	0.32	-
Hentriacontane, C$_{31}$H$_{64}$	9.68	16.69	19.27	7.12	13.45	27.84	4.57	11.41	0.26	13.20	-
1-Triacontanol, C$_{30}$H$_{62}$O	1.03	4.14	2.85	2.12	3.92	1.89	7.24	2.34	-	2.22	-

Separations **2022**, *9*, 80

Table 1. *Cont.*

Compound Identified	Chamomile	Basil	Ginger	Jasmine	Lavender	Tobacco	Marjoram	Tangerine	Cannabis	Rosemary	Clove Buds
Dotriacontane, $C_{32}H_{66}$	0.61	0.96	0.76	0.17	0.52	0.89	0.30	0.16	0.07	0.38	-
Tritriacontane, $C_{33}H_{68}$	1.13	1.23	1.06	0.52	0.84	1.36	0.54	0.49	0.56	0.62	-
Methyldotriacontane, $C_{33}H_{68}$	-	0.50	0.16	-	1.41	0.34	0.30	0.82	-	0.13	-

4. Conclusions

In the present work, a detailed study on the composition of cuticular waxes extracted and fractionated by SFE is reported. GC-MS analysis confirmed that the separation from the other extractable materials was accurate, and these products can be considered a sort of fingerprint of the specific vegetable matter. C_{27}, C_{29} and C_{31} were the most abundant compounds found in the investigated vegetable materials, in line with the previous findings reported in the literature. Moreover, the specific selectivity of SC-CO_2 extraction towards non-polar or slightly polar compounds makes these cuticular waxes suitable for higher added-value applications, such as in the medical and pharmaceutical field, in which purity and biocompatibility are key features that justify the selection of a more complex extraction process with respect to the traditional ones.

Author Contributions: Conceptualization, E.R.; methodology, M.S.; validation, L.B. and E.R.; formal analysis, M.S.; investigation, L.B. and M.S.; resources, E.R.; data curation, L.B. and M.S.; writing—original draft preparation, L.B. and E.R.; writing—review and editing, L.B.; supervision, E.R. All authors have read and agreed to the published version of the manuscript.

Funding: This research received no external funding.

Conflicts of Interest: The authors declare no conflict of interest.

References

1. Cheng, G.; Huang, H.; Zhou, L.; He, S.; Zhang, Y.; Cheng, X. Chemical composition and water permeability of the cuticular wax barrier in rose leaf and petal: A comparative investigation. *Plant Physiol. Biochem.* **2019**, *135*, 404–410. [CrossRef] [PubMed]
2. Trivedi, P.; Nguyen, N.; Klavins, L.; Kviesis, J.; Heinonen, E.; Remes, J.; Jokipii-Lukkari, S.; Klavins, M.; Karppinen, K.; Jaakola, L.; et al. Analysis of composition, morphology, and biosynthesis of cuticular wax in wild type bilberry (*Vaccinium myrtillus* L.) and its glossy mutant. *Food Chem.* **2021**, *354*, 129517. [PubMed]
3. Ahmad, H.M.; Rahman, M.-U.; Ali, Q.; Awan, S.I. Plant cuticular waxes: A review on functions, composition, biosyntheses mechanism and transportation. *Life Sci. J.* **2015**, *12*, 60–67.
4. Busta, L.; Jetter, R. Moving beyond the ubiquitous: The diversity and biosynthesis of specialty compounds in plant cuticular waxes. *Phytochem. Rev.* **2018**, *17*, 1275–1304. [CrossRef]
5. Wang, X.; Kong, L.; Zhi, P.; Chang, C. Update on cuticular wax biosynthesis and its roles in plant disease resistance. *Int. J. Mol. Sci.* **2020**, *21*, 5514.
6. Martin, L.B.B.; Rose, J.K.C. There's more than one way to skin a fruit: Formation and functions of fruit cuticles. *J. Exp. Bot.* **2014**, *65*, 4639–4651. [CrossRef] [PubMed]
7. Al Bulushi, K.; Attard, T.M.; North, M.; Hunt, A.J. Optimisation and economic evaluation of the supercritical carbon dioxide extraction of waxes from waste date palm (*Phoenix dactylifera*) leaves. *J. Clean. Prod.* **2018**, *186*, 988–996. [CrossRef]
8. Attard, T.M.; Bukhanko, N.; Eriksson, D.; Arshadi, M.; Geladi, P.; Bergsten, U.; Budarin, V.L.; Clark, J.H.; Hunt, A.J. Supercritical extraction of waxes and lipids from biomass: A valuable first step towards an integrated biorefinery. *J. Clean. Prod.* **2018**, *177*, 684–698. [CrossRef]
9. Trivedi, P.; Nguyen, N.; Hykkerud, A.L.; Häggman, H.; Martinussen, I.; Jaakola, L.; Karppinen, K. Developmental and environmental regulation of cuticular wax biosynthesis in fleshy fruits. *Front. Plant Sci.* **2019**, *10*, 431. [CrossRef]
10. Sin, E.H.K.; Marriott, R.; Hunt, A.J.; Clark, J.H. Identification, quantification and Chrastil modelling of wheat straw wax extraction using supercritical carbon dioxide. *C. R. Chim.* **2014**, *17*, 293–300. [CrossRef]
11. Guo, Y.; Jetter, R. Comparative analyses of cuticular waxes on various organs of potato (*Solanum tuberosum* L.). *J. Agric. Food Chem.* **2017**, *65*, 3926–3933. [CrossRef] [PubMed]
12. Jetter, R.; Schäffer, S.; Riederer, M. Leaf cuticular waxes are arranged in chemically and mechanically distinct layers: Evidence from *Prunus laurocerasus* L. *Plant Cell Environ.* **2000**, *23*, 619–628. [CrossRef]
13. Silvestroni Pimentel, B.; Negri, G.; Cordeiro, I.; Barbosa Motta, L.; Salatino, A. Taxonomic significance of the distribution of constituents of leaf cuticular waxes of Croton species (Euphorbiaceae). *Biochem. Syst. Ecol.* **2020**, *92*, 104106. [CrossRef]
14. Simões, R.; Rodrigues, A.; Ferreira-Dias, S.; Miranda, I.; Pereira, H. Chemical composition of cuticular waxes and pigments and morphology of leaves of *Quercus suber* trees of different provenance. *Plants* **2020**, *9*, 1165. [CrossRef] [PubMed]
15. Canizares, D.; Angers, P.; Ratti, C. Organogelation capacity of epicuticular and cuticular waxes from flax and wheat straws. *J. Am. Oil Chem. Soc.* **2021**, *98*, 329–339. [CrossRef]
16. Lefebvre, T.; Destandau, E.; Lesellier, E. Selective extraction of bioactive compounds from plants using recent extraction techniques: A review. *J. Chromatogr. A* **2021**, *1635*, 461770. [CrossRef]
17. Costa, R.; Albergamo, A.; Arrigo, S.; Gentile, F.; Dugo, G. Solid-phase microextraction-gas chromatography and ultra-highperformance liquid chromatography applied to the characterizationof lemon wax, a waste product from citrus industry. *J. Chromatogr. A* **2019**, *1603*, 262–268. [CrossRef] [PubMed]

18. Pham, T.-C.-T.; Angers, P.; Ratti, C. Extraction of wax-like materials from cereals. *Can. J. Chem. Eng.* **2018**, *96*, 2273–2281. [CrossRef]

19. Sökmen, M.; Demir, E.; Alomar, S.Y. Optimization of sequential supercritical fluid extraction (SFE) of caffeine and catechins from green tea. *J. Supercrit. Fluids* **2018**, *133*, 171–176. [CrossRef]

20. Pimentel-Moral, S.; Borrás-Linares, I.; Lozano-Sánchez, J.; Arráez-Román, D.; Martínez-Férez, A.; Segura-Carretero, A. Supercritical CO_2 extraction of bioactive compounds from *Hibiscus sabdariffa*. *J. Supercrit. Fluids* **2019**, *147*, 213–221. [CrossRef]

21. Fuentes-Gandara, F.; Torres, A.; Fernández-Ponce, M.T.; Casas, L.; Mantell, C.; Varela, R.; Martínez de la Ossa-Fernández, E.J.; Macías, F.A. Selective fractionation and isolation of allelopathic compounds from *Helianthus annuus* L. leaves by means of high-pressure techniques. *J. Supercrit. Fluids* **2019**, *143*, 32–41. [CrossRef]

22. Campalani, C.; Chioggia, F.; Amadio, E.; Gallo, M.; Rizzolio, F.; Selva, M.; Perosa, A. Supercritical CO_2 extraction of natural antibacterials from low value weeds and agro-waste. *J. CO_2 Utiliz.* **2020**, *40*, 101198. [CrossRef]

23. Gomes Silva, S.; Santana de Oliveira, M.; Neves Cruz, J.; Almeida da Costa, W.; da Silva, S.H.M.; Barreto Maia, A.A.; Lopes de Sousa, R.; Carvalho Junior, R.N.; de Aguiar Andrade, E.H. Supercritical CO_2 extraction to obtain *Lippia thymoides* Mart. & Schauer (Verbenaceae) essential oil rich in thymol and evaluation of its antimicrobial activity. *J. Supercrit. Fluids* **2021**, *168*, 105064.

24. Yousefi, M.; Rahimi-Nasrabadi, M.; Mirsadeghi, S.; Mahdi Pourmortazavi, S. Supercritical fluid extraction of pesticides and insecticides from food samples and plant materials. *Crit. Rev. Anal. Chem.* **2021**, *51*, 482–501. [CrossRef] [PubMed]

25. Shukla, A.; Naik, S.N.; Goud, V.V.; Das, C. Supercritical CO_2 extraction and online fractionation of dry ginger for production of high-quality volatile oil and gingerols enriched oleoresin. *Ind. Crops Prod.* **2019**, *130*, 352–362. [CrossRef]

26. Baldino, L.; Reverchon, E. *Artemisia annua* organic solvent extract, processed by supercritical CO_2. *Chem. Technol. Biotechnol.* **2018**, *93*, 3171–3175. [CrossRef]

27. Baldino, L.; Reverchon, E. Supercritical fluid extraction of compounds of pharmaceutical interest from *Wendita calysina* (Burrito). *Processes* **2020**, *8*, 1023. [CrossRef]

28. Gaspar, F. Extraction of essential oils and cuticular waxes with compressed CO_2: Effect of extraction pressure and temperature. *Ind. Eng. Chem. Res.* **2002**, *41*, 2497–2503. [CrossRef]

29. Sovova, H.; Stateva, R.P. New approach to modeling supercritical CO_2 extraction of cuticular waxes: Interplay between solubility and kinetics. *Ind. Eng. Chem. Res.* **2015**, *54*, 4861–4870. [CrossRef]

30. Baldino, L.; Della Porta, G.; Reverchon, E. Supercritical CO_2 processing strategies for pyrethrins selective extraction. *J. CO_2 Utiliz.* **2017**, *20*, 14–19. [CrossRef]

31. Baldino, L.; Adami, R.; Reverchon, E. Concentration of *Ruta graveolens* active compounds using SC-CO_2 extraction coupled with fractional separation. *J. Supercrit. Fluids* **2018**, *131*, 82–86. [CrossRef]

32. Subra, P.; Vega-Bancel, A.; Reverchon, E. Breakthrough curves and adsorption isotherms of terpene mixtures in supercritical carbon dioxide. *J. Supercrit. Fluids* **1998**, *12*, 43–57. [CrossRef]

33. Reverchon, E.; Della Porta, G. Supercritical CO_2 extraction and fractionation of Lavender essential oil and waxes. *J. Agric. Food Chem.* **1995**, *43*, 1654–1658. [CrossRef]

34. Reverchon, E.; Senatore, F. Supercritical carbon dioxide extraction of Chamomile essential oil and its analysis by gas chromatography-mass spectrometry. *J. Agric. Food Chem.* **1994**, *42*, 154–158. [CrossRef]

35. Reverchon, E.; Sesti Osseo, L. Supercritical CO_2 extraction of basil oil: Characterization of products and process modelling. *J. Supercrit. Fluids* **1994**, *7*, 185–190. [CrossRef]

36. Reverchon, E.; Della Porta, G. Supercritical CO_2 fractionation of Jasmine concrete. *J. Supercrit. Fluids* **1995**, *8*, 60–65. [CrossRef]

37. Reverchon, E. Fractional separation of SCF extracts from Marjoram leaves: Mass transfer and optimization. *J. Supercrit. Fluids* **1992**, *5*, 256–261. [CrossRef]

38. Baldino, L.; Scognamiglio, M.; Reverchon, E. Supercritical fluid technologies applied to the extraction of compounds of industrial interest from *Cannabis sativa* L. and to their pharmaceutical formulations: A review. *J. Supercrit. Fluids* **2020**, *165*, 104960. [CrossRef]

39. Karğılı, U.; Aytaç, E. Supercritical fluid extraction of cannabinoids (THC and CBD) from four different strains of cannabis grown in different regions. *J. Supercrit. Fluids* **2022**, *179*, 105410. [CrossRef]

40. Szakiel, A.; Pączkowski, C.; Pensec, F.; Bertsch, C. Fruit cuticular waxes as a source of biologically active triterpenoids. *Phytochem. Rev.* **2012**, *11*, 263–284. [CrossRef]

41. Han, N.; Bakovic, M. Biologically active triterpenoids and their cardioprotective and antiInflammatory effects. *J. Bioanal. Biomed.* **2015**, *S12*, 1–11.

42. Francini, A.; Pintado, M.; Manganaris, G.A.; Ferrante, A. Editorial: Bioactive compounds biosynthesis and metabolism in fruit and vegetables. *Front. Plant Sci.* **2020**, *11*, 129. [CrossRef] [PubMed]

43. Haliński, Ł.P.; Paszkiewicz, M.; Gołębiowski, M.; Stepnowski, P. The chemical composition of cuticular waxes from leaves of the gboma eggplant (*Solanum macrocarpon* L.). *J. Food Compos. Anal.* **2012**, *25*, 74–78. [CrossRef]

44. Wang, Y.; Su, S.; Chen, G.; Mao, H.; Jiang, Y. Relationship between cuticular waxes and storage quality parameters of Korla pear under different storage methods. *J. Plant Growth Regul.* **2021**, *40*, 1152–1165. [CrossRef]

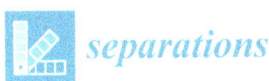 *separations*

Article

Systematic Identification of Bioactive Compositions in Leaves of *Morus* Cultivars Using UHPLC-ESI-QTOF-MS/MS and Comprehensive Screening of High-Quality Resources

Xiang-Yue Zou [1,†], Ying-Jie He [2,*,†], Yi-Hui Yang [1], Xin-Pei Yan [1], Zhang-Bao Li [1] and Hua Yang [3,*]

1   The Sericultural Research Institute of Hunan Province, Changsha 410127, China; xiangyuezou@163.com (X.-Y.Z.); yangyihui0626@163.com (Y.-H.Y.); yanxinpei1224@163.com (X.-P.Y.); lzb1165@163.com (Z.-B.L.)
2   School of Chemical Science and Technology, Yunnan University, Kunming 650091, China
3   College of Bioscience and Biotechnology, Hunan Agricultural University, Changsha 410128, China
*   Correspondence: yingjiehe272@163.com (Y.-J.H.); yhua7710@hunau.edu.cn (H.Y.)
†   These authors contributed equally to this work.

Abstract: *Morus* spp. leaves (MSLs) show various beneficial effects in the treatment of metabolic-related diseases, which have created a growing interest in MSL development as dietary supplements and functional foods. The illustration of chemical compositions and screening of high-quality MSL resources are therefore necessary for further application. This study developed a new UHPLC-ESI-QTOF-MS/MS strategy of in-source collision-induced dissociation (IS-CID) and target collision-cell CID (TCC-CID) to quickly capture analogues with consistent skeleton, and combined global natural product social molecular networking (GNPS) to efficiently annotate bioactive phytochemicals in MSLs. For the results, 49 bioactive ingredients, including quercetin-type flavonoids, kaempferol-type flavonoids, chlorogenic acid isomers, 1-deoxynojirimycin, γ-aminobutyric acid, amino acids, and unsaturated fatty acids, were systematically identified in MSLs for the first time. Quantification for the typical components was simultaneously carried out in MSLs of 90 *Morus* resources collected from different locations. Partial least squares discriminant analysis (PLS-DA) indicated that quercetin-3-*O*-(6″-*O*-malonyl)-glucoside, rutin, kaempferol-3-*O*-(6″-*O*-malonyl)-glucoside, kaempferol-3-*O*-rutinoside, and chlorogenic acid showed high variable importance in the project (VIP > 1) that were significant constituents for the differences between MSL species. Then, high-quality MSLs were comprehensively screened in multiple *Morus* cultivars based on the criteria importance through intercriteria correlation (CRITIC) method. This study presented an efficient strategy to annotate bioactive compounds, revealed the difference of bioactive components in MSLs, and provided important information for the high-value production of *Morus* cultivars in food and supplement fields.

Keywords: *Morus* spp. leaves; high-resolution mass spectrometry; bioactive compounds; GNPS; PLS-DA; CRITIC method

Citation: Zou, X.-Y.; He, Y.-J.; Yang, Y.-H.; Yan, X.-P.; Li, Z.-B.; Yang, H. Systematic Identification of Bioactive Compositions in Leaves of *Morus* Cultivars Using UHPLC-ESI-QTOF-MS/MS and Comprehensive Screening of High-Quality Resources. *Separations* 2022, 9, 76. https://doi.org/10.3390/separations9030076

Academic Editor: Ernesto Reverchon

Received: 23 February 2022
Accepted: 14 March 2022
Published: 15 March 2022

Publisher's Note: MDPI stays neutral with regard to jurisdictional claims in published maps and institutional affiliations.

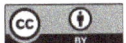

1. Introduction

Morus spp. (also commonly named mulberry) belong to the family Moraceae and are natively cultivated in China, as well as distributed in Japan and Korea [1]. For 5000 years, the mulberry plant (leaves) has been the sole fodder for silkworms (*Bombyx mori*) for the production of silk in China, and sericulture is one of the most important symbols of ancient China [2]. The major mulberry species, such as *Morus alba* L., *Morus multicaulis* Pitter., and *Morus atropurpurea* Roxb., are extensively used to produce mulberry leaves for silkworms after thousands of years of improvement and domestication. These species are generally divided into eight cultivar types according to their geographical distribution in China: Pearl River Basin type, Taihu Basin type, Sichuan Basin type, Middlestream of the Yangtze River type, Downstream of the Yellow River type, Loess Plateau type, Xinjiang type, and Northeast type [3].

In addition to application as plant fodder in traditional sericulture, mulberry leaves possess great developmental potential and utilization value in relation to medicine, food, and ecological protection [2]. For example, the dry leaves of *M. alba* are a traditional Chinese medicine recorded as Mori Folium in the *Chinese Pharmacopoeia* (2020 edition) to treat anemopyretic cold, lung cough, headache, and dizziness [4]. In particular, its fresh leaves serve as a general food due to enriched nutrients such as carbohydrates, protein, fats, fiber, and vitamins [5,6], which are an essential part of a healthy lifestyle. They also possess numerous essential compounds with various bioactivities that are important for the health of organisms. Previous research suggested that flavonoids, alkaloids, chlorogenic acid, free amino acids, some organic acids, etc., were the main bioactive constituents in *M.* spp. leaves (MSLs) [7–10]. The preclinical and clinical studies indicated that MSLs possessed beneficial functions, such as antidiabetic, antihyperglycemic, antioxidant, and antiobesity functions [11].

The multiple beneficial functions of MSLs explain their extensive application in food products, such as mulberry leaf tea and beverages [12–14]. MSLs are also usually pulverized as an additive to improve the flavor and nutritional value of food. Mulberry leaf kueh (桑叶粿) is a delicious pastry made of homogenized liquid of fresh MSLs and glutinous rice, which has been popular in the Chaoshan region of China for hundreds of years [15]. Nevertheless, bioactive compositions of different MSL resources have not yet been illustrated clearly or compared comprehensively by researchers. Even the same variety of MSL usually shows great variation in widely cultivated regions. Therefore, it is very important to systematically analyze the compositions in different MSL resources for screening of highly valuable *Morus* cultivars.

Liquid chromatography coupled with high-resolution mass spectrometry (LC-HRMS) methods, such as ultrahigh-performance liquid chromatography–electrospray ionization quadrupole time-of-flight mass spectrometry (UHPLC-ESI-QTOF-MS/MS), have been successfully used for efficient annotation and rapid quantification of organic ingredients in complex matrices [16–21]. These improved LC-HRMS technologies have made it easier to study bioactive components in foods and plants. This study developed an improved LC-HRMS strategy to systematically identify the main components and construct chemical profiles of MSLs using UHPLC-ESI-QTOF-MS/MS coupled with global natural product social molecular networking (GNPS). Furthermore, multiple MSL resources collected from different geographical areas were evaluated by semiquantitation of these typical components. High-quality *Morus* cultivars were finally screened based on multivariate statistical analysis methods.

2. Materials and Methods

2.1. Materials and Chemicals

A total of 90 *Morus* resources that mainly originated from eight geographical areas, including three major species, namely *Morus alba* L., *Morus multicaulis* Perr., and *Morus atropurpurea* Roxb., along with *Morus cathayana* Hemsl., *Morus bombycis* Koidz., *Morus australis* Poir., and *Morus mizuho* Hotta., were cultivated in the Mulberry Variety Resources Nursery of Sericultural Research Institute in Changsha City, the Mulberry Experimental Base in Lixian County, and the Donghuang Mulberry Seedling Base in Ningxiang City, China. The leaves of each of them were collected in June 2021. The fresh weight of mulberry leaves of each sample was first calculated and then dried at 50 °C to constant dry weight. The dried leaf samples were milled with a grinder and then screened through a 100-mesh sieve. The filtered powder was stored in a desiccator at room temperature in the dark before the experiment.

Commercial standards comprising isoleucine, leucine, phenylalanine, tryptophan, valine, 1-deoxynojirimycin (1-DNJ), γ-aminobutyric acid (GABA), chlorogenic acid, rutin, isoquercitrin, quercetin, and kaempferol were purchased from Yuanye Bio-Technology Co., Ltd. (Shanghai, China) and had over 98% purity as detected by high-performance liquid chromatography (HPLC). Acetonitrile, methanol, and formic acid were of chromatographic grade for LC-HRMS analysis (Merck KGaA Co., Ltd., Darmstadt, Germany). Analytical ethanol and other reagents were purchased from Sinopharm Chemical Reagent Co., Ltd. (Shanghai, China). Wahaha purified water was used in the study.

2.2. Preparation Solutions of Standards and Samples for LC-HRMS Analysis

In total, 12 reference standards, isoleucine (1.06 mg), leucine (1.04 mg), phenylalanine (1.03 mg), tryptophan (1.01 mg), valine (1.07 mg), 1-DNJ (0.81 mg), GABA (0.98 mg), chlorogenic acid (1.17 mg), rutin (1.07 mg), isoquercitrin (0.90 mg), quercetin (0.77 mg), and kaempferol (0.83 mg), were each dissolved in 1.0 mL acetonitrile/methanol (1:1, v/v) to prepare individual stock solutions. Each solution was diluted at appropriate concentrations of 5.0−10.0 μg/mL for qualitative analysis. All the stock solutions were mixed and further diluted into a series of appropriate concentrations at a range of 0.03−100.0 μg/mL for quantitative analysis.

Next, 0.15 g powder of each sample was added to 3.0 mL 60% ethanol solution and extracted for 20 min using an ultrasonic instrument with consistent power (200 W, 40 Hz; Kunshan Ultrasonic Instrument Co., Ltd., Kunshan, China). The extract was centrifuged at 12,000 rpm for 15 min, and then 1.0 mL of supernatant was filtered by a 0.22 μm membrane and then used for LC-HRMS analysis. All of the tests on the sample were carried out in triplicate.

2.3. LC-HRMS Conditions

An Agilent 1290 UHPLC coupled with a 6545B ESI-Q-TOF/MS system (Agilent Technologies, Palo Alto, CA, USA) was employed for the qualitative and quantitative analysis of mulberry leaves. An SB C18 column (2.1 × 100 mm, 1.8 μm, Agilent Technologies, Palo Alto, CA, USA) at a consistent temperature condition of 35 °C was used for the chromatographic separation. A two-phase system composed of phase A (ultrapure water containing 0.1% formic acid) and phase B (acetonitrile) was adopted with a flow rate of 0.15 mL/min, and an optimized gradient elution condition was created (0–2 min, 2% B; 2–3 min, 2–10% B; 3–5 min, 10% B; 5–8 min, 10–25% B; 8–10 min, 25% B; 10–13 min, 25–55% B; 13–16 min, 55% B; 16–19 min, 55–90% B; 19–21 min, 90–98% B; 21–30 min, 98% B). The injection volume for individual samples and standard solutions was 2.0 μL.

The mass-spectrometric conditions were improved in positive and negative ESI modes. The drying gas temperature was 325 °C with a flow rate was 9 L/min, the nebulizer pressure was 50 psi, the sheath gas temperature was 365 °C with a flow rate of 11 L/min, the nozzle voltage was 0.5 kV, the VCAP voltage was 4.0 kV, the fragmentor voltage was from 80 to 200 V, the OCT1 RF Vpp was 750 V, and the skimmer voltage was 65 V. The mass data were obtained at a range of between m/z 50 and m/z 1000 Da. Fragment ions of individual mass peaks were acquired under collision energies from 5 to 40 eV. Data acquisition and processing were carried out with Agilent Acquisition software and Agilent MassHunter Qualitative Analysis (version B.08.00), respectively.

2.4. GNPS Library Help to Identification of Compounds

The ".d" data were converted into ".MGF" file format by Agilent MassHunter Quantitative Navigator (version B.08.00), and the dedicated module "Create Molecular Networking" was used to create a network on the GNPS web platform to match potential compounds by comparing MS/MS spectra in the GNPS library. This work can be accessed via the GNPS website at https://gnps.ucsd.edu/ProteoSAFe/status.jsp?task=8d05eff8ec5e4fb3a8786c501 8600d49 (25 December 2021).

2.5. Quality Evaluation by Multivariate Statistical Analysis

The SIMCA tool (14.1) was employed to analyze responsible markers in MSL samples. The criteria importance through intercriteria correlation (CRITIC) method was used to comprehensively evaluate the MSL quality [22].

3. Results and Discussion

One type of bioactive analogue generally possessed a certain kind of skeleton and was found extensively in complex matrices. Thus, it is important to rapidly mark and effectively identify these substances. However, some compounds were found to have the same m/z of skeleton (isomeric structures) when MS/MS analysis was carried out. It is necessary to discriminate fragments of skeleton ions to avoid the possible misattribution of homologues. The identification of compounds was undertaken using the strategy of combining in-source collision-induced dissociation (IS-CID) with target collision-cell CID (TCC-CID) to quickly catch analogues with the same skeleton (Figure 1).

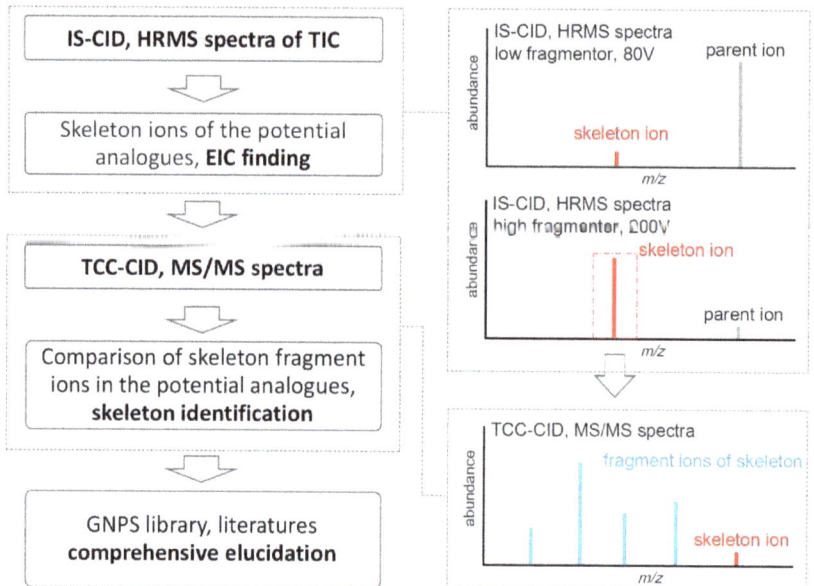

Figure 1. An improved strategy combining IS-CID with TCC-CID to screen analogues with the same skeleton.

The fragmentor (80–200 V) has traditionally been selected according to the structural characteristics of compounds to obtain HRMS spectra with low dissociation for parent ions. In this study, a strategy that combined IS-CID with TCC-CID based on UHPLC-ESI-QTOF-MS/MS was successfully established for fast annotation of analogues with the same skeleton. In brief, TIC containing the HRMS spectrum of a sample solution was first collected under a higher fragmentor voltage (200 V) after liquid chromatography separation. The intensity of the skeleton ion dissociated from the parent ions generally increased after improving the fragmentor, and then the RT for each potential analogue was marked by an EIC finding. Subsequently, TCC-CID at a specific collision energy (CE) was performed for the potential skeleton ion (with consistent mass to charge, m/z) to capture the MS/MS spectrum. These MS/MS spectra were compared with each other to accurately label the skeleton with unanimous fragment ions and intensity to screen analogues.

3.1. Characterization of Morus Leaves

To quickly acquire more abundant mass data of bioactive components present in these *Morus* leaves, a QC sample was prepared by mixing an equal solution of each MSL sample, and the mass information was collected by the IS-CID−TCC-CID strategy (Figure 2a,b). The typical mass characteristics of total ion chromatograms (TICs) under ESI positive and negative modes indicated that multiple bioactive compositions in MSLs potentially exist

(Table 1). Efficient identification of these bioactive ingredients is the basic foundation for understanding the beneficial effects. Therefore, GNPS was introduced to assist in the identification of potential compounds by comparison with MS/MS spectra in the online library.

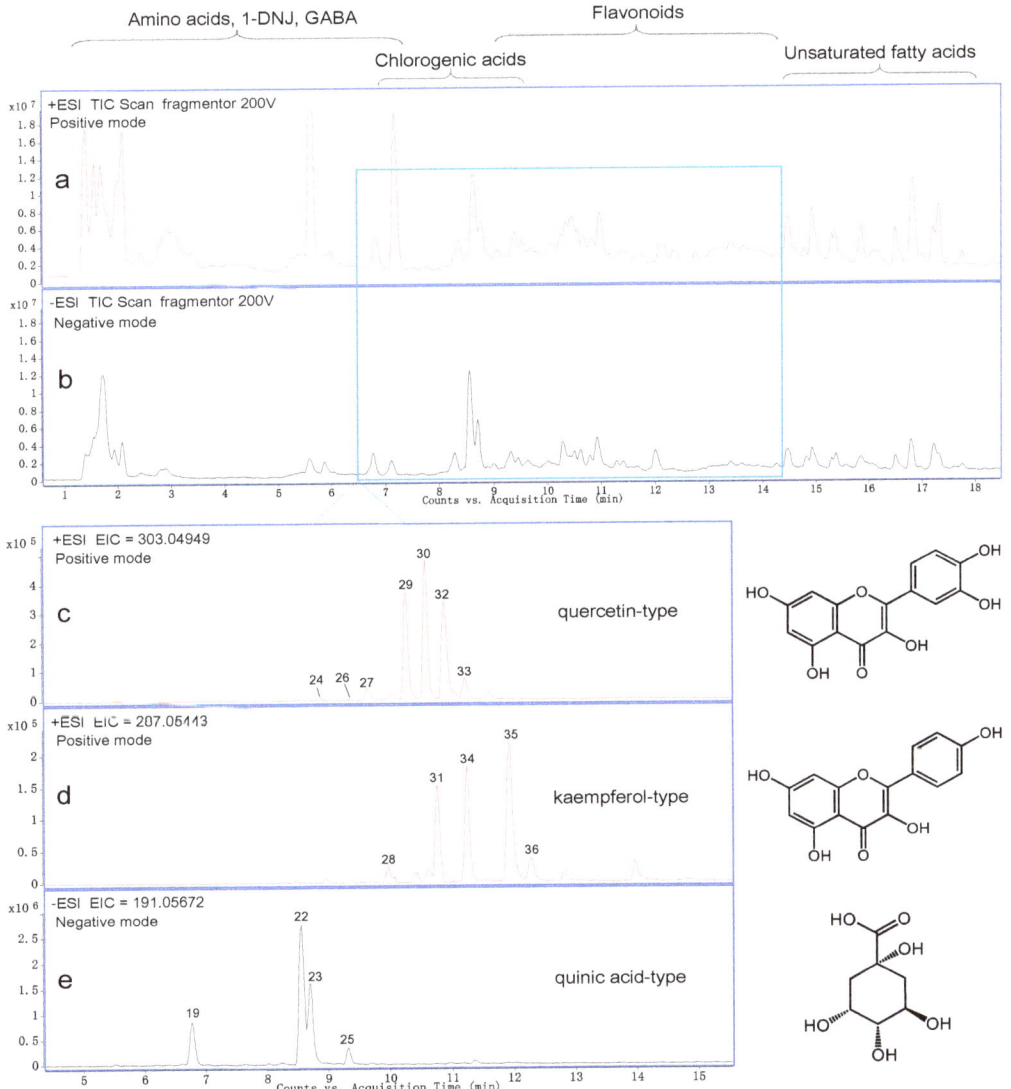

Figure 2. TICs of *Morus* spp. leaves (QC) in −ESI (**a**) an d +ESI (**b**) modes, EIC finding potential skeletons of quercetin, kaempferol, and quinic acid at *m/z* 303.05 (**c**), *m/z* 287.05 (**d**), and *m/z* 191.05 (**e**), respectively.

Table 1. Bioactive and nutritive compositions in 90 samples of *Morus* leaves under UHPLC-ESI-QTOF-MS/MS investigation in positive and negative ESI modes.

Peak No.	RT	Precursor Ion Type	Precursor Ion (*m/z*)	Formula	Δppm	Fragment Ions (*m/z*)	Identification
Quercetin-type flavonoids							
24	8.92	[M + H]⁺	713.15743	C30H32O20	−1.92	551, 465, 303	quercetin-3-*O*-(6″-*O*-malonyl)-glucose-7-*O*-glucoside (que-mal-glu-glu) [bc]
26	9.39	[M + H]⁺	697.16142	C30H32O19	−0.63	611, 465, 303	quercetin-3-*O*-(6″-*O*-malonyl)-glucose-7-*O*-rhamnoside (que-mal-glu-rha) [b]
27	9.68	[M + H]⁺	757.22036	C33H40O20	−1.81	611, 465, 303	quercetin-3-*O*-rutinoside-7-*O*-rhamnoside (que-rut-rha) [b]
29	10.32	[M + H]⁺	611.16102	C27H30O16	−0.39	465, 303	rutin (que-3-rut) [abc]
30	10.62	[M + H]⁺	465.10302	C21H20O12	−0.42	303	isoquercitrin (que-3-glu) [abc]
32	10.95	[M + H]⁺	551.10476	C24H22O15	−2.72	303	quercetin-3-*O*-(6″-*O*-malonyl)-glucoside (que-mal-glu 1) [bc]
33	11.30	[M + H]⁺	551.10375	C24H22O15	−1.02	303	quercetin-3-*O*-(2″-*O*-malonyl)-glucoside (que-mal-glu 2) [b]
37	14.07	[M + H]⁺	303.05002	C15H10O7	−0.04	285, 257, 229, 165, 153, 137	quercetin [ac]
Kaempferol-type flavonoids							
28	10.10	[M + H]⁺	741.22479	C33H40O19	−0.98	595, 449, 287	kaempferol-3-*O*-rutinoside-7-*O*-rhamnoside (kae-rut-rha) [b]
31	10.80	[M + H]⁺	595.16694	C27H30O15	−1.80	449, 287	kaempferol-3-*O*-rutinoside (kae-rut) [bc]
34	11.32	[M + H]⁺	449.10847	C21H20O11	−1.36	287	kaempferol-3-*O*-glucoside (kae-glu) [bc]
35	12.05	[M + H]⁺	535.10956	C24H22O15	−2.20	287	kaempferol-3-*O*-(6″-*O*-malonyl)-glucoside (kae-mal-glu 1) [b]
36	12.42	[M + H]⁺	535.10956	C24H22O15	−1.49	287	kaempferol-3-*O*-(2″-*O*-malonyl)-glucoside (kae-mal-glu 2) [b]
40	14.86	[M + H]⁺	287.05499	C15H10O6	0.07	213, 165, 153, 121	kaempferol [ac]
Chlorogenic acids							
19	6.79	[M - H]⁻	353.0887	C16H18O9	−2.55	191, 175, 135	neochlorogenic acid [b]
22	8.61	[M - H]⁻	353.0886	C16H18O9	−1.90	191	chlorogenic acid [ac]
23	8.75	[M - H]⁻	353.0888	C16H18O9	−2.60	191, 175, 173, 135	cryptochlorogenic acid [b]
25	9.32	[M - H]⁻	353.0884	C16H18O9	−1.52	191	1-caffeoylquinic acid [b]
Amino acids							
1	1.43	[M + H]⁺	147.11284	C6H14N2O2	−0.23	130, 84	lysine [d]
2	1.44	[M + H]⁺	156.07686	C6H9N3O2	−1.26	110, 95, 83	histidine [d]
4	1.53	[M + H]⁺	175.11944	C6H14N4O2	−2.79	158, 130, 116, 70, 60	arginine [d]
5	1.54	[M + H]⁺	133.06391	C4H8N2O3	−1.22	116, 87, 74	asparagine [d]
6	1.57	[M + H]⁺	147.07687	C5H10N2O3	−3.07	130, 84	glutamine [d]
7	1.56	[M + H]⁺	120.06571	C4H9NO3	−1.76	102, 84, 74, 56	threonine [d]
8	1.58	[M + H]⁺	148.06073	C5H9NO4	−1.99	130, 102, 84	glutamic acid [d]
10	1.66	[M + H]⁺	146.08170	C6H11NO3	−3.46	128, 100	*N*-isobutyrylglycine [d]
11	1.69	[M + H]⁺	116.07081	C5H9NO2	−1.96	70	proline [c]
12	1.83	[M + H]⁺	118.08648	C5H11NO2	−1.90	72, 55	valine [a]

Table 1. *Cont.*

Peak No.	RT	Precursor Ion Type	Precursor Ion (*m/z*)	Formula	Δppm	Fragment Ions (*m/z*)	Identification
13	2.15	[M + H]$^+$	150.05820	C5H11NO2S	−0.05	133, 104, 61, 56	methionine [d]
14	3.02	[M + H]$^+$	182.08159	C9H11NO3	−2.11	165, 147, 136, 123, 119	tyrosine [c]
15	3.05	[M + H]$^+$	132.10215	C6H13NO2	−1.86	86, 69, 44	isoleucine [ac]
16	3.40	[M + H]$^+$	132.10212	C6H13NO2	−1.68	86, 69, 44	leucine [a]
17	5.60	[M + H]$^+$	166.08622	C9H11NO2	0.10	149, 131, 120, 107, 103	phenylalanine [ac]
21	7.23	[M + H]$^+$	205.09744	C11H12N2O2	−1.17	188, 170, 159, 146, 132, 118	tryptophan [ac]
Unsaturated fatty acids							
38	14.46	[M + Na]$^+$	351.21477	C18H32O5	−2.13	333, 315	C18:2, trihydroxy- [d]
39	14.81	[M + Na]$^+$	353.22999	C18H34O5	−0.24	335, 317	C18:1, trihydroxy- [d]
41	14.93	[M + Na]$^+$	351.21470	C18H32O5	−2.06	333, 315	C18:2, trihydroxy- [d]
42	15.29	[M + Na]$^+$	333.20394	C18H30O4	−1.80	315, 297	C18:3, dihydroxy- [d]
43	15.36	[M + Na]$^+$	333.20374	C18H30O4	−1.05	315, 297	C18:3, dihydroxy- [d]
44	15.83	[M + Na]$^+$	331.18826	C18H28O4	−0.97	313, 295	C18:4, dihydroxy- [d]
45	16.04	[M + Na]$^+$	331.18843	C18H28O4	−1.21	313, 295	C18:4, dihydroxy- [d]
46	16.49	[M + Na]$^+$	333.20429	C18H30O4	−1.90	315, 297	C18:3, dihydroxy- [d]
47	16.78	[M + H]$^+$	353.26920	C21H36O4	−1.63	335, 279, 261	C21:3, dihydroxy- [d]
48	17.19	[M + H]$^+$	353.26881	C21H36O4	−0.33	335, 279, 261, 243	C21:3, dihydroxy- [d]
49	17.75	[M + Na]$^+$	333.20379	C18H30O4	−0.39	315, 297	C18:3, dihydroxy- [d]
Others							
3	1.47	[M + H]$^+$	164.09195	C6H13NO4	−1.26	146, 128, 110, 82, 80, 69	1-deoxynojirimycin (1-DNJ) [a]
9	1.59	[M + H]$^+$	104.07077	C4H9NO2	−1.88	87, 69, 45	γ-aminobutyric acid (GABA) [a]
18	5.94	[M + H]$^+$	220.11824	C9H17NO5	−1.24	-	pantothenic acid [c]
20	7.05	[M + H]$^+$	298.09732	C11H15N5O3S	−1.54	163, 145, 136	vitamin L2 [d]

[a] confirmed by standard substances; [b] annotated by the IS-CID−TCC-CID strategy; [c] identified by comparison through GNPS library; [d] tentatively identified.

3.1.1. Identification of Quercetin-Type Flavonoids (QTFs)

The general nomenclature of the aglycone fragments is shown in Figure 3a. The IS-CID technique was first performed to dissociate the QTFs with a fragmentor at 200 V, and the potential QTFs were screened by EIC finding with *m/z* 303.05 (skeleton ion of potential quercetin) as shown in Figure 2c. Then, these skeleton ions were measured with target MS/MS by the TCC-CID technique, resulting in MS/MS spectra of individual skeleton ions (Figure 3b), which were compared with MS/MS spectra of the standard quercetin (Figure 3c). The MS/MS spectra of quercetin exhibited the consecutive loss of the neural ions of H_2O and CO (Figure 3c), resulting in typical fragment ions at *m/z* 257.04 [M + H - H_2O - CO]$^+$, *m/z* 229.05 [M + H - H_2O - 2 × CO]$^+$, and *m/z* 201.05 [M + H - 2 × H_2O - 2 × CO]$^+$. Simultaneously, *m/z* 165.02 [^{0,2}A]$^+$, *m/z* 153.02 [^{1,3}A]$^+$, and *m/z* 137.02 [^{0,2}B]$^+$ showed the typical fractures of quercetin. Therefore, aglycones of compounds **24**, **26**, **27**, **29**, **30**, **32**, **33**, and **37** showed consistent fragment ions with quercetin that were undoubtedly classified as QTFs. The next step was to assign the linkage between quercetin aglycone and a sugar unit, which was performed under a moderate fragmentor voltage (100 V) to capture HRMS spectra of TIC with low dissociation of parent ions. QTFs possess a basic quercetin skeleton that generally joins glucoside, rutinoside, or malonyl-glucoside with C3, which were confirmed as the major phytochemicals in MSLs. The C7 position would link to some other sugar unit when C3 was occupied.

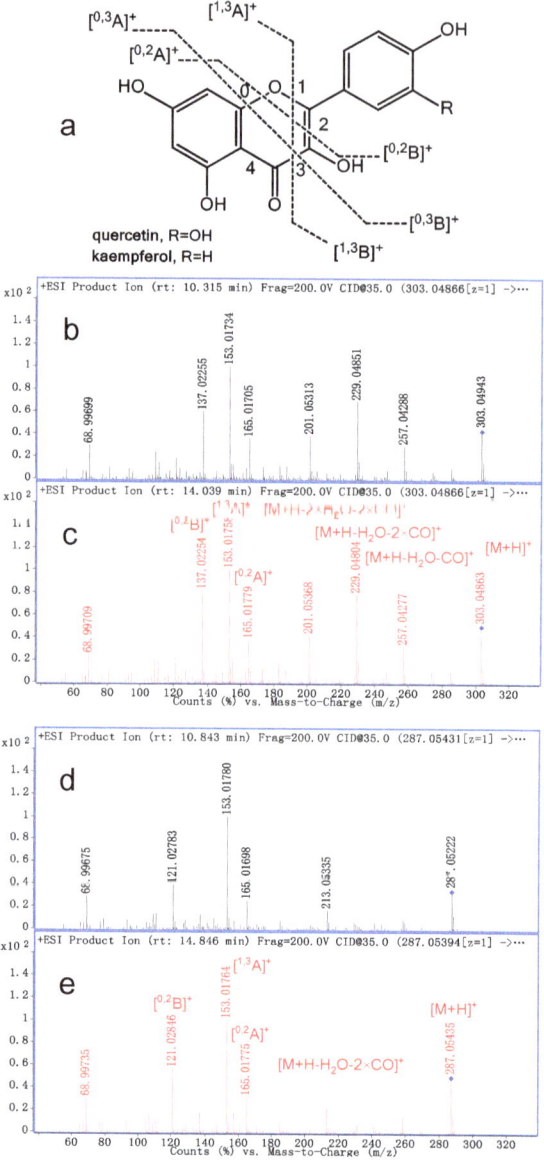

Figure 3. General nomenclature of the aglycone fragments (**a**); comparison of MS/MS spectrum between potential quercetin skeleton (**b**) and authorized quercetin substance (**c**); comparison of MS/MS spectrum between potential kaempferol skeleton (**d**) and authorized kaempferol substance (**e**).

Compounds **29**, **30**, and **37** were identified as rutin (que-3-rut), isoquercitrin (que-3-glu), and quercetin, respectively, by comparison with the authorized substances. Compound **24** showed a parent ion at m/z 713.16 [M + H]$^+$, and fragment ions at m/z 551.10 [M + H - glu]$^+$, m/z 465.10 [M + H - glu - mal]$^+$, and m/z 303.05 [M + H - glu - mal - glu]$^+$ were identified as quercetin-3-*O*-(6″-*O*-malonyl)-glucose-7-*O*-glucoside (que-mal-glu-glu) by referring to the GNPS library. Similarly, compound **26** had a parent ion and m/z 697.16 [M + H]$^+$ and possessed fragment ions at m/z 611.16 [M + H - mal]$^+$, m/z 465.10 [M +

H - mal - rha]$^+$, and m/z 303.05 [M + H - mal - rha - glu]$^+$. Compound **27** possessed parent ion and m/z 757.22 [M + H]$^+$ and possessed fragment ions at m/z 611.16 [M + H - rha]$^+$, m/z 465.10 [M + H - rha - rha]$^+$, m/z 449.11 [M + H - rut]$^+$, and m/z 303.05 [M + H - rha - rut]$^+$. Compounds **26** and **27** were identified as quercetin-3-*O*-(6″-*O*-malonyl)-glucose-7-*O*-rhamnoside (que-mal-glu-rha) and quercetin-3-*O*-rutinoside-7-*O*-rhamnoside (que-rut-rha), respectively, by comparing MS/MS data. Compounds **32** and **33** showed the same parent ion and fragment ion at m/z 551.10 and m/z 303.05, respectively, which indicated the existence of malonyl-glucoside in conjunction with quercetin aglycone, and both were empirically identified as quercetin-3-*O*-(6″-*O*-malonyl)-glucoside (que-mal-glu 1) and quercetin-3-*O*-(2″-*O*-malonyl)-glucoside (que-mal-glu 2), respectively.

3.1.2. Identification of Kaempferol-Type Flavonoids (KTFs)

KTFs are also important bioactive compounds in MSLs that contain kaempferol agly-cone and show the same sugar connection mode as QTFs. Potential KTFs were screened by an EIC finding with m/z 287.05 (skeleton ion of potential kaempferol) using the IS-CID technique with a fragmentor at 200 V (Figure 2d). Similarly, TCC-CID was performed to compare MS/MS spectra of these skeleton ions with the standard kaempferol (Figure 3d,e). The MS/MS spectra of kaempferol showed similar fragment patterns to quercetin and had diagnostic ions at m/z 121.03 [^{0,2}B]$^+$, which had been confirmed in our previous study [23].

As results, compounds **28**, **31**, **34**, **35**, and **36** accurately belonged to KTFs compared with MS/MS spectra of the standard kaempferol (**40**). Compound **28** had a parent ion at m/z 741.22 [M + H]$^+$ and fragment ions at m/z 595.17 [M + H - rha]$^+$, m/z 449.18 [M + H - rha - rha]$^+$, and m/z 287.05 [M + H - rha - rut]$^+$; compound **31** exhibited a parent ion at m/z 595.17 [M + H]$^+$ and fragment ions at m/z 449.18 [M + H - rha]$^+$ and m/z 287.05 [M + H - rut]$^+$; compound **34** showed a parent ion and m/z 449.18 [M + H]$^+$ and a fragment ion at m/z 287.05 [M + H - glu]$^+$. These three compounds were annotated as kaempferol-3-*O*-rutinoside-7-*O*-rhamnoside (kae-rut-rha), kaempferol-3-*O*-rutinoside (kae-rut), and kaempferol-3-*O*-glucoside (kae-glu), respectively. Compounds **35** and **36** showed the same parent ion and typical fragment ion at m/z 535.11 and m/z 287.05, respectively, which indicated the existence of malonyl-glucoside in conjunction with kaempferol aglycone, and both were empirically assigned as kaempferol-3-*O*-(6″-*O*-malonyl)-glucoside (kae-mal-glu 1) and kaempferol-3-*O*-(2″-*O*-malonyl)-glucoside (kae-mal-glu 2), respectively.

3.1.3. Identification of Chlorogenic Acids (CAs)

IS-CID with a fragmentor at 200 V in ESI negative mode showed a consistent skeleton ion of four potential quinic acid homologues at m/z 191.06 (Figure 2e). One of them was identified as chlorogenic acid by standard reference (compound **22**). The skeleton ions (m/z 191.06) of the other three peaks showed consistent MS/MS spectra with the skeleton ion of chlorogenic acid under TCC-CID, which indicated that they were isomers due to the variety of different substituted positions of the caffeoyl unit on quinic acid (Figure 4a).

It is very difficult to accurately annotate these positional isomers. Fortunately, Jia-Yu Zhang et al. reported these four CA isomers [24], and MS/MS spectra in this study showed consistent retention behaviors and fragment ions with them. CAs **19**, **23**, and **25** were identified as neochlorogenic acid, cryptochlorogenic acid, and 1-caffeoylquinic acid, respectively, which exhibited similar fragment patterns. For cryptochlorogenic acid, for example, the parent ion (m/z 353.09 [M - H]$^-$) was dissociated from m/z 179.04 by loss of quinic acid and subsequently generated m/z 135.05 by loss of CO_2, or was dissociated from m/z 191.06 by loss of caffeoyl unit and then generated m/z 173.05 by loss of H_2O (Figure 4b). These similar fragment ions might lead to uncertain annotation; therefore, this study calculated the ratio of parent ion to skeleton ion at a specific collision energy (10 eV), and each CA isomer was efficiently discriminated in complex matrices (Figure 4c).

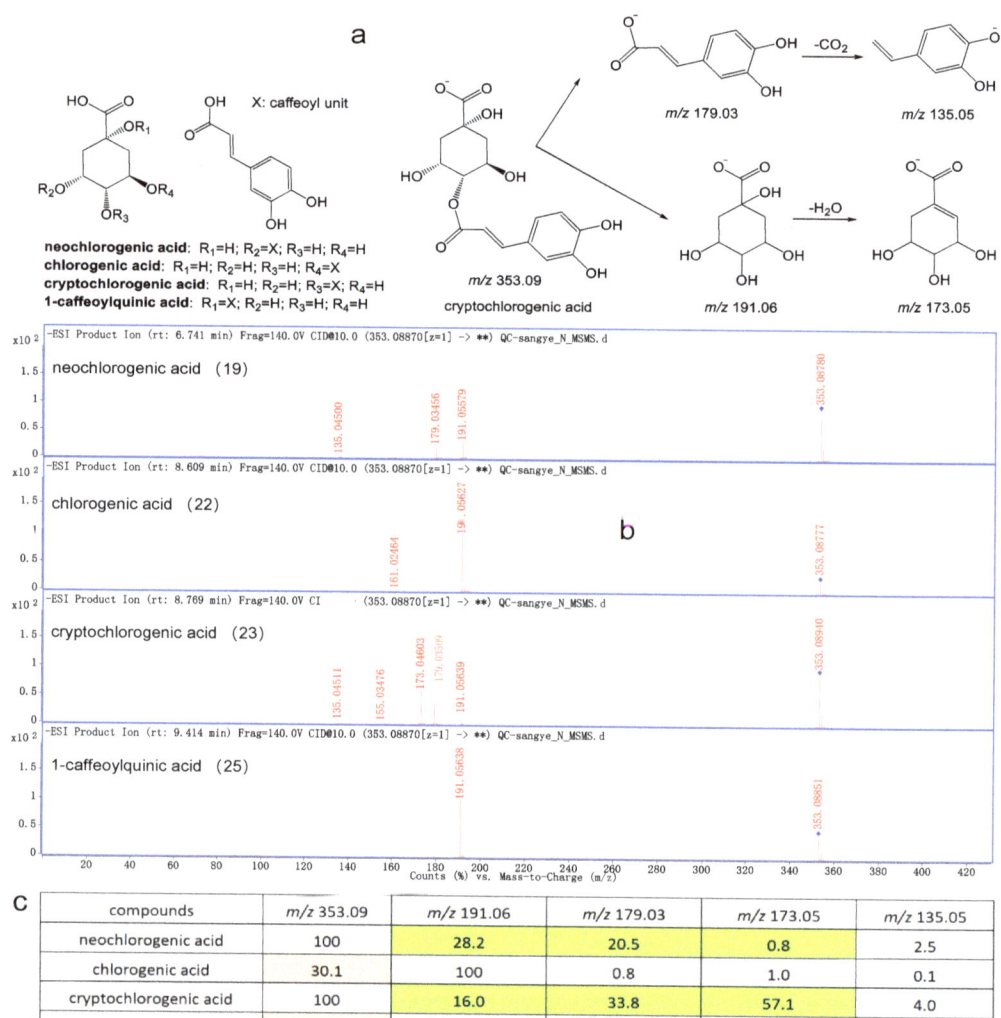

Figure 4. Fragmentation patterns (**a**), MS/MS spectrum (**b**) and ion ratios of four chlorogenic acid isomers (**c**).

3.1.4. Identification of 1-DNJ, GABA, Amino Acids, and Unsaturated Fatty Acids

1-DNJ (**3**) and GABA (**9**) were typical bioactive compounds in MSLs and were accurately identified by referring to the authorized compounds. In total, 16 amino acids (AAs), including the standard substances valine, isoleucine, leucine, phenylalanine, and tryptophan, and the initial identified AAs by accurate mass, MS/MS spectra, GNPS library, were determined. A pair of AA isomers, isoleucine and leucine, showed close RT and fragment ions. This study also provided an effective identification method that showed that isoleucine generally exhibited a higher fragment ion at m/z 69.07 than leucine in one consistent LC-HRMS setting in ESI positive mode. Additionally, unsaturated fatty acids and the other compounds in MSLs were also tentatively elucidated referring to accurate mass and fragment ions (Table 1).

3.2. Qualification of Bioactive Compounds

Semiquantitative analysis was performed using mixed standard solutions by Agilent MassHunter Quantitative Analysis (version 10.2). The calibration curve of each compound with correlation coefficients (R^2) higher than 0.997 in appropriate concentration ranges was determined. Limits of detection (LOD) and quantification (LOQ) were obtained accordingly. RSD values of precision, reproducibility, and stability of the 12 compounds within 2.9% indicated that the method was suitable for the qualified requirement. Analogous or isomeric compounds that do not have standard substances were tentatively quantified using a similar authorized structure [19,25]. Specifically, the identified AAs, flavonoids, and CAs were quantified by referring to isoleucine, rutin, and chlorogenic acid, respectively.

The contents of 36 identified bioactive and nutritive compounds were quantified in 90 MSLs from different *Morus* cultivars. For the sum of 16 nutritive AAs, S55, S16, S34, S61, S40, S38, S53, S27, S05, S46, S59, S04, S20, and S37 showed higher values from 10.00 to 13.45 mg/g. Heat map analysis suggested that phenylalanine, leucine tyrosine, isoleucine, valine, proline, tryptophan, and asparagine possessed the major contents in the MSL samples (Figure 5a).

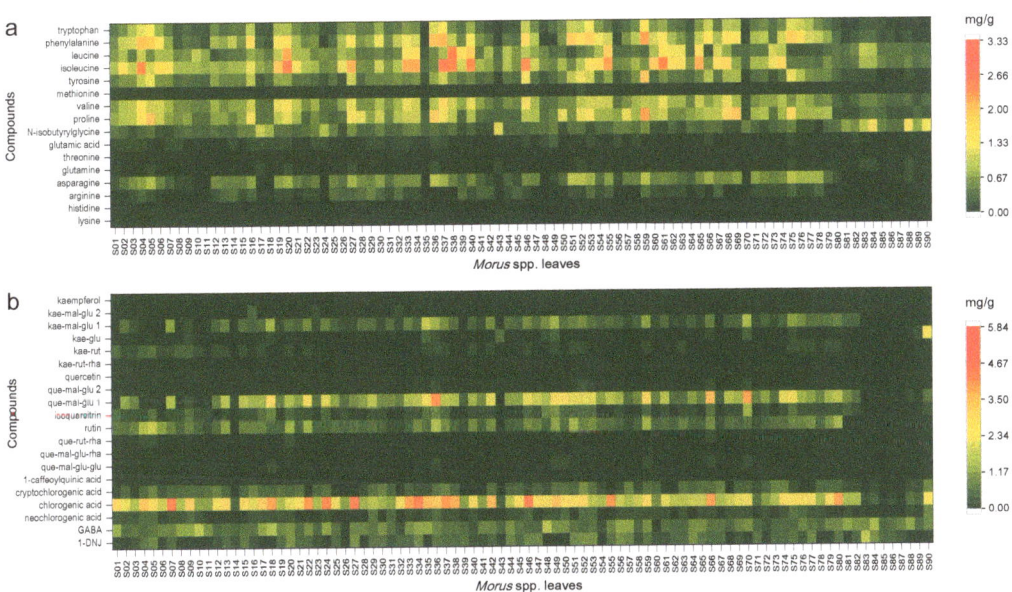

Figure 5. Amino acids (**a**) and typical bioactive compounds (**b**) in different *Morus* spp. leaves.

The concentrations of 20 bioactive compositions in different MSLs were calculated as shown in Figure 5b. The unique bioactive compound in MSLs was 1-DNJ, which showed over 1.00 mg/g in S64, S84, S20, S53, S56, S52, S27, and S83, from 1.00 to 1.83 mg/g. GABA had values over 1.50 mg/g in S84, S18, S10, and S48, from 1.54 to 1.82 mg/g. Chlorogenic acid possessed high content compared to all qualified compounds, and 80 of the 90 MSL samples had chlorogenic acid content of over 1.10 mg/g. Chlorogenic acid above 5.00 mg/g was detected in S34, S27, and S46 (Figure 5b). Rutin, quercetin-3-*O*-(6"-*O*-malonyl)-glucoside (que-mal-glu 1), and kaemferol-3-*O*-(6"-*O*-malonyl)-glucoside (kae-mal-glu 1) were the main flavonoids in MSLs. In particular, que-mal-glu 1 showed values of more than 1.50 mg/g in 35 MSL samples, and it showed high content in S66, S70, and S36 from 3.51 to 4.38 mg/g. Most of the wild MSLs (S81–S90) showed low contents of the qualified bioactive compounds. For the sum of 20 bioactive compounds, S33, S27, S20, S50, S75, S42, S51, S24, S80, S34, S37, S52, S07, S35, S22, S59, S70, S18, S66, S49, S46, and S36 exhibited higher values from 10.27 to 15.60 mg/g. As a result, S20, S37, S46, and S59 were screened with high values of nutritive AAs and bioactive compounds that all exceeded 10.00 mg/g in MSL samples.

3.3. Important Variables of M. spp. Leaves

The fact that there were several quantified datasets made the interpretation of MSL quality difficult. Therefore, partial least squares discriminant analysis (PLS-DA) was initially introduced to find important variables in these samples. First, 90 MSL samples were divided according to the species (cultivars), and the PLS-DA score scatter plot was presented (Figure 6a). The corresponding score plot combined with variable importance in the project (VIP > 1) values screened out compounds, namely quercetin-3-*O*-(6″-*O*-malonyl)-glucoside (que-mal-glu 1), chlorogenic acid, kaempferol-3-*O*-rutinoside (kae-rut), rutin, kaempferol-3-*O*-(6″-*O*-malonyl)-glucoside (kae-mal-glu 1), isoleucine, valine, *N*-isobutyrylglycine, and phenylalanine, which were significant constituents of the differences between MSL species (Figure 6b). Then, these samples were divided based on geographical distribution in a PLS-DA score scatter plot (Figure 6c). Similarly, these compounds mentioned above, along with proline and asparagine, were important variables (VIP > 1) for the differences between MSL original types (Figure 6d). The combined results of the PLS-DA data demonstrated that these important variables could serve as key values in evaluating the quality of different MSL samples.

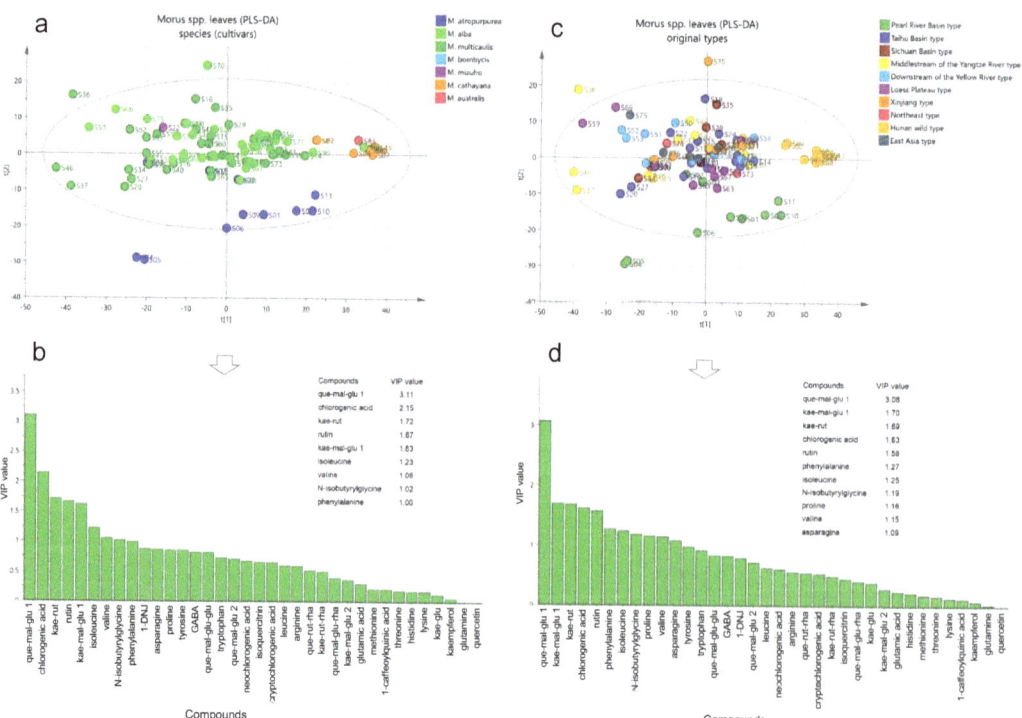

Figure 6. PLS-DA score scatter plot for different species of *Morus* spp. leaves (**a**) and VIP value of compounds (**b**); PLS-DA score scatter plot for different original types of *Morus* spp. leaves (**c**) and VIP value of compounds (**d**).

3.4. Quality Evaluation of M. spp. Leaves

To comprehensively evaluate the quality of MSL samples according to the screened important variables obtained in PLS-DA analysis, the objective weight (W_j) of each compound was calculated according to the CRITIC method that was based on characteristic conflict (R_j), correlation of indicators (r_{ij}), amount of information (C_j), and standard deviation or intensity (σ_j). In short, the data matrix was established according to the standardized data and formulas (experimental values − experimental minimum)/(experimental maximum − experimental minimum), and the objective weight of each indicator was obtained (Table 2). The calculated formulas are depicted as follows [22]:

$$R_j = \sum_{i=1}^{n} \left(1 - r_{ij}\right) \tag{1}$$

$$C_j = \sigma_j R_j \tag{2}$$

$$W_j = \frac{C_j}{\sum_{j=1}^{n} C_j} \tag{3}$$

Table 2. Comparison of intensity, conflict, information, and objective weight of each indicator.

Indicator	Intensity (σ_j)	Conflict (R_j)	Information (C_j)	Objective Weight (W_j)
chlorogenic acid	0.212	6.305	1.337	0.079
rutin	0.203	5.567	1.130	0.067
que-mal-glu 1	0.212	7.067	1.497	0.088
kae-rut	0.186	7.195	1.337	0.079
kae-mal-glu 1	0.203	7.638	1.549	0.091
asparagine	0.278	6.017	1.675	0.099
N-isobutyrylglycine	0.198	12.683	2.511	0.148
proline	0.229	5.974	1.369	0.081
valine	0.239	6.032	1.439	0.085
isoleucine	0.228	7.314	1.667	0.098
phenylalanine	0.266	5.501	1.463	0.086

This objective method resulted in a comprehensive evaluation of MSL resources from different species and areas of origin (Table 3). Samples S46 (M. multicaulis), S37 (M. multicaulis), S36 (M. multicaulis), S59 (M. alba), S20 (M. multicaulis), S34 (M. multicaulis), S27 (M. multicaulis), S66 (M. alba), S33 (M. alba), S52 (M. multicaulis), etc., had a higher score in the 90 MSL samples, which indicated the excellent potential of these *Morus* cultivars for higher value application of MSLs in the field of medicine and food.

Table 3. Comprehensive evaluation of M. spp. leaves from different areas using the CRITIC method.

Original Type	Species	Region	Sample	Score	Rank
Pearl River Basin type	*M. atropurpurea* Roxb.	Guangdong Province	S01	64.72	63
	M. atropurpurea Roxb.	Guangdong Province	S02	88.59	36
	M. atropurpurea Roxb.	Guangdong Province	S03	75.34	51
	M. atropurpurea Roxb.	Guangdong Province	S04	119.49	12
	M. atropurpurea Roxb.	Guangdong Province	S05	110.40	18
	M. atropurpurea Roxb.	Guangdong Province	S06	80.54	47
	M. atropurpurea Roxb.	Guangdong Province	S07	114.56	15
	M. atropurpurea Roxb.	Guangxi Province	S08	44.76	79
	M. atropurpurea Roxb.	Guangxi Province	S09	69.75	57
	M. atropurpurea Roxb.	Guangxi Province	S10	36.22	83
	M. atropurpurea Roxb.	Guangxi Province	S11	34.25	85

Table 3. *Cont.*

Original Type	Species	Region	Sample	Score	Rank
Taihu Basin type	*M. multicaulis* Perr.	Zhejiang Province	S12	76.38	49
	M. multicaulis Perr.	Zhejiang Province	S13	92.16	31
	M. multicaulis Perr.	Zhejiang Province	S14	46.94	77
	M. multicaulis Perr.	Zhejiang Province	S15	90.87	34
	M. multicaulis Perr.	Zhejiang Province	S16	104.50	23
	M. multicaulis Perr.	Zhejiang Province	S17	86.44	41
	M. multicaulis Perr.	Zhejiang Province	S18	100.66	25
	M. multicaulis Perr.	Zhejiang Province	S19	90.96	33
	M. multicaulis Perr.	Zhejiang Province	S20	133.94	5 #
	M. multicaulis Perr.	Zhejiang Province	S21	87.67	38
	M. mizuho Hotta.	Zhejiang Province	S22	109.64	20
	M. alba L.	Jiangsu Province	S23	65.88	62
	M. alba L.	Jiangsu Province	S24	93.98	30
	M. alba L.	Jiangsu Province	S25	67.57	60
	M. alba L.	Jiangsu Province	S26	57.00	71
	M. multicaulis Perr.	Jiangsu Province	S27	131.86	7 #
Sichuan Basin type	*M. bombycis* Koidz.	Sichuan Province	S28	70.41	56
	M. multicaulis Perr	Sichuan Province	S29	74.46	52
	M. alba L.	Sichuan Province	S30	82.96	46
	M. alba L.	Sichuan Province	S31	56.00	73
	M. alba L.	Yunnan Province	S32	75.70	50
	M. alba L.	Sichuan Province	S33	123.31	9 #
	M. multicaulis Perr.	Chongqing City	S34	133.29	6 #
	M. multicaulis Perr.	Chongqing City	S35	84.16	44
Middlestream of the Yangtze River type	*M. multicaulis* Perr.	Anhui Province	S36	151.37	3 #
	M. multicaulis Perr.	Anhui Province	S37	156.11	2 #
	M. multicaulis Perr.	Anhui Province	S38	118.48	14
	M. multicaulis Perr.	Hunan Province	S39	49.17	76
	M. multicaulis Perr.	Hunan Province	S40	112.53	16
	M. multicaulis Perr.	Hunan Province	S41	55.39	74
	M. multicaulis Perr.	Hunan Province	S42	87.51	40
	M. cathayana Hemsl.	Hunan Province	S43	32.97	86
	M. alba L.	Hunan Province	S44	61.96	67
	M. alba L.	Hunan Province	S45	60.35	68
	M. multicaulis Perr.	Hubei Province	S46	157.84	1 #
	M. alba L.	Hubei Province	S47	98.17	26
	M. multicaulis Perr.	Hunan Province	S48	66.92	61
	M. multicaulis Perr.	Hunan Province	S49	96.80	27
Downstream of the Yellow River type	*M. alba* L.	Henan Province	S50	94.17	29
	M. multicaulis Perr.	Hebei Province	S51	109.13	21
	M. multicaulis Perr.	Hebei Province	S52	119.92	10 #
	M. multicaulis Perr.	Hebei Province	S53	111.54	17
	M. multicaulis Perr.	Shandong Province	S54	87.52	39
	M. multicaulis Perr.	Shandong Province	S55	119.89	11
	M. multicaulis Perr.	Shandong Province	S56	60.09	69
	M. multicaulis Perr.	Shandong Province	S57	64.29	64
	M. alba L.	Shandong Province	S58	76.40	48
Loess Plateau type	*M. alba* L.	Shanxi Province	S59	144.93	4 #
	M. alba L.	Shanxi Province	S60	73.76	54
	M. alba L.	Shanxi Province	S61	110.22	19
	M. alba L.	Shanxi Province	S62	69.29	58
	M. alba L.	Shanxi Province	S63	70.67	55
	M. alba L.	Shanxi Province	S64	63.22	65
	M. multicaulis Perr.	Shanxi Province	S65	88.33	37
	M. alba L.	Shaanxi Province	S66	126.12	8 #
	M. alba L.	Shaanxi Province	S67	74.01	53

Table 3. *Cont.*

Original Type	Species	Region	Sample	Score	Rank
Xinjiang type	*M. alba* L.	Xinjiang U. A. R.	S68	104.05	24
	M. alba L.	Xinjiang U. A. R.	S69	91.04	32
	M. alba L.	Xinjiang U. A. R.	S70	88.81	35
	M. alba L.	Xinjiang U. A. R.	S71	56.76	72
	M. alba L.	Xinjiang U. A. R.	S72	68.42	59
Northeast type	*M. multicaulis* Perr.	Jilin Province	S73	58.84	70
	M. alba L.	Liaoning Province	S74	105.29	22
East Asia type	*M. alba* L.	Japan	S75	118.83	13
	M. alba L.	Japan	S76	95.88	28
	M. alba L.	Japan	S77	84.08	45
	M. alba L.	Japan	S78	62.92	66
	M. alba L.	Japan	S79	84.51	43
	M. multicaulis Perr.	Korea	S80	85.24	42
Hunan wild type	*M. cathayana* Hemsl.	Hunan Province	S81	44.44	80
	M. cathayana Hemsl.	Hunan Province	S82	43.13	82
	M. australis Poir.	Hunan Province	S83	35.94	84
	M. cathayana Hemsl.	Hunan Province	S84	46.42	78
	M. cathayana Hemsl.	Hunan Province	S85	20.63	88
	M. cathayana Hemsl.	Hunan Province	S86	17.89	89
	M. cathayana Hemsl.	Hunan Province	S87	16.19	90
	M. alba L.	Hunan Province	S88	43.24	81
	M. cathayana Hemsl.	Hunan Province	S89	23.64	87
	M. alba L.	Hunan Province	S90	53.15	75

Top ten high-quality MSL samples evaluated by the CRITIC method.

4. Conclusions

There have been many studies on the chemical composition of mulberry leaves. However, due to the potential existence of isomeric skeletons in MSLs, there were possible attribution errors in the identification of homologous compounds. This study constructed an IS-CID−TCC-CID strategy based on UHPLC-ESI-QTOF-MS/MS that showed the advantage of being able to solve this problem by accurately comparing the skeleton MS/MS spectra of analogous compounds. Meanwhile, semiquantitative determination combined with PLS-DA analysis showed that the major flavonoids (rutin, que-mal-glu 1, kae-rut, and kae-mal-glu 1), chlorogenic acid, and amino acids (isoleucine, phenylalanine, valine, *N*-isobutyrylglycine, proline, and asparagine) were important indicators of qualitative differences between MSL cultivars. Then, the high-quality MSLs were comprehensively screened in 90 *Morus* cultivars based on the CRITIC method, which will provide excellent genetic resources for further utilization of MSLs in food and supplement fields.

Author Contributions: Y.-J.H. and X.-Y.Z. conceived and designed the experiments; X.-Y.Z. and Y.-J.H. performed the experiments, analyzed the data, and wrote the paper; Y.-H.Y. and Z.-B.L. prepared the materials; X.-P.Y. participated in the coordination of the experiments; H.Y. helped revise the manuscript. All authors have read and agreed to the published version of the manuscript.

Funding: This research was supported by the Natural Science Foundation of Hunan Province (grant number: 2020JJ4043).

Institutional Review Board Statement: Not applicable.

Informed Consent Statement: Not applicable.

Data Availability Statement: Data are available in the article.

Conflicts of Interest: The authors declare no conflict of interest.

References

1. Chan, W.C.; Lye, P.Y.; Wong, S.K. Phytochemistry, pharmacology, and clinical trials of *Morus alba*. *Chin. J. Nat. Med.* **2016**, *14*, 17–30. [PubMed]
2. Jiao, F.; Luo, R.; Dai, X.; Liu, H.; Yu, G.; Han, S.; Lu, X.; Su, C.; Chen, Q.; Song, Q.; et al. Chromosome-level reference genome and population genomic analysis provide insights into the evolution and improvement of domesticated mulberry (*Morus alba*). *Mol. Plant* **2020**, *13*, 1001–1012. [CrossRef] [PubMed]
3. Lu, C.; Ji, D.F. *Mulberry Cultivars in China*; Southwest Normal University Press: Chongqing, China, 2017; Chapter 1.
4. National Pharmacopoeia Commission. *Chinese Pharmacopeia*; China Medical Science Press: Beijing, China, 2020.
5. Srivastava, S.; Kapoor, R.; Thathola, A.; Srivastava, R.P. Nutritional quality of leaves of some genotypes of mulberry (*Morus alba*). *Int. J. Food Sci. Nutr.* **2006**, *57*, 305–313. [CrossRef] [PubMed]
6. Butt, M.S.; Nazir, A.; Sultan, M.T.; Schroen, K. *Morus alba* L. nature's functional tonic. *Trends Food Sci. Technol.* **2008**, *19*, 505–512. [CrossRef]
7. Gryn-Rynko, A.; Bazylak, G.; Olszewska-Slonina, D. New potential phytotherapeutics obtained from white mulberry (*Morus alba* L.) leaves. *Biomed. Pharmacother.* **2016**, *84*, 628–636. [CrossRef]
8. Sanchez-Salcedo, E.M.; Tassotti, M.; Del Rio, D.; Hernandez, F.; Martinez, J.J.; Mena, P. (Poly)phenolic fingerprint and chemometric analysis of white (*Morus alba* L.) and black (*Morus nigra* L.) mulberry leaves by using a non-targeted UHPLC-MS approach. *Food Chem.* **2016**, *212*, 250–255. [CrossRef]
9. Nastic, N.; Linares, I.; Sanchez, J.; Gajic, J.; Carretero, A. Optimization of the extraction of phytochemicals from black mulberry (*Morus nigra* L.) leaves. *J. Ind. Eng. Chem.* **2018**, *68*, 282–292. [CrossRef]
10. He, X.R.; Fang, J.C.; Ruan, Y.L.; Wang, X.X.; Sun, Y.; Wu, N.; Zhao, Z.F.; Chang, Y.; Ning, N.; Guo, H.; et al. Structures, bioactivities and future prospective of polysaccharides from *Morus alba* (white mulberry): A review. *Food Chem.* **2018**, *245*, 899–910. [CrossRef]
11. Thaipitakwong, T.; Numhom, S.; Aramwit, P. Mulberry leaves and their potential effects against cardiometabolic risks: A review of chemical compositions, biological properties and clinical efficacy. *Pharm. Biol.* **2018**, *56*, 109–118. [CrossRef]
12. Katsube, T.; Yamasaki, Y. Apoptosis-inducing activity of ethanol extracts from the tea of mulberry (*Morus alba*) leaves in HL-60 cells. *J. Jpn. Soc. Food Sci.* **2002**, *49*, 195–198. [CrossRef]
13. Pothinuch, P.; Tongchitpakdee, S. Melatonin contents in mulberry (*Morus* spp.) leaves: Effects of sample preparation, cultivar, leaf age and tea processing. *Food Chem.* **2011**, *128*, 415–419. [CrossRef] [PubMed]
14. Charunuch, C.; Tangkanakul, P.; Limsangouan, N.; Sonted, V. Effects of extrusion conditions on the physical and functional properties of instant cereal beverage powders admixed with mulberry (*Morus alba* L.) leaves. *Food Sci. Technol. Res.* **2008**, *14*, 421–430. [CrossRef]
15. Zhang, G.Q.; Cai, X.Y.; Zhang, Y.J. Research development of mulberry leaf food. *Farm Prod. Process* **2017**, *435*, 43–45.
16. He, Y.J.; Zhou, Y.; Qin, Y.; Zhou, Z.S.; Zhu, M.; Zhu, Y.Y.; Wang, Z.J.; Xie, T.Z.; Zhao, L.X.; Luo, X.D. Development of a LC-HRMS based approach to boost structural annotation of isomeric citrus flavanones. *Phytochem. Anal.* **2021**, *32*, 749–756. [CrossRef]
17. He, Y.J.; Zhu, M.; Zhou, Y.; Zhao, K.H.; Zhou, J.L.; Qi, Z.H.; Zhu, Y.Y.; Wang, Z.J.; Xie, T.Z.; Tang, Q.; et al. Comparative investigation of phytochemicals among ten citrus herbs by ultra high performance liquid chromatography coupled with electrospray ionization quadrupole time-of-flight mass spectrometry and evaluation of their antioxidant properties. *J. Sep. Sci.* **2020**, *43*, 3349–3358. [CrossRef]
18. Tang, Q.; Zhang, R.Y.; Zhou, J.L.; Zhao, K.H.; Lu, Y.; Zheng, Y.J.; Wu, C.Q.; Chen, F.; Mu, D.T.; Ding, Z.X.; et al. The levels of bioactive ingredients in Citrus aurantiumL. at different harvest periods and antioxidant effects on H_2O_2-induced RIN-m5F cells. *J. Sci. Food Agr.* **2021**, *101*, 1479–1490. [CrossRef]
19. He, Y.J.; Qin, Y.; Zhang, T.L.; Zhu, Y.Y.; Wang, Z.J.; Zhou, Z.S.; Xie, T.Z.; Luo, X.D. Migration of (non-) intentionally added substances and microplastics from microwavable plastic food containers. *J. Hazard. Mater.* **2021**, *417*, e126074. [CrossRef]
20. Trovato, E.; Arigo, A.; Vento, F.; Micalizzi, G.; Dugo, P.; Mondello, L. Influence of citrus flavor addition in brewing process: Characterization of the volatile and non-volatile profile to prevent frauds and adulterations. *Separations* **2021**, *8*, 18. [CrossRef]
21. Almalki, A.H.; Ali, N.A.; Elroby, F.A.; El Ghobashy, M.R.; Emam, A.A.; Naguib, I.A. ESI-LC-MS/MS for therapeutic drug monitoring of binary mixture of pregabalin and tramadol: Human plasma and urine applications. *Separations* **2021**, *8*, 21. [CrossRef]
22. He, Y.J.; Chen, Y.; Shi, Y.T.; Zhao, K.H.; Tan, H.Y.; Zeng, J.G.; Tang, Q.; Xie, H.Q. Multiresponse optimization of ultrasonic-assisted extraction for Aurantii Fructus to obtain high yield of antioxidant flavonoids using a response surface methodology. *Processes* **2018**, *6*, 258. [CrossRef]
23. Lu, Y.; Zhu, S.; He, Y.; Mo, C.; Wu, C.; Zhang, R.; Zheng, X.; Tang, Q. Systematic characterization of flavonoids from Siraitia grosvenorii leaf extract using an integrated strategy of high-speed counter-current chromatography combined with ultra high performance liquid chromatography and electrospray ionization quadrupole time-of-flight mass spectrometry. *J. Sep. Sci.* **2020**, *43*, 852–864. [PubMed]
24. Zhang, J.Y.; Zhang, Q.; Li, N.; Wang, Z.J.; Lu, J.Q.; Qiao, Y.J. Diagnostic fragment-ion-based and extension strategy coupled to DFIs intensity analysis for identification of chlorogenic acids isomers in Flos Lonicerae Japonicae by HPLC-ESI-MS(n). *Talanta* **2013**, *104*, 1–9. [CrossRef] [PubMed]
25. Kruve, A. Strategies for drawing quantitative conclusions from nontargeted liquid chromatography-high-resolution mass spectrometry analysis. *Anal. Chem.* **2020**, *92*, 4691–4699. [CrossRef] [PubMed]

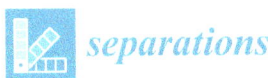 *separations*

Article

DES Based Efficient Extraction Method for Bioactive Coumarins from *Angelica dahurica (Hoffm.) Benth. & Hook.f. ex Franch. & Sav.*

Ting Wang and Qian Li *

Gansu Provincial Key Laboratory of Aridland Crop Science, College of Agronomy, Gansu Agricultural University, Lanzhou 730070, China; wangting2021echo@163.com
* Correspondence: liqian1984@gsau.edu.cn

Abstract: In this study, a simple and environmentally friendly method was developed for the extraction of seven active coumarins from *Angelica dahurica (Hoffm.) Benth. & Hook.f. ex Franch. & Sav.* (*A. dahurica*) based on deep eutectic solvents (DESs). Among the 16 kinds of DES based on choline chloride, the DES system with the molar ratio of choline chloride, citric acid, and water as 1:1:2 had the best extraction effect. Ultrasonic-assisted response surface methodology (RSM) was used to investigate the optimal extraction scheme. The results showed that the optimal extraction conditions were a liquid–solid ratio of 10:1 (mL/g), an extraction time of 50 min, an extraction temperature of 59.85 °C, and a moisture content of 49.28%. Under these conditions, the extraction yield reached 1.18%. In addition, scanning electron microscopy (SEM) was used to observe the degree of powder fragmentation before and after extraction with different solvents. The cells of *A. dahurica* medicinal materials obtained by DES ultrasonic-assisted treatment were the most seriously broken, indicating that DES had the highest efficiency in the treatment of *A. dahurica*. The 1,1-diphenyl-2-picrylhydrazyl (DPPH) DPPH radical scavenging model was used to evaluate the biological activity of DES extract. The results showed that DES extract had better scavenging ability of DPPH free radical. Therefore, DES is a green solvent suitable for extracting coumarin compounds of *A. dahurica*, with great potential to replace organic solvents.

Keywords: deep eutectic solvents; *Angelicae dahuricae*; coumarins; response surface methodology

Citation: Wang, T.; Li, Q. DES Based Efficient Extraction Method for Bioactive Coumarins from *Angelica dahurica (Hoffm.) Benth. & Hook.f. ex Franch. & Sav. Separations* **2022**, *9*, 5. https://doi.org/10.3390/separations 9010005

Academic Editor: Ki Hyun Kim

Received: 30 November 2021
Accepted: 21 December 2021
Published: 23 December 2021

Publisher's Note: MDPI stays neutral with regard to jurisdictional claims in published maps and institutional affiliations.

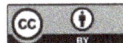
1. Introduction

Angelica dahurica (Hoffm.) Benth. & Hook.f. ex Franch. & Sav. (A. dahuricae) is the dry root belonging to umbelliferaceae. *A. dahuricae* has been frequently used as a food additive and a folk medicinal herb in Asian countries [1]. *A. dahuricae* has a wide range of pharmacological activities, including analgesia, anti-inflammatory, antibacterial, vascular dilation, anti-cancer, and central excitatory properties, and so on [2]. It has been used as an anodyne, and is very effective at relieving neuralgic pain [3]. *A. dahuricae* is known to contain a large number of compounds, including volatile oil, coumarins, and glycosides. Among these compounds, coumarins are generally considered the major components; so far, more than 20 kinds of coumarins have been isolated from this crude drug, such as oxypeucedanin, imperatorin, cnidilin, isoimperatorin, xanthotoxol, byakangelicin, bergapten, etc. [4]. Therefore, the efficient extraction of coumarins is important and desirable.

As known to us, a major disadvantage of conventional methods such as impregnation, percolation, and soxhlet extraction using alcohol or other common organic solvents is the use of a large number of flammable, non-degradable, or toxic organic solvents in the extraction process. In order to solve this problem, a new green natural deep eutectic solvents (NADESs) has been studied [5]. Compared to traditional organic solvents, NADES is a promising alternative to traditional organic solvents because of its green, non-toxic, biodegradable, and recyclable properties [6].

At present, DESs are widely used in science to extract the following types of biologically-active substances (BASs): flavonoids, alkaloids, anthocyanins, flavors, saponins, etc. [7]. DESs are mostly composed of primary metabolites such as sugars, sugar alcohols, organic acids, amino acids, and amines and additionally often contain water in certain molar ratios [8]. Compared with traditional extraction solvents, DESs could improve the extraction rate of products, which is an effective method to extract bioactive products [9]. Owing to these unique properties, DESs have been widely used in catalysis, organic synthesis, and analytical chemistry [10,11]. DESs have been widely used in liquid–liquid extraction, solid-phase microextraction, and other fields [12]. Recently, several studies used DESs for the extraction and separation of different types of bioactive compounds, such as phenolic acids, flavonoids, and alkaloids from various plant materials [13]. In general, the extraction capacity of DESs for biologically active natural products is related to their physicochemical properties, including H-bond interactions, polarity, pH, and viscosity. The polarity of DESs is an important factor affecting the extraction efficiency. Due to the high polarity of synthesized DESs, they have been used for the extraction of polar natural compounds like alkaloids, anthocyanins, polysaccharides, and glycosides. In general, as for natural compounds with low polarity, such as anthraquinones, their extraction rate is low [6,14]. In addition, the solid–liquid ratio of the sample to the DES, the extraction time, and even the molecular weight of the DES may affect the extraction effect. A high-efficiency and green extraction approach by DESs prepared by inexpensive and natural components was successfully developed for the extraction of coumarins in Cortex Fraxini by Wang et al. [15].

Ultrasonic-assisted extraction (UAE) UAE can significantly improve the efficiency of the classical extraction process, and the combination of UAE with NADESs can also be effective [16]. Compared with the conventional method using 96% ethanol as solvent, the NADES-UAE method had higher extraction efficiency for trans-cinnamaldehyde and coumarin from C. burmanni by Widya Dwi ARYATI [17,18]. Chen et al. established a liquid chromatography–tandem mass spectrometry (LC-MS /MS) method for simultaneous quantification of nine furanocoumarins, which could separate nine furanocoumarins within 6 min [19]. Pfeifer et al. detected coumarin in *A. dahurica* roots by supercritical fluid chromatography [20]. However, as known to us, the method of extracting bioactive compound coumarins by DESs is still limited, and the efficiency of extracting coumarin from *A. dahuricae* is not clear.

In this study, a series of DESs based on choline chloride was developed to evaluate the extraction effect on coumarin of *A. dahurica*. A Box–Behnken design (BBD) and the response surface method (RSM) were used to optimize the extraction conditions of DESs. Scanning electron microscopy (SEM) was used to study the degree of crushing of medicinal powder by ultrasonic-assisted DES and conventional extraction. Finally, the scavenging effect of DES extract on DPPH free radical was studied.

2. Experimental

2.1. Materials and Reagents

A. dahurica was purchased from Suining City, Qing Mountain sulphur free food store (Sichuan, China). An appropriate amount of medicinal materials was taken and baked in an oven at 60 °C for 24 h. Then, they were crushed through a 40-mesh sieve and the coarse powder of *A. dahurica* root was obtained, which was put into a zipper bag for use.

All the chemicals for the preparation of the DES and coumarins were purchased from companies in several Chinese cities mentioned later. Analytical reagents such as choline chloride, sucrose, xylitol, citric acid, glucose, ethylene glycol, 1,2-propanediol, 1,4-butanediol, 1,3-butanediol, glycerol, fructose, and urea were purchased from Sinopharm Chemical Reagent Co., Ltd. (Shanghai, China); malic acid was purchased from Shanghai Sanpu Chemical Co., Ltd. (Shanghai, China); acetic acid was purchased from Tianjin Beichenfang Reagent., Ltd. (Tianjin, China) and lactic acid was purchased from Yantai Shuangshuang Chemical Co., Ltd. (Yantai, China). All the above reagents are analytically pure.

Oxypeucedanin (lot: Y29S9S65152 ≥ 98%), isoimperatorin (lot: 18062202 ≥ 98%), bergapten (lot: 17120501 ≥ 98%), psoralen (lot: 19101703 ≥ 98%), imperatorin (lot: 1805150 ≥ 98%), and xanthotoxol (lot: 19111602 ≥ 99%) were purchased from Chengdu Pufeide Biological Technology Co., Ltd. (Sichuan, China)Byakangelicin (lot: B-005-180921 ≥ 98%) was purchased from Chengdu Ruifensi Biological Technology Co., Ltd. (Sichuan, China) The deionized water used in this study was obtained from a Milli-Q water purification system (Bedford, NY, USA). All other reagents and chemicals used were of analytical grade. The chemical structures of coumarins used in this study are shown in Figure 1.

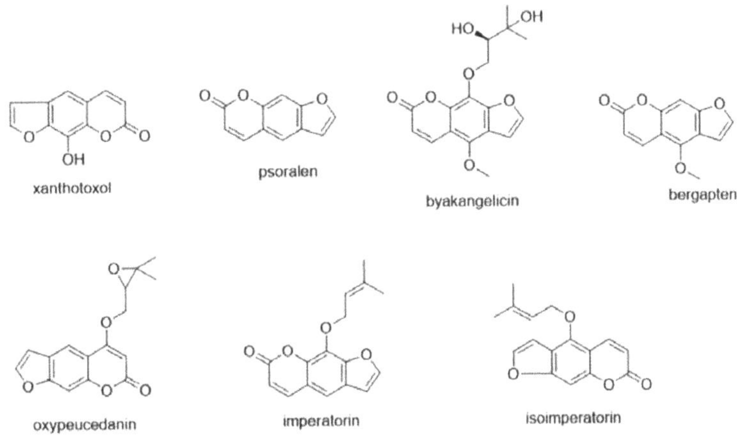

Figure 1. Chemical structures of xanthotoxol, psoralen, byakangelicin, bergapten, oxypeucedanin, imperatorin, and isoimperatorin.

2.2. Preparation of DESs

The direct synthesis method of DESs is easy to operate and has few equipment requirements. The mixture with a certain molar ratio was put into a small beaker of 100 mL and stirred in an oil bath at a certain temperature (80–90 °C) until a uniform and stable transparent liquid was formed (generally 120–180 min). Because some components have high viscosity and a high melting point, it was difficult to obtain an ideal solvent by the direct heating synthesis method. A certain proportion of water should be added before heating to reduce the viscosity. Five kinds of three-phase DESs and 11 kinds of two-phase DESs were prepared by the above method, which are shown in the following Table 1.

Table 1. List of DESs synthesized in this study.

No.	Hydrogen Bond Acceptors (HBAs)	Hydrogen Bond Donors (HBDs)	HBA/HBD (Water) Ratio	Appearance at Room Temperature
1	Choline chloride	Sucrose	1:1:(2)	Transparent liquid
2	Choline chloride	Xylitol	1:1:(1)	Transparent liquid
3	Choline chloride	Citric acid	1:1:(2)	Transparent liquid
4	Choline chloride	D-Glucose	1:1:(2)	Transparent liquid
5	Choline chloride	DL-Malic acid	1:1:(2)	Transparent yellow liquid
6	Choline chloride	Acetic acid	1:2	Transparent liquid
7	Choline chloride	Lactic acid	1:3	Transparent liquid
8	Choline chloride	Lactic acid	1:2	Transparent liquid
9	Choline chloride	Ethylene glycol	1:2	Transparent liquid
10	Choline chloride	1,2-Propanediol	1:2	Transparent liquid
11	Choline chloride	1,4-Butanediol	1:2	Viscous liquid

Table 1. *Cont.*

No.	Hydrogen Bond Acceptors (HBAs)	Hydrogen Bond Donors (HBDs)	HBA/HBD (Water) Ratio	Appearance at Room Temperature
12	Choline chloride	1,3-Butanediol	1:2	Viscous liquid
13	Choline chloride	Glycerol	1:2	Transparent liquid
14	Choline chloride	Glycerol	1:3	Transparent liquid
15	Choline chloride	Fructose	1:2	Transparent liquid
16	Choline chloride	Urea	1:2	Transparent liquid

2.3. Experimental Design

2.3.1. Preparation of Standard Solution

A certain amount of standard was precisely weighed, placed in a 10 mL volumetric flask, and then filled with methanol to the scale line to obtain 7 standard solutions of varying concentrations. Then, 1 mL of each standard solution was precisely sucked and added to the same volumetric flask to obtain a mixed standard solution. After filtration with 0.45 μm microporous membrane, the mixed standard solution was injected into high-performance liquid chromatography (HPLC) at different volumes (4, 8, 10, 12, 16, 20 μL), and the peak area was recorded for each.

2.3.2. Preparation of Sample Solution

In the initial screening, 1 g *A. dahurica* herb powder was accurately weighted and added to a 150 mL conical flask with a certain proportion of DES solvent. After vortexing, the mixture was put into an ultrasonic bath at 60 °C, 300 W power, and 50 Hz for 60 min, then the solution was collected and centrifuged at 6000 RPM for 15 min. A total of 1 mL of the preparation solution was added to a 5 mL volumetric flask and the volume was fixed with methanol to the scale line. Then it was filtered through a 0.45 μm filter and quantified by HPLC analysis. Each experiment was performed three times.

2.3.3. Traditional Extraction Method Comparison

Compared with traditional extraction methods, 75% ethanol and methanol were used for an ultrasonic bath (300 W, 50 Hz, 60 °C, 60 min). After filtration with a 0.45 μm microporous membrane, 10 μL of filtrate were injected into HPLC for analysis, and the yield of total coumarins was calculated.

2.4. Single-Factor Experimental Analysis of Extraction of Coumarins from A. dahurica

2.4.1. Effect of Liquid–Solid Ratio

As shown in Figure 2, the extraction rates of different liquid–solid ratios (10, 20, 30, 40, 50 mL/g) were investigated under ultrasonic bath conditions (300 W, 50 Hz, 60 min, 60 °C) and 30% DES moisture content. When the liquid–solid ratio was 20:1, the extraction rate reached the highest value of 2.06%. When the liquid–solid ration continued to increase, the extraction rate showed a decreasing trend, because the increase in the liquid–solid ratio can make the system have higher solubility and promote the breakdown of cell walls, aiming to increase the overflow ratio of the content. However, when the solubility is large enough, there will be a saturation phenomenon, which would lead to some components not being dissolved, resulting in waste of extraction solvent and complexity of the extraction process, thus affecting the extraction effect.

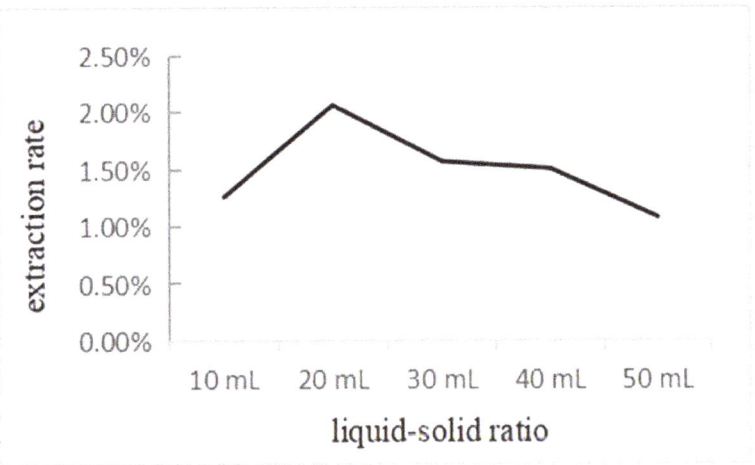

Figure 2. Effect of liquid–solid ratio on the extraction yield of coumarins.

2.4.2. Effect of Extraction Temperature

Extraction rates at different temperatures (40, 50, 60, 70, 80 °C) were investigated under ultrasonic bath conditions (300 W, 50 Hz, 60 min), a liquid–solid ratio of 10:1, and 30% DES moisture content. Extraction temperature is the key factor affecting extraction rate. The target compound is adsorbed on the sample matrix by physical adsorption and chemical interaction, which would be reduced by high temperatures, thereby increasing the leaching of the target compound in the extraction solvent. In addition, a high extraction temperature can greatly reduce the viscosity of the extraction solvent, increase the diffusion of the extraction solvent, and accelerate the mass transfer of the target compound. Figure 3 shows that the extraction temperature of 50 °C provided a higher extraction rate than the other test extraction temperatures. Although a higher extraction temperature may improve extraction yield, it may not be able to avoid the thermal degradation of active ingredients at high temperatures [21]. Therefore, the extraction temperature of 50 °C was selected as the optimal extraction temperature in this study.

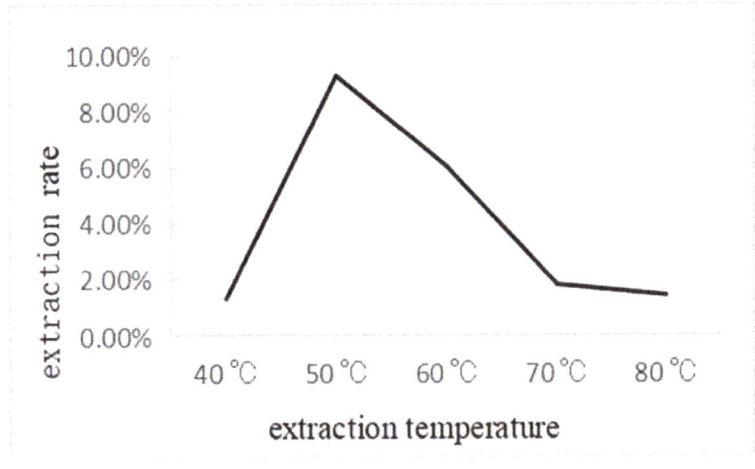

Figure 3. Effect of extraction temperature on the extraction yield of coumarins.

2.4.3. Effect of Extraction Time

To some extent, the extraction rate is always proportional to the extraction time [22]. As shown in Figure 4, different extraction times (30, 40, 50, 60 min) were investigated under the conditions of an ultrasonic bath (300 W, 50 Hz, 60 °C), a liquid–solid ratio of 10:1, and a DES moisture content of 30%. The extraction rate showed an upward trend at 30–40 min, and a downward trend at 40–60 min. This may have been because the longer the time, the greater the energy generated by ultrasonic waves, forming a strong cavitation effect in the solution, which will cause more damage to the cell wall of medicinal materials, which means the extraction rate is also greater [23,24]. However, with the extension of the ultrasonic action time, the amount of extraction decreases, which may be because when the sample is under long-term ultrasonic action and a high temperature of 60 °C, the system is affected by ultrasonic radiation and thermal effect, which may produce double degradation. Therefore, 40 min was selected as the optimal extraction time at 60 °C. The extraction time was 20 min less than that of the traditional extraction method.

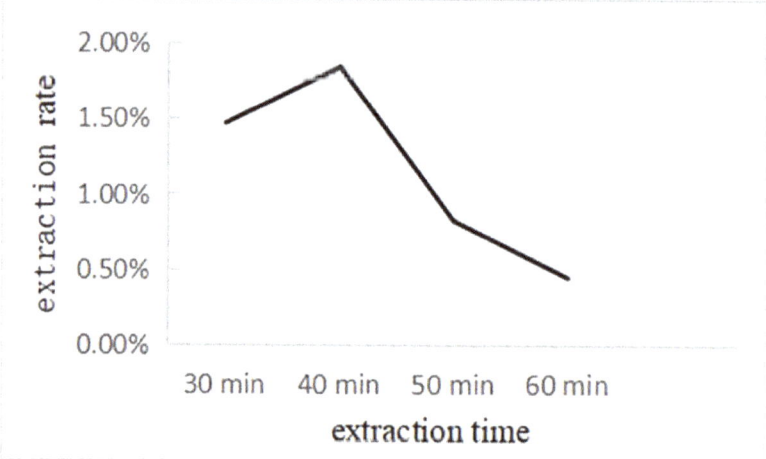

Figure 4. Effect of extraction time on the extraction yield of coumarins.

2.4.4. Effect of DES Moisture Content

There are extensive hydrogen bond networks among DES components, resulting in high viscosity and weak mobility. Its viscosity and fluidity must be altered to obtain good permeability of the pores in the sample matrix and to facilitate mass transfer from the plant matrix to the solution. Adding water to DES can significantly reduce the viscosity and improve the extraction rate. In addition, the DES–water mixture is more alkaline and has a lower cost of extracting the target compound than the normal DES solvent [10]. Therefore, the extraction rate appears to be strongly dependent on the water content of the DES solution. As can be seen from Figure 5, different DES moisture counts were investigated under the conditions of an ultrasonic bath (300 W, 50 Hz, 60 min, 60 °C), and a liquid–solid ratio of 10:1. The extraction rate increased in the range of a 0–50% volume ratio and decreased in the range of 50–60%. It is possible that the excess water content increased the polarity of the mixture and reduced the interaction between the compounds. Therefore, a 50% DES moisture content was identified as the best choice during subsequent extraction.

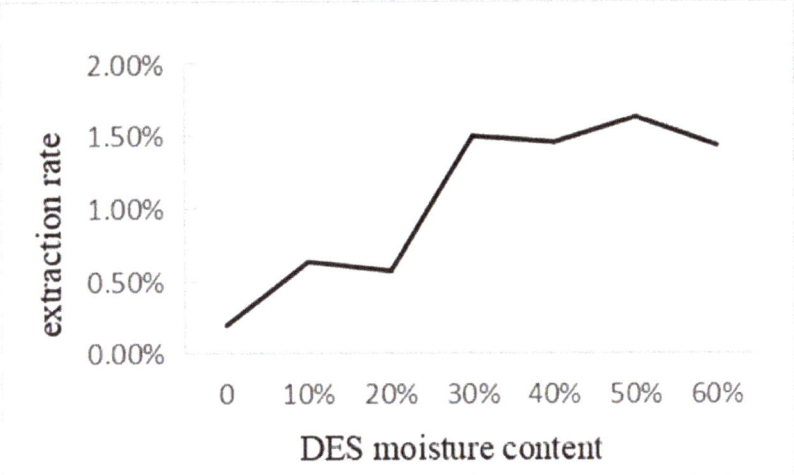

Figure 5. Effect of DES moisture content on the extraction yield of coumarins.

On the basis of the preliminary single-factor experiments, the extraction process parameters were optimized by BBD with the ratio of liquid to solid, extraction time, ultrasonic temperature, and DES moisture content as four independent variables. The total extraction rate of 7 coumarin compounds was used as the response of the design experiment. Regression analysis was performed on the experimental data and additional validation experiments were performed to verify the effectiveness of the statistical experimental strategy. Software Design-Expert 12 was used to generate and evaluate experimental designs.

2.5. HPLC Conditions and Method Validation

The HPLC system consists of a Waters quad gradient high-performance liquid chromatography (ACQUITY Arc), a 122 Rheodyne injector (20 µL sample loop), and a full wavelength (200–600nm) diode array detector. The chromatographic analysis was performed on a C18 column (1.6 × 250 mm, 5.0 µm). The linear gradient elution was performed used methanol (A) and water (B) as mobile phases. The gradient elution procedure was as follows: 0–5 min: A-B (35:65), 15 min: A-B (65:35), 17 min: A-B (85:15), 30 min: A-B (90:10), 35 min: A-B (35:65), 37 min: A-B (35:65). The detection wavelength was set at 268 nm, the flow rate was 1 mL/min, the column temperature was 30 °C, and the injection volume was 10 µL. Sampling was started 10 min after system equilibrium, and all samples were analyzed by HPLC after passing through a 0.45 µm microporous membrane. The HPLC chromatogram of 7 coumarin standard substances and 7 coumarin compounds extracted from *A. dahurica* are shown in Figure 6.

The quantitative analysis of 7 coumarins in *A. dahurica* was verified by method validation. The linearity, precision, repeatability, and stability were verified. The calibration curves of 7 coumarins were performed with 6 standard solutions of different concentrations in triplicate. All calibration curves were well linear with high correlation coefficients ($R^2 > 0.9948$) over the test range. The accuracy of the method was determined by intra-day and inter-day testing. Intra-day testing means the same sample was analyzed 6 times in the same day. Inter-day test was repeated testing of 3 samples obtained by the same extraction method for 3 consecutive days. The relative standard deviations of intra-day and inter-day precision were less than 1.24% and 2.13%, respectively. Six replicates of the same sample were prepared and analyzed for the repeatability test. In stability tests, the same sample was stored at room temperature and analyzed repeatedly at 0, 4, 6, 8, 12, and 24 h. The repeatability expressed by relative standard deviation was less than 1.37%, and the stability was less than 1.23%. The results showed that the established method was accurate and sensitive for the quantitative analysis of 7 components of *A. dahuricae*. All of the above data are shown in Table 2.

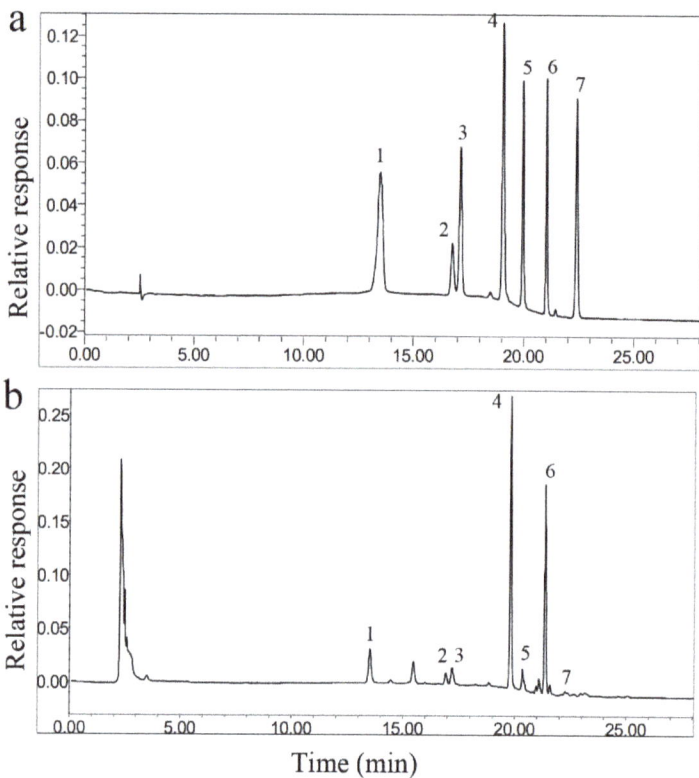

Figure 6. The typical HPLC chromatograms: (**a**) 7 coumarin reference standards and (**b**) *A. dahurica* sample (1. xanthotoxol, 13.48 min; 2. psoralen, 16.76 min; 3. byakangelicin, 17.13 min; 4. bergapten, 19.04 min; 5. oxypeucedanin, 19.95 min; 6. imperatorin, 21.02 min; and 7. isoimperatorin, 22.38 min) and separation degree of chromatographic peak: 5.86%, 1.27%, 4.17%, 1.87%, 3.36%, 1.82%.

Table 2. Validation of linear regression equation, linear range, precision, repeatability, and stability of 7 coumarins.

No.	Analyte	Regression Equation	R^2	Linear Range (mg/mL)	Precision Intra-Day RSD (%)	Inter-Day RSD (%)	Repeatability RSD (%)	Stability RSD (%)
1	Xanthotoxol	Y = 9286.6X + 43348	0.9948	0.040–0.200	0.26	1.46	1.13	0.22
2	Psoralen	Y = 2232.3X − 8340.4	0.9998	0.036–0.180	0.54	1.74	1.37	1.23
3	Byakangelicin	Y = 5192.5X − 3041.4	0.9996	0.040–0.200	0.47	1.62	0.57	1.09
4	Bergapten	Y = 8584.5X + 21114	0.9998	0.040–0.200	0.83	2.13	0.47	0.68
5	Oxypeucedanin	Y = 4801.5X + 2149.1	0.9996	0.040–0.200	1.24	1.82	0.44	0.34
6	Imperatorin	Y = 4442.6X − 7511.1	0.9999	0.040–0.200	0.20	1.78	0.45	0.94
7	Isoimperatorin	Y = 5522.3X − 10479	0.9999	0.040–0.200	0.23	1.57	0.47	0.95

2.6. Determination of Antioxidant Activity of Plant Extracts

Oxidation is one of the most important processes in food spoilage. Antioxidants can protect against the harmful effects of free radicals in the body and prevent the oxidation of fats and other food components [25]. The widely documented 1,1-diphenyl-2-

pyrylhydrazyl (DPPH) radical was used to assess antioxidant activity, because it is a stable free radical that can accept electrons or hydrogen radicals to form stable chemicals [26].

In this study, the antioxidant activities of two different extraction methods were compared (75% ethanol traditional heating reflux extraction and DES ultrasonic extraction). The concentration of the solution varied from 0.1 to 27 mg/mL for each sample. In addition, the vitamin C (VC) solution of the corresponding concentration was prepared by deionized water as a control test of antioxidant activity. The absorbance was measured at 517 nm relative to the blank. The percentage of scavenging activity was calculated as follows: $(1 - (A_1 - A_2)/A_0) \times 100\%$, where A_0 is the absorbance of the control, A_1 is the absorbance of the sample, and A_2 is the absorbance of the blank sample without DPPH free radical. The scavenging activity of the sample is expressed as the IC_{50} value, which is the concentration required to remove 50% DPPH free radicals [27].

2.7. Microstructure of Plant Material

In order to study the microscopic effects of different extraction methods on the fragmentation degree of *A. dahuricae* powder, the microstructure changes in the powder before and after extraction by three different extraction methods were observed by scanning electron microscope. The dried powder was secured to the sample table with double-sided tape and gilded. Then the morphology of the powders extracted with different solvents was observed by scanning electron microscope at 10 kV accelerating voltage.

3. Results and Discussion

3.1. Screening of DESs

The total yield of coumarins in each extraction solvent was the sum of seven kinds of coumarin compounds. The results showed that the total extraction rate of seven coumarin compounds was affected by different solvents. In order to understand the advantages of DESs in extracting coumarin compounds from *A. dahurica*, the extraction rates of different organic solvents (methanol and 75% ethanol) and different DESs were compared. As shown in Figure 7, compared with the traditional extraction method, the extraction rate of DES-3 was significantly higher than that of other DES solvents and traditional organic solvents.

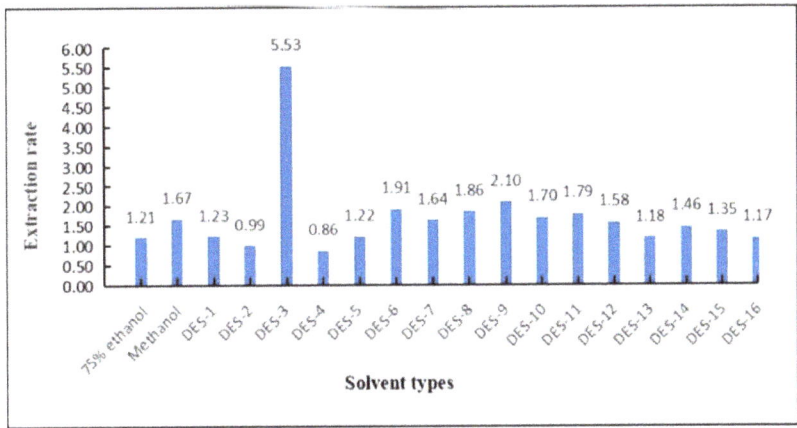

Figure 7. The yield of total coumarins extracted with different organic solvents and DES. Note: The yield of total coumarins was the sum of 7 kinds of coumarins.

The composition of DES could influence the hydrogen bond between the hydrogen bond donor and the hydrogen bond acceptor, thus determining its viscosity and polarity. The high viscosity of DES restricts its application in extraction compared to conventional solvents. High viscosity may reduce extraction efficiency because of slow mass transfer, whereas low-viscosity DES results in high diffusivity and therefore improved extraction performance. Most DESs showed a low total extraction rate for the seven coumarins, but DES prepared with choline chloride, citric acid, and water at a molar ratio of 1:1:2 produced a higher extraction efficiency. This may be because citric acid has higher hydrogen-bonding capacity and more electrostatic interaction with choline chloride than other hydrogen bond donors. Therefore, this type of DES was chosen as the best extraction solvent for coumarins compounds and applied in further tests based on the initial screening results.

3.2. Optimization of the Extraction Conditions by Response Surface Methodology

The above extraction studies show that the molar ratio of choline chloride, citric acid, and water of 1:1:2 was the best DES. In order to obtain the best extraction rate, RSM was used to optimize several extraction conditions that affected the extraction rate. Four-factor and three-level BBD were used to investigate the influence of four independent variables—liquid–solid ratio (A), extraction temperature (B), extraction time (C), and DES moisture content (D)—on the extraction yield (Y), which is shown in Table 3.

Table 3. Factors and levels in response surface analysis.

Factors	Level		
	−1	0	1
A Liquid–solid ratio (mg/mL)	10	20	30
B Extraction temperature (°C)	40	50	60
C Extraction time (min)	30	40	50
D DES moisture content (%)	40	50	60

The extraction process parameters of ultrasonic assisted DES extraction were systematically investigated, and the optimal extraction conditions of coumarin compounds in *A. dahurica* were determined. The solid-liquid ratio, ultrasonic temperature, extraction time and DES moisture content were investigated by single factor test. As shown in Table 4, on the basis of single factor test, RSM and BBD were used to determine the optimal combination of solid-liquid ratio, extraction temperature, extraction time and DES moisture content.

Table 4. Experimental order, variable levels, and response values in Box–Behnken designs.

Run	Liquid–Solid Ratio (A, mL/g)	Extraction Temperature (B, °C)	Extraction Time (C, min)	DES Moisture Content (D, %)	Total Extraction Yields (mg/g)
1	0	−1	−1	0	0.92
2	0	0	1	−1	1.17
3	0	0	−1	1	1.07
4	−1	0	1	0	1.13
5	−1	0	0	−1	1.07
6	0	1	1	0	1.31
7	0	0	0	0	1.02
8	0	0	1	1	1.24
9	−1	1	0	0	1.26
10	1	0	0	−1	0.5
11	1	0	1	0	0.71
12	1	0	−1	0	0.75
13	0	1	−1	0	1.26
14	0	0	−1	−1	0.88
15	0	1	0	−1	0.46
16	0	0	0	0	0.94
17	1	0	0	1	1.07
18	0	0	0	0	0.88
19	0	−1	0	1	0.95
20	0	1	0	1	1.04

Table 4. *Cont.*

Run	Liquid–Solid Ratio (A, mL/g)	Extraction Temperature (B, °C)	Extraction Time (C, min)	DES Moisture Content (D, %)	Total Extraction Yields (mg/g)
21	−1	0	−1	0	0.95
22	1	−1	0	0	0.68
23	0	−1	0	−1	0.52
24	1	1	0	0	0.85
25	0	−1	1	0	1.19
26	−1	0	0	1	0.98
27	−1	−1	0	0	0.89
28	0	0	0	0	1.09
29	0	0	0	0	1.11

The above tests were performed in three replicates. Design-Expert 12 was used to carry out multiple regression of BBD data to obtain the second-order polynomial model.

3.3. Fitting the Response Surface Model

The effects of four parameters on the yield of total coumarins in *A. dahurica* were investigated at the levels of −1, 0, and +1. A total of 29 different tests were carried out, and the mean values were fitted using a second-order polynomial model, as follows:

$$Y = 1.01 - 0.14A + 0.086B + 0.077C + 0.15D - 0.050AB - 0.055AC + 0.17AD - 0.055BC + 0.038BD - 0.030CD - 0.10A^2 - 0.040B^2 + 0.12C^2 - 0.087D^2$$

Analysis of variance was used to evaluate the optimal conditions for ultrasonic-assisted DES extraction and the relationship between the reaction and the variables. Table 5 shows the analysis of variance for the quadratic model. The F-value in analysis of variance ANOVA was used to estimate differences between groups. The F-value represents the significance of the whole fitting equation. The larger the F value is, the more significant the equation is and the better the fitting degree is. The *p*-value is a measure of the size of the difference. $p < 0.05$ indicates significant difference. $p < 0.01$ indicates extremely significant difference.

Table 5. The analysis of variance (ANOVA) results of the quadratic multiple regression model for total coumarin yield.

Variables	Sum of Squares	df	Mean Square	F-Value	*p*-Value	
Model	1.06	14	0.076	2.66	0.0388	significant
A-Liquid-solid ratio	0.25	1	0.25	8.62	0.0108	
B-Extraction temperature	0.088	1	0.088	3.09	0.1005	
C-Extraction time	0.071	1	0.071	2.47	0.1386	
D-DES moisture content	0.26	1	0.26	8.93	0.0098	
AB	0.010	1	0.010	0.35	0.5636	
AC	0.012	1	0.012	0.42	0.5258	
AD	0.11	1	0.11	3.81	0.0713	
BC	0.012	1	0.012	0.42	0.5258	
BD	0.006	1	0.006	0.20	0.6641	
CD	0.004	1	0.004	0.13	0.7280	
A^2	0.066	1	0.066	2.32	0.1501	
B^2	0.010	1	0.010	0.36	0.5581	
C^2	0.088	1	0.088	3.08	0.1013	
D^2	0.049	1	0.049	1.73	0.2095	
Residual	0.40	14	0.029			
Lake of fit	0.36	10	0.036	3.78	0.1058	Not significant
R^2	0.974					
Adj R^2	0.817					

According to the F-value of the analysis of variance in Table 3, the influence degree of the four factors on the extraction rate of coumarins of *A. dahurica* was DES moisture content (D) > liquid–solid ratio (A) > extraction temperature (B) > extraction time (C), which is visually expressed by the Pareto diagram in Figure 8. The *p*-value of the model < 0.05, indicating that the regression relationship between the total rate of coumarins of *A. dahuricae* and their respective variables is significant, which can better simulate the real surface. The loss of fitting term *p* = 0.1058 > 0.05, and the influence was not significant, indicating that the experimental data and the model were significantly consistent. This model can be used to analyze and predict the extraction rate of coumarins in *A. dahuricae*, and it is true and reliable. In this model, primary term D had a highly significant effect on the total extraction rate of coumarins (*p* < 0.01), and primary term A had a significant effect on the total extraction rate of coumarins in *A. dahuricae* (*p* < 0.05); the interaction effect was not significant. The correlation coefficient R^2 = 0.974 and the adjusted determination coefficient adjustment R^2 (Adj R ^{2}) = 0.817, indicating that this model can be used to explain the change in the extraction rate of coumarin components in 81.7% of *A. dahuricae*.

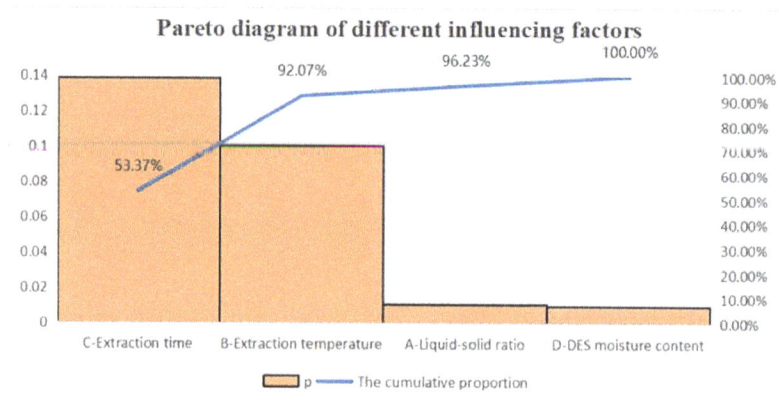

Figure 8. Pareto diagram of different influencing factors.

3.4. Verification of Predictive Model

Using Design-Expert software, the optimal values of independent and dependent variables were as follows: liquid–solid ratio (A) was 10 mL/g, extraction temperature (B) was 59.85 °C, extraction time (C) was 50 min, and DES moisture content (D) was 49.28%. The maximum predicted extraction rate was 1.34%. Under the optimal extraction conditions, three verification experiments were carried out, and the average extraction rate was 1.18%. The results showed that the regression model was appropriate for predicting the extraction yield of coumarins from *A. dahuricae*. In addition, compared with the reported methods, the extraction time and solid–liquid ratio in this study were greatly reduced. The traditional solvent extraction time of coumarins is 4.23 h. Compared to the traditional extraction time, the extraction time used in this study was reduced by 5 times, only 50 min. Therefore, this model can save cost and is suitable for the optimization of the ultrasonic-assisted extraction process based on DESs.

3.5. 3D Response Surface

For the response surface test, the three-dimensional surface of the interaction term of two factors is shown in Figure 9. The steeper the slope change of the 3D surface, the denser the contour line, and more like an oval or saddle shape, the more significant the interaction between the two factors. As shown in Figure 9, the contour lines of the AB, AC, AD, BC, BD, and CD interaction terms were basically saddle-shaped or elliptic, and the contour map of the AD interaction terms was typical elliptic. The contour map of the AC, AD, BC, BD, and CD interaction terms was elliptic, but the slope change of the 3D surface of the interaction terms in group BD was relatively gentle compared to those in groups AB, AC, AD, and BC. This is consistent with the results of the analysis of variance in Table 5.

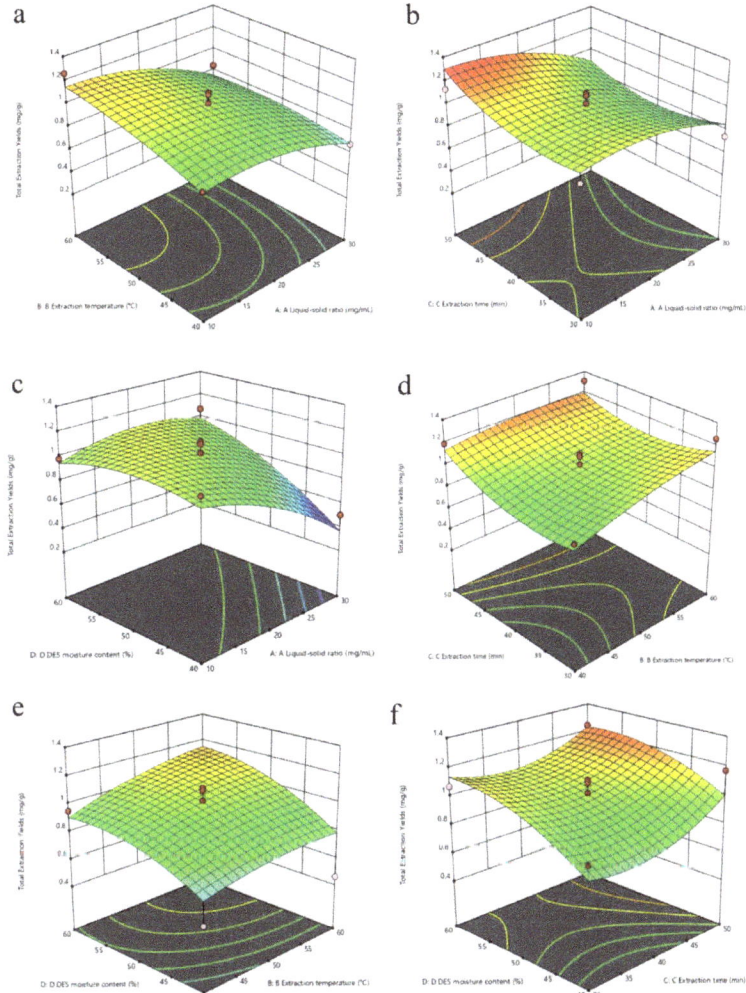

Figure 9. 3D response surface. Notes: (**a**) the reciprocal response of A and B, (**b**) the reciprocal response of A and C, (**c**) the reciprocal response of A and D, (**d**) the reciprocal response of B and C, (**e**) the reciprocal response of B and D, (**f**) the reciprocal response of C and D.

3.6. Microstructure of Plant Material

The residues of different extraction methods were observed by scanning electron microscopy (SEM). As shown in Figure 10, it can be seen that the cells of *A. dahurica* medicinal materials obtained by DES ultrasonic assisted treatment were the most seriously broken, indicating that DES had the highest efficiency in the treatment of *A. dahurica*. This result is the same as that shown in Section 3.1. The degree of cell fragmentation was proportional to the extraction rate. By contrast, the outer surface of the sample powder was significantly cracked by pulsed ultrasonic treatment, and loose and broken structures could be observed. This is similar to what Sukor et al. observed when extracting phenolic acids using ultrasonic processing of an ionic liquid probe [28], and Chen et al. used ultrasound-assisted extraction methods for imperatorin and isoimperatorin from *A. dahurica* roots [22].

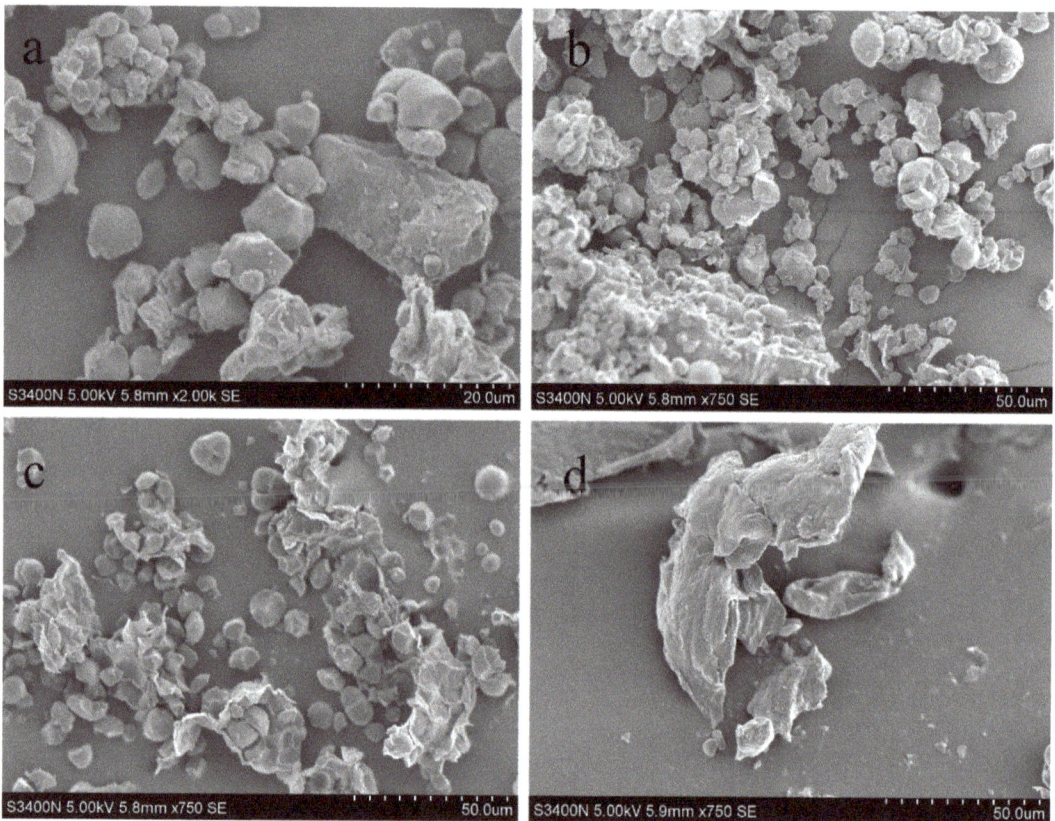

Figure 10. The field emission scanning electron microscope images: (**a**) unextracted *A. dahurica* powder, (**b**) 75% ethanol ultrasound, (**c**) methanol ultrasonic, and (**d**) the selected DES ultrasound.

Organic solvent extraction, microwave-assisted extraction, and ultrasonic extraction have been widely used in the extraction of single medicinal materials [29]. In addition, Feng et al. combined ultrasonic-assisted extraction and microwave-assisted extraction technology to rapidly determine the essential oil of *A. dahurica* [30]. Ultrasonic-assisted extraction is a technique based on cavitation phenomena or mechanical waves generated by high-frequency impulses [31]. This force can break down plant cell walls and reduce particle size, promote swelling, and extract solvents to penetrate cells and release bioactive compounds from vacuoles [32,33]. Therefore, ultrasound-assisted extraction of coumarins compounds from *A. dahuricae* with DESs can replace the traditional organic solvent extraction method, becoming a green and efficient extraction method.

3.7. Antioxidant Activity of Extracts

DPPH has been widely used to determine the antioxidant capacity of biological samples, pure compounds, and extracts in vitro. This method is simple and can be used to evaluate the antioxidant activity of the samples [28]. With VC as the control, the DPPH radical scavenging activities of the two different treated solutions are shown in Figure 11.

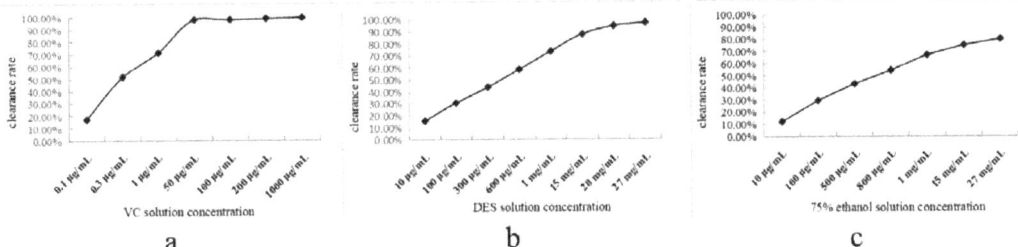

Figure 11. Comparison of DPPH radical scavenging activity in different solutions. (**a**) VC reference solution; (**b**) DES solution; (**c**) 75% ethanol solution.

As shown in Figure 11, with the increase in the concentration of different sample solutions, the scavenging ability of antioxidants in different solutions on DPPH free radical gradually increased, and gradually leveled off after reaching a certain concentration. The clearance rate of VC to DPPH tended to be stable when the concentration was 50 µg/mL, and reached the maximum at 100 µg/mL, with a maximum clearance rate was 99.54%. The DPPH clearance rate of DES extract tended to be stable at 20 mg/mL, and the maximum clearance rate was 97.22%. When reflux extraction with a concentration of 75% ethanol reached the specified concentration, its clearance rate was lower than that of DES solution (79.83%). According to SPSS software analysis, the IC_{50} values of VC extract, DES extract, and 75% ethanol heated reflux extract were 0.289 µg/mL, 0.477 mg/mL, and 0.772 mg/mL, respectively. In conclusion, VC control solution has the strongest DPPH radical scavenging ability. The scavenging ability of DES extract was better than that of 75% ethanol extract. The antioxidant capacity of 75% ethanol extract was not as good as that of DES solution, but it still had a significant effect.

4. Conclusions

This study aimed to provide a more green, efficient, economic, and environmentally protective target ingredient extraction method, which could better promote the in-depth development of Chinese herbal *A. dahurica* resources and provide data support for the development of green chemistry and the study of natural products in China. DESs were used to extract coumarin compounds from *A. dahurica* with ultrasonic assistance. A rapid and green extraction method for coumarins such as xanthotoxol, psoralen, byakangelicin, bergapten, oxypeucedanin, imperatorin, and isoimperatorin from *A. dahuricae* was developed. Experiments showed that the ultrasonic-assisted DES system is an effective system for extracting coumarin compounds from *A. dahurica*, which solves the problems of environmental pollution and solvent residue in extracting natural active ingredients of traditional Chinese medicine with traditional organic solvents.

Author Contributions: Conceptualization, T.W. and Q.L.; data curation, T.W.; formal analysis, T.W.; investigation, T.W. and Q.L.; methodology, T.W. and Q.L.; project administration, Q.L.; supervision, T.W. and Q.L.; validation, T.W.; writing—original draft, T.W.; writing—review and editing, T.W. and Q.L. All authors have read and agreed to the published version of the manuscript.

Funding: This work was supported by the Discipline Construction Fund Project of Gansu Agricultural University (GSAU-XKJS-2018-086), the National Science Foundation of China (31860102), Young Talents introduction projects (GSU-RCZX201704), the research program sponsored by Gansu Provincial Key Laboratory of Aridland Crop Science, Gansu Agricultural University (No.GSCS-2018-3), and the Outstanding Graduate Student Innovation Star Project in Gansu Province (2021CXZX-399).

Institutional Review Board Statement: Not applicable.

Informed Consent Statement: Not applicable.

Data Availability Statement: The data presented in this study are available on request from the corresponding author.

Conflicts of Interest: There are no conflict of interest to declare.

Sample Availability: Samples of the compounds are available from the authors.

References

1. Bai, Y.; Li, D.; Zhou, T.; Qin, N.; Li, Z.; Yu, Z.; Hua, H. Coumarins from the roots of *Angelica dahurica* with antioxidant and antiproliferative activities. *J. Funct. Foods* **2016**, *20*, 453–462. [CrossRef]
2. Chen, Y.; Fan, G.; Chen, B.; Xie, Y.; Wu, H.; Wu, Y.; Yan, C.; Wang, J. Separation and quantitative analysis of coumarin compounds from *Angelica dahurica* (Fisch. ex Hoffm) Benth. et Hook. f by pressurized capillary electrochromatography. *J. Pharm. Biomed. Anal.* **2006**, *41*, 105–116. [CrossRef] [PubMed]
3. Kim, S.H.; Kang, S.S.; Kim, C.M. Coumarin glycosides from the roots of *Angelica dahurica*. *Arch. Pharmacal Res.* **1992**, *15*, 73–77. [CrossRef]
4. Zheng, X.; Zhang, X.; Sheng, X.; Yuan, Z.; Yang, W.; Wang, Q.; Zhang, L. Simultaneous characterization and quantitation of 11 coumarins in Radix Angelicae Dahuricae by high performance liquid chromatography with electrospray tandem mass spectrometry. *J. Pharm. Biomed. Anal.* **2010**, *51*, 599–605. [CrossRef]
5. Fu, X.; Wang, D.; Belwal, T.; Xu, Y.; Li, L.; Luo, Z. Sonication-synergistic natural deep eutectic solvent as a green and efficient approach for extraction of phenolic compounds from peels of Carya cathayensis Sarg. *Food Chem.* **2021**, *355*, 129577. [CrossRef]
6. Obluchinskaya, E.; Pozharitskaya, O.; Zakharova, L.; Daurtseva, A.; Flisyuk, E.; Shikov, A. Efficacy of Natural Deep Eutectic Solvents for Extraction of Hydrophilic and Lipophilic Compounds from Fucus vesiculosus. *Molecules* **2021**, *26*, 4198. [CrossRef] [PubMed]
7. Boyko, N.; Zhilyakova, E.; Malyutina, A.; Novikov, O.; Pisarev, D.; Abramovich, R.; Potanina, O.; Lazar, S.; Mizina, P.; Sahaidak-Nikitiuk, R. Studying and Modeling of the Extraction Properties of the Natural Deep Eutectic Solvent and Sorbitol-Based Solvents in Regard to Biologically Active Substances from Glycyrrhizae Roots. *Molecules* **2020**, *25*, 1482. [CrossRef] [PubMed]
8. Dai, Y.; Witkamp, G.-J.; Verpoorte, R.; Choi, Y.H. Tailoring properties of natural deep eutectic solvents with water to facilitate their applications. *Food Chem.* **2015**, *187*, 14–19. [CrossRef]
9. Zhang, L.; Wang, M. Optimization of deep eutectic solvent-based ultrasound-assisted extraction of polysaccharides from Dioscorea opposita Thunb. *Int. J. Biol. Macromol.* **2017**, *95*, 675–681. [CrossRef]
10. Bi, W.; Tian, M.; Row, K.H. Evaluation of alcohol-based deep eutectic solvent in extraction and determination of flavonoids with response surface methodology optimization. *J. Chromatogr. A* **2013**, *1285*, 22–30. [CrossRef]
11. Peng, X.; Duan, M.H.; Yao, X.H.; Zhang, Y.H.; Zhao, C.G.; Zu, Y.G.; Fu, Y.J. Green extraction of five target phenolic acids from Lonicerae japonicae Flos with deep eutectic solvent. *Sep. Purif. Technol.* **2016**, *157*, 249–257. [CrossRef]
12. Skarpalezos, D.; Detsi, A. Deep Eutectic Solvents as Extraction Media for Valuable Flavonoids from Natural Sources. *Appl. Sci.* **2019**, *9*, 4169. [CrossRef]
13. Yang, G.-Y.; Song, J.-N.; Chang, Y.-Q.; Wang, L.; Zheng, Y.-G.; Zhang, D.; Guo, L. Natural Deep Eutectic Solvents for the Extraction of Bioactive Steroidal Saponins from Dioscoreae Nipponicae Rhizoma. *Molecules* **2021**, *26*, 2079. [CrossRef] [PubMed]
14. Duan, L.; Dou, L.-L.; Guo, L.; Li, P.; Liu, E.-H. Comprehensive evaluation of deep eutectic solvents in extraction of bioactive natural products. *ACS Sustain. Chem. Eng.* **2016**, *4*, 2405–2411. [CrossRef]
15. Wang, Y.; Hu, Y.; Wang, H.; Tong, M.; Gong, Y. Green and enhanced extraction of coumarins from Cortex Fraxini by ultrasound-assisted deep eutectic solvent extraction. *J. Sep. Sci.* **2020**, *43*, 3441–3448. [CrossRef] [PubMed]
16. Razboršek, M.I.; Ivanović, M.; Krajnc, P.; Kolar, M. Choline Chloride Based Natural Deep Eutectic Solvents as Extraction Media for Extracting Phenolic Compounds from Chokeberry (*Aronia melanocarpa*). *Molecules* **2020**, *25*, 1619. [CrossRef]
17. Ahmad, I.; Arifianti, A.E.; Sakti, A.S.; Saputri, F.C.; Mun'im, A. Simultaneous Natural Deep Eutectic Solvent-Based Ultrasonic-Assisted Extraction of Bioactive Compounds of Cinnamon Bark and Sappan Wood as a Dipeptidyl Peptidase IV Inhibitor. *Molecules* **2020**, *25*, 3832. [CrossRef]
18. Aryati, W.D.; Nadhira, A.; Febianli, D.; Fransisca, F.; Mun'im, A. Natural deep eutectic solvents ultrasound-assisted extraction (NADES-UAE) of trans-cinnamaldehyde and coumarin from cinnamon bark [*Cinnamomum burmannii* (Nees T. Nees) Blume]. *J. Res. Pharm.* **2020**, *24*, 389–398. [CrossRef]
19. Chen, L.; Jian, Y.; Wei, N.; Yuan, M.; Zhuang, X.; Li, H. Separation and simultaneous quantification of nine furanocoumarins from Radix Angelicae dahuricae using liquid chromatography with tandem mass spectrometry for bioavailability determination in rats. *J. Sep. Sci.* **2016**, *38*, 4216–4224. [CrossRef]
20. Pfeifer, I.; Murauer, A.; Ganzera, M. Determination of coumarins in the roots of *Angelica dahurica* by supercritical fluid chromatography. *J. Pharm. Biomed. Anal.* **2016**, *129*, 246–251. [CrossRef]
21. Xu, D.-P.; Zheng, J.; Zhou, Y.; Li, Y.; Li, S.; Li, H.-B. Ultrasound-assisted extraction of natural antioxidants from the flower of Limonium sinuatum: Optimization and comparison with conventional methods. *Food Chem.* **2017**, *217*, 552–559. [CrossRef] [PubMed]
22. Chen, Y.; Yang, S.Y.; Li, N.; Zhang, L.J.; Qian, Y. Ultrasound-Assisted Extraction of Imperatorin and Isoimperatorin from Roots of *Angelica dahurica*. *Adv. Mater. Res.* **2012**, *550–553*, 1845–1851. [CrossRef]

23. Živković, J.; Šavikin, K.; Janković, T.; Ćujić, N.; Menković, N. Optimization of ultrasound-assisted extraction of polyphenolic compounds from pomegranate peel using response surface methodology. *Sep. Purif. Technol.* **2018**, *194*, 40–47. [CrossRef]
24. Kazemi, M.; Karim, R.; Mirhosseini, H.; Hamid, A.A. Optimization of pulsed ultrasound-assisted technique for extraction of phenolics from pomegranate peel of Malas variety: Punicalagin and hydroxybenzoic acids. *Food Chem.* **2016**, *206*, 156–166. [CrossRef]
25. Musa, K.H.; Abdullah, A.; Al-Haiqi, A. Determination of DPPH free radical scavenging activity: Application of artificial neural networks. *Food Chem.* **2016**, *194*, 705–711. [CrossRef]
26. Bishnoi, A.; Chawla, H.M.; Pant, N.; Mrig, S.; Kumar, S. Evaluation of the radical scavenging activity of resorcinarenes by DPPH• free radical assay. *J. Chem. Res.* **2010**, *34*, 440–444. [CrossRef]
27. Shi, H.; Yang, H.; Zhang, X.; Yu, L. Identification and Quantification of Phytochemical Composition and Anti-inflammatory and Radical Scavenging Properties of Methanolic Extracts of Chinese Propolis. *J. Agric. Food Chem.* **2012**, *60*, 12403–12410. [CrossRef]
28. Xu, Z.; Cai, Y.; Ma, Q.; Zhao, Z.; Yang, D.; Xu, X. Optimization of Extraction of Bioactive Compounds from Baphicacanthus cusia Leaves by Hydrophobic Deep Eutectic Solvents. *Molecules* **2021**, *26*, 1729. [CrossRef]
29. Duan, H.; Zhai, K.F.; Cao, W.G.; Gao, G.Z.; Shan, L.L.; Zhao, L. The Optimum Extraction Process for Radix glycyrrhizae and *Angelica dahurica* (Fisch.) Benth.et Hook with Orthogonal Design. *Indian J. Pharm. Educ. Res.* **2017**, *51*, S631–S636. [CrossRef]
30. Feng, X.-F.; Jing, N.; Li, Z.-G.; Wei, D.; Lee, M.-R. Ultrasound-Microwave Hybrid-Assisted Extraction Coupled to Headspace Solid-Phase Microextraction for Fast Analysis of Essential Oil in Dry Traditional Chinese Medicine by GC–MS. *Chromatographia* **2014**, *77*, 619–628. [CrossRef]
31. Calderón-Oliver, M.; Ponce-Alquicira, E. Environmentally Friendly Techniques and Their Comparison in the Extraction of Natural Antioxidants from Green Tea, Rosemary, Clove, and Oregano. *Molecules* **2021**, *26*, 1869. [CrossRef] [PubMed]
32. He, X.; Yang, J.; Huang, Y.; Zhang, Y.; Wan, H.; Li, C. Green and Efficient Ultrasonic-Assisted Extraction of Bioactive Components from Salvia miltiorrhiza by Natural Deep Eutectic Solvents. *Molecules* **2019**, *25*, 140. [CrossRef] [PubMed]
33. Oomen, W.W.; Begines, P.; Mustafa, N.R.; Wilson, E.G.; Verpoorte, R.; Choi, Y.H. Natural Deep Eutectic Solvent Extraction of Flavonoids of Scutellaria baicalensis as a Replacement for Conventional Organic Solvents. *Molecules* **2020**, *25*, 617. [CrossRef] [PubMed]

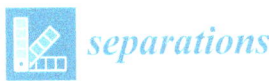

MDPI

Article

What You Extract Is What You Get: Different Methods of Protein Extraction from Hemp Seeds

Annalisa Givonetti [†], Chiara Cattaneo [*,†] and Maria Cavaletto

Dipartimento di Scienze e Innovazione Tecnologica-DiSIT, Università del Piemonte Orientale, 13100 Vercelli, Italy; annalisa.givonetti@uniupo.it (A.G.); maria.cavaletto@uniupo.it (M.C.)
* Correspondence: chiara.cattaneo@uniupo.it
† These authors contributed equally to the work.

Abstract: *Cannabis sativa* L. seeds are rich in essential polyunsaturated fatty acids and highly digestible proteins, with a good nutritional value. Proteomics studies on hempseed reported so far have mainly been conducted on processed seeds and, to our knowledge, no optimization of protein extraction from hemp seeds has been performed. This study investigates the SDS-PAGE profile of hempseed proteins comparing different methods of extraction, (Osborne sequential extraction, TCA/acetone, MTBE/methanol, direct protein solubilization of defatted hempseed flour), two conditions to keep low temperature during seed grinding (liquid nitrogen or ice) and two solubilization buffers (urea-based or Laemmli buffer). Among the tested conditions, the combination of liquid nitrogen + TCA/acetone + Laemmli buffer was not compatible with SDS-PAGE of proteins. On the other hand, urea-based buffer achieved more reproducible results if combined with all the other conditions. TCA/acetone, MTBE/methanol, and direct protein solubilization of defatted hempseed flour demonstrated a good overview of protein content, but less abundant proteins were poorly represented. The Osborne sequential separation was helpful in diluting abundant proteins thus enhancing the method sensitivity.

Keywords: protein extraction; hempseed; seed storage proteins; SDS-PAGE

Citation: Givonetti, A.; Cattaneo, C.; Cavaletto, M. What You Extract Is What You Get: Different Methods of Protein Extraction from Hemp Seeds. *Separations* **2021**, *8*, 231. https://doi.org/10.3390/separations8120231

Academic Editor: Ernesto Reverchon

Received: 25 October 2021
Accepted: 30 November 2021
Published: 2 December 2021

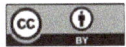
1. Introduction

Cannabis sativa L. is an anemophilous annual plant, one of the oldest cultivable plants in history, and its use is mainly due to the great versatility of this plant. It has been, and still is, used for the production of paper, textile fibres, paints, building products, and also for cosmetics and medicines due to the presence of bioactive compounds. Secondary metabolites, such as phytocannabinoids, as well as proteins and peptides could act as natural antioxidants and can be used in the preparation of food supplements [1–4]. Despite the numerous uses of this plant, its cultivation was banned in the first half of the twenty-first century, due to its widespread use as a recreational drug. Only recently, the cultivation of *Cannabis sativa* with a low THC content has been approved, therefore increasing the diffusion of hemp varieties suitable for the production of fibre and food [5]. If in the recent past hemp seeds were used as animal feed and considered a waste product, recently their properties have been recognized for human nutrition, although their use as a food date back to more than 3000 years ago. Hempseed is considered nutritionally complete, containing 25–35% lipids, 20–25% proteins, 20–30% carbohydrates, mostly represented by fibre, and a valuable source of vitamins and minerals [6]. Hempseed oil is rich in polyunsaturated fatty acids (PUFA), especially linoleic acid (omega-6) and alpha-linolenic acid (omega-3), which are essential for mammals and must be introduced with the diet [4].

The most abundant proteins in seeds are the storage proteins that provide amino acids during the germination of the seed [7]. Based on their solubility properties, seeds storage proteins can be classified into four different classes: albumins include water-soluble proteins; then there is the class of globulins which are salt-soluble proteins; prolamin class groups hydro-alcoholic soluble proteins; and finally, glutelins, which are soluble in alkali or acid solution [8]. The globulin family is divided into two groups based on sedimentation coefficients: 7S, called vicilins, and 11S, called legumins. The main 11S globulin present in hempseed is edestin in its 3 isoforms: edestin 1, edestin 2 and edestin 3, which are composed of subunits of 50 kDa, which are post translationally cleaved to obtain acid (30 kDa) and basic (20–22 kDa) chains, linked by a disulphide bond [9]. Globulins account for 80% of proteins present in hemp seeds, followed by albumins with 13% [10]. Despite being low in lysine, the proteins present in these seeds are easily digestible and rich in many essential amino acids, and have a low amount of anti-nutritional factors, making them suitable for infant and pre-school children nutrition [11,12]. Protein extraction is one of the most critical steps in sample preparation and gel-based proteomic techniques are strongly influenced by the conditions used during this step, with changes in both quantity and quality of the final protein profile and related information regarding protein composition and association. Another critical step of sample preparation is low temperature maintenance to prevent protein degradation by proteases. The use of liquid nitrogen is often the first choice, since it also facilitates the disruption of plant samples while keeping them frozen. However, liquid nitrogen must be handled with care, as it is expensive and not always available in a laboratory, so a low-cost alternative is implemented by sample refrigeration on ice. This latter option does not reach temperatures as low as with liquid nitrogen and a check on the quality of protein extracts is necessary when this condition is applied for the first time to the sample. A large amount of literature on hemp proteins refers to processed hemp seeds, such as hemp protein meal obtained after oil removal, hemp protein isolate resulting from isoelectric protein precipitation, or hemp protein hydrolysates, but few proteomics studies consider hemp seeds in their natural conformation [13,14]. In this study, we aim at filling this gap by comparing different protein extraction methods from hemp seeds in attempt to find which conditions are best-suited to their SDS-PAGE analysis and show higher sustainability.

2. Materials and Methods

2.1. Experimental Design

We tested two conditions to keep low temperatures during seed grinding (liquid nitrogen or ice). The powders were fractionated following the Osborne sequential extraction or directly extracted with three methods to obtain "total" proteins (TCA/acetone, MTBE:MeOH, direct protein solubilization of defatted hempseed flour) and solubilized with two buffers (2D and Laemmli buffer) to optimize a method that is best-suited to the proteomic analysis of hempseed (Figure 1). Three independent sample extractions were performed to test each condition.

2.2. Protein Extraction

Hemp seeds of the variety Finola were kindly provided by ArsUniVCO, an association for the development of culture for university studies and research in the Verbano Cusio Ossola area (Italy). Hemp seed flour was obtained by grinding five grams of frozen seeds with a mortar and pestle. Two conditions for sample maintenance at cold temperatures were tested: seeds grinding in liquid nitrogen or keeping the mortar on ice. Fifty milligrams of powder were aliquoted in 2 mL centrifuge tubes.

Sequential fractions were extracted as indicated in [15] with some modifications. Briefly, hempseed powder was mixed with 1 mL of hexane to delipidate the samples. The tubes were incubated overnight at room temperature keeping the samples stirred at 250 rpm on an orbital shaker (Multi-functional Orbital Shaker PSU-20i, bioSan, Riga, Latvia). The supernatant was removed, and the pellets were dried (Concentrator plus, Eppendorf). The albumin fraction was extracted by adding 0.5 mL of ultrapure water to the pellet; this step was repeated twice. The globulin fraction was obtained extracting the pellet with 0.5 mL of 5% (w/v) NaCl solution. The prolamin fraction was extracted with 0.5 mL of 60% (v/v) ethanol and 2% dithiothreitol (DTT). After this step, the pellets were dried and the glutelin fraction was extracted with a 0.1 M NaOH solution (pH 11–11.5). Each extraction step started by vortex mixing for 5 min and then shaking for 55 min at 4 °C (albumins and globulins) or at room temperature (prolamins and glutelins). The protein extracts were obtained after a centrifuge step (12,000× *g*, 10 min). The supernatant containing the different protein fractions were stored at −20 °C until analysis. After each extraction step, the pellets were washed twice with the previous extraction solution, vortexed 5 min and centrifuged at 12,000× *g* for 10 min.

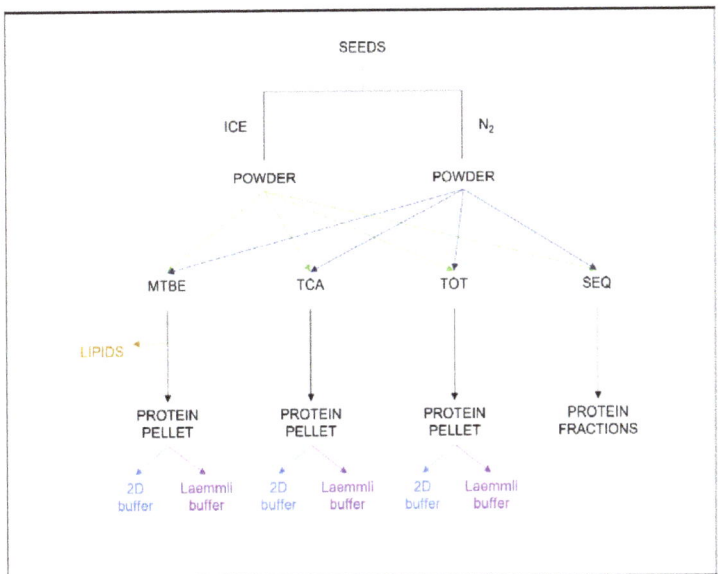

Figure 1. Workflow of experiments. ICE: powder produced by holding the mortar on ice (4 °C), N$_2$: powder produced in the presence of liquid nitrogen. MTBE: total protein extraction after delipidation with MTBE: MeOH; TCA: total protein extraction after precipitation in TCA/acetone; TOT: total protein extraction after delipidation with hexane; SEQ: sequential protein extraction after delipidation with hexane.

TCA/Acetone protein extracts were obtained as indicated in [16]. The hempseed powder was mixed with 1 mL of 10% TCA in cold acetone (−20 °C), 20 mM DTT and 1% protease inhibitors cocktail (P9599, Sigma Aldrich). The homogenate was then incubated overnight at −20 °C to allow protein precipitation. The samples were centrifuged (18,000× *g*, 1 h, 4 °C) and the pellet was washed three times with cold acetone and finally dried. The samples were stored at −20 °C until analysis.

Protein extracts were obtained after methyl tert-butyl ether (MTBE) lipid extraction as indicated in [17]. Briefly, the powder was mixed with 1 mL of MTBE and methanol (MTBE:MeOH 3:1, vol/vol) refrigerated solution. The samples were vortexed for 1 min and then shaken (100 rpm) for 45 min at room temperature. The samples were sonicated for 15 min in an ultrasonic bath, then 0.65 mL of water and methanol (3:1, vol/vol) solution were added to each tube, followed by vortexing for 1 min and centrifuging (20,000× *g*, 5′, 4 °C). We transferred 0.5 mL of the superficial phase containing lipids into new tubes, removed the rest of the lipid phase, and dried the remaining phase. The pellets were stored at −20 °C until analysis.

Total proteins were extracted after hemp seed powder delipidation with 1 mL of hexane. The sample: hexane mixtures were incubated overnight at room temperature under stirring at 250 rpm on an orbital shaker. After hexane removal, the pellet was dried and stored at −20 °C until analysis.

2.3. Solubilization

Protein pellets were solubilized using two different buffers: the first one was a urea containing buffer, often used for 2-D electrophoresis (7 M urea, 2 M thiourea, 4% *w/v* CHAPS, 100 mM DTT, IPG-buffer (pH 3–10)) which we named the "2D buffer". The second one was a Reducing Laemmli buffer (2% *w/v* SDS, 10% glycerol, 5% 2-mercaptoethanol, 62 mM Tris–HCl pH 6.8), named as "LB1X-R". Irrespective of the buffer used, protein solubilization took place at room temperature for 1 h, shaking the samples at 100 rpm on an orbital shaker. The samples were centrifuged ($18,000 \times g$, 10', 4 °C) and the supernatant was transferred to new tubes.

The protein content of samples resulting from sequential extraction and 2D buffer solubilization was estimated using the Bradford assay [18] with bovine serum albumin (BSA) as the protein standard.

2.4. Protein Analysis

Hempseed proteins resulting from different extraction methods were analysed in triplicate by sodium dodecyl sulphate–polyacrylamide gel electrophoresis (SDS-PAGE): 10 μg of protein extracts solubilized in 2D buffer were mixed with Laemmli buffer (2% *w/v* SDS, 10% glycerol, 5% 2-mercaptoethanol, 62 mM Tris–HCl pH 6.8) and 0.6 μL (the same volume loaded for 2D buffer extracts) of protein extracts solubilized in LB1X-R were loaded onto 10 × 8 cm vertical 12% polyacrylamide gels. Protein standards (Precision Plus Protein Dual Color Standards, Biorad) were loaded in order to estimate the apparent molecular weight of proteins.

Due to the low protein content of the prolamin fraction, we dried 50 μL of this fraction in speedvac and solubilized the pellet in 5 μL of LB1X-R. The samples, together with 3 μL of protein standards (Precision Plus Protein Dual Xtra Standards, Biorad) were loaded onto 10 × 8 cm vertical a 15% polyacrylamide gel.

SDS-PAGE was performed at 15 mA for 30 min and 30 mA with a Mini Protean System (BioRad). The running buffer was 25 mM Tris–HCl, 200 mM glycine, 0.1% *w/v* SDS. Gel staining was performed with Colloidal Coomassie brilliant blue G250 and the gel image was acquired by a GS-900 densitometer and image analysis of protein bands was performed by using the software ImageLab (BioRad). Results are presented as mean ± SD of the mean (n = 3). Statistical analysis was performed with RStudio (version 1.3.1093) using one-way ANOVA, followed by Tukey post hoc test, Bonferroni adjustment. *p*-value < 0.05 was considered significant.

3. Results and Discussion

The protein profile of samples obtained with TCA/acetone (TCA), MTBE:methanol (MTBE) and direct protein solubilization of defatted flour (TOT) methods are shown in Figure 2.

Regarding the two cooling methods (ICE vs. N_2), no signs of protein degradation were observed, which could be revealed by an increase in the number of low MW bands. However, ICE extracts show minor bands that are less evident in N_2 extracts. Besides, the ICE method was more efficient than N_2 when combined with TCA/acetone precipitation and LB1X-R solubilization, where the protein profile is almost absent. In fact, after solubilization, these samples had a pH of 3 and needed to be neutralized with NaOH, but this procedure did not provide an efficient protein separation.

Thus, the production of hempseed powder for the purpose of extracting proteins seems to work best on ice.

Considering the same method of powder production and protein extraction, the 2D buffer extracts showed higher molecular weight bands (over 75 kDa) compared to the LB1X-R buffer ones.

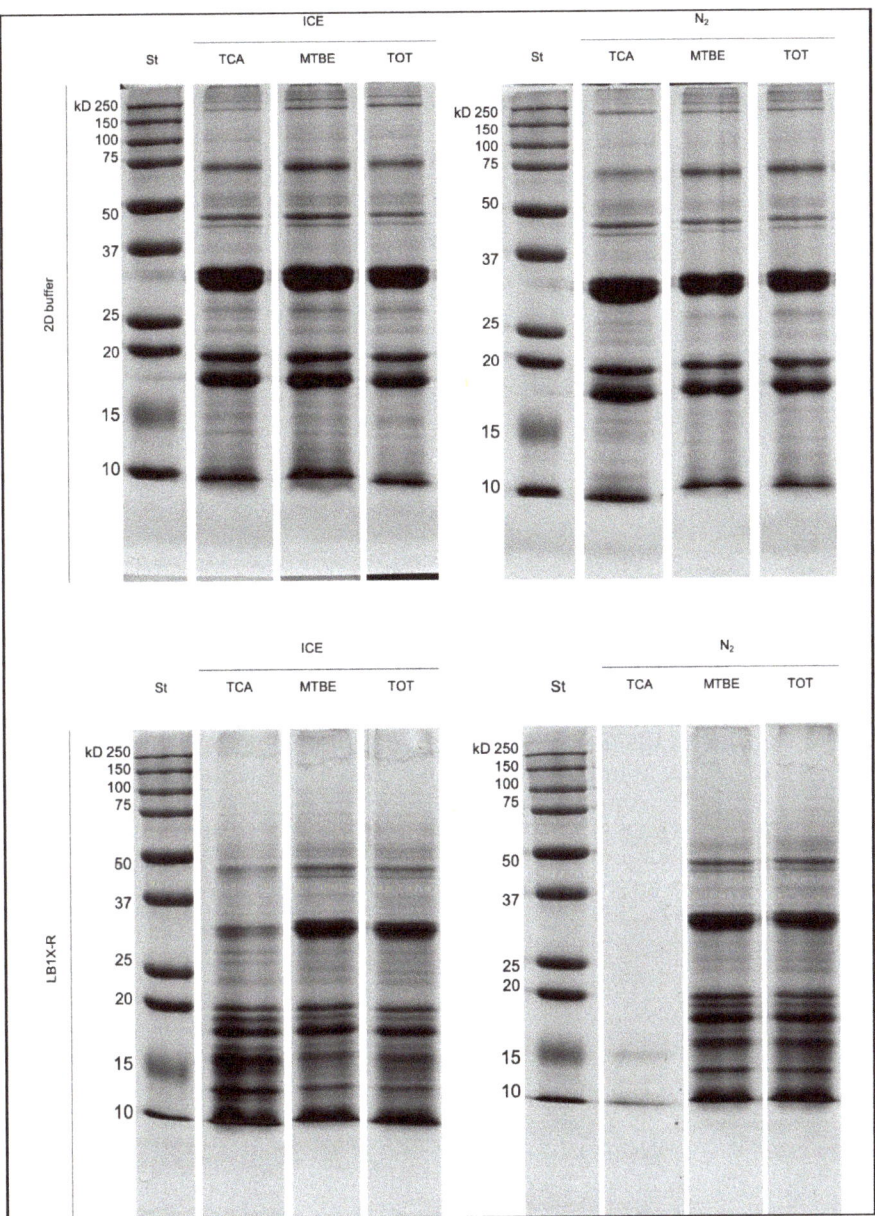

Figure 2. SDS PAGE of ICE + 2D buffer extracts and N$_2$ + 2D buffer extracts, ICE + LB1X-R buffer extracts and N$_2$ + LB1X-R buffer extracts. Three different methods are compared: TCA/Acetone precipitation (TCA), MTBE:MeOH delipidation (MTBE), hexane delipidation (TOT).

The molecular weight bands at about 75 kDa of 2D buffer extracts can be ascribed to edestin 1, vicilin C72-like, heat shock 70 kDa protein-as identified in [4]. The appearance of such bands depending on the solubilizing buffer is in accordance with the observations of Mamone [19], where the presence of edestin at 50 kDa was observed after 2D-electrophoresis under reducing conditions.

On the other hand, the profile of the LB1X-R extracts is similar to that obtained from hemp flour by [19], with highly intense bands at about 30 and 20 kDa, where the acid and basic subunits of the three isoforms of edestin can be identified.

To compare the performance of the methods, image analysis of the bands was conducted, and the optical density (OD) mean and standard deviation, together with statistic parameters, are reported in Supplementary Material 1. The most significant bands, presenting at least 2-fold differences in the OD values, are shown in Figure 3 and here discussed.

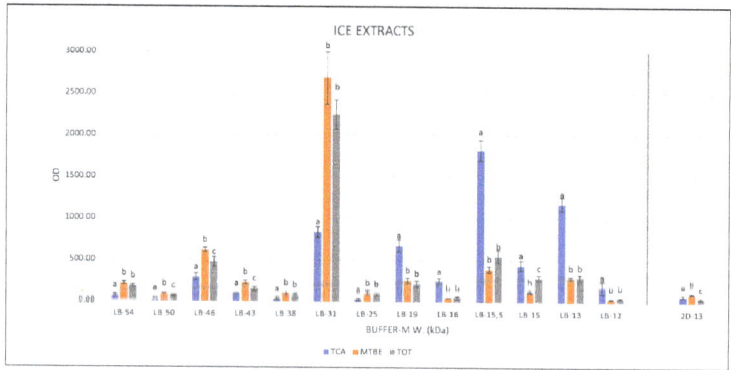

Figure 3. Histogram representing the optical density (mean ± standard deviation), of SDS-PAGE protein bands with at least 2-fold differences among ICE extracts obtained with TCA, MTBE and TOT methods. The grey vertical bar divides LB1X-R (left side) from 2D-buffer solubilized samples (right side). Significant different values (*p*-value < 0.05) are indicated by different letters.

We can observe that the TCA, MTBE and TOT profiles of 2D buffer extracts are quite similar to each other, except for the 13 kDa band observed in ICE-2D extracts, which is less intense in TOT samples.

On the other hand, ICE-TCA-LB1X-R extracts show a decrease in band intensity over 20 kDa and an increase under the same MW compared with the other two methods.

The result of sequential extraction is shown in Figure 4. The pattern of the albumin fraction of N_2 extracts has fewer bands above 100 kDa, between 30–25 and 20–15 kDa when compared with ICE extracts.

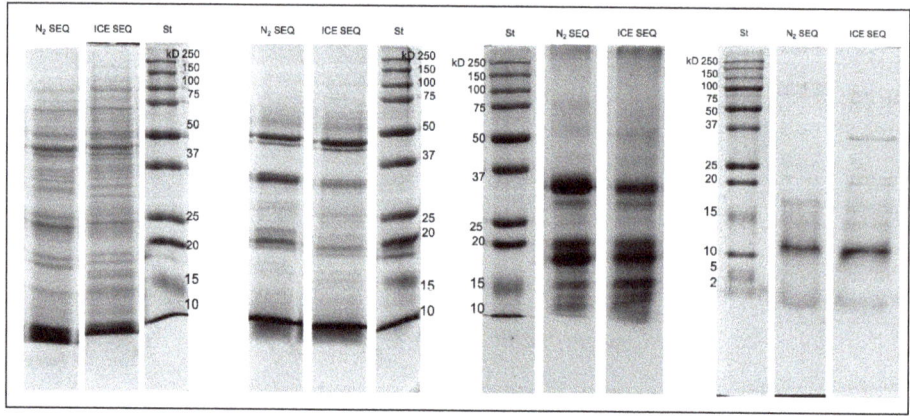

Figure 4. SDS PAGE of different protein fractions, from left to right: N_2 and ICE albumins, N_2 and ICE globulins, N_2 and ICE glutelins. N_2 and ICE prolamins.

The protein pattern of the globulin and glutelin fractions is quite similar in both conditions. The electrophoretic profile of the prolamin fraction of the two samples differs in the distribution of bands above10 kDa: the N_2 extracts have no bands above 18 kDa, while ICE extracts show two bands at about 37 kDa.

Three bands at about 30, 20 and 18 kDa are evident in the glutelin fraction. In this case, the band intensity is higher in N_2 than in ICE extracts. As previously mentioned, in this MW range the acid and basic chains of edestin are usually identified. As found in the literature, the solubility of globulins increases with the increase in pH [20]. Probably, edestin aggregates were more strongly associated after the N_2 treatment and could be efficiently extracted only under alkaline conditions. It is thus evident that the sequential extraction does not uniquely separate the proteins based on their solubility but helps to fractionate the sample to make the proteins present in small quantities that otherwise would not be possible to identify from a total extract more visible. The electrophoretic profile of the prolamin fraction of the two samples differs in the distribution of bands above 10 kDa: the N_2 extracts and have no bands above 18 kDa, while ICE extracts show two bands at about 37 kDa.

4. Conclusions

The ICE method seems to be the one that gives the best results, being simpler and safer and preserving the sample from degradation.

Reducing the Laemmli buffer showed a greater denaturing and reducing action compared to the urea-based buffer. The presence of high MW bands only in 2D-buffer extracts could be a sign of inefficient removal of protein aggregates and needs to be taken into account when performing 2D-electrophoresis. However, 2D-buffer extracts showed minor variability in the OD of bands, giving more reproducible results among the methods tested.

The MTBE method was comparable to the others with the advantage of preserving the lipid fraction for the specific analysis. Moreover, with this method it is possible to obtain a good representation of hempseed proteins using both urea-based and Laemmli solubilization buffers.

TCA/acetone, MTBE/methanol, and direct solubilization of defatted hemp seed flour demonstrated a good overview of protein content, but the detection of less abundant proteins can be enhanced by the use of the Osborne sequential separation.

Supplementary Materials: The following are available online at https://www.mdpi.com/article/10.3390/separations8120231/s1.

Author Contributions: Conceptualization, A.G. and C.C.; methodology, A.G. and C.C.; writing—review and editing, A.G. and C.C.; supervision, M.C. All authors have read and agreed to the published version of the manuscript.

Funding: This research was supported by the University of Piemonte Orientale, grant: bando ateneo ricerca FAR17.

Institutional Review Board Statement: Not applicable.

Informed Consent Statement: Not applicable.

Data Availability Statement: The data can be available upon reasonable request.

Acknowledgments: We thank ArsUniVCO for the recruitment of hemp seeds and Nigel Joyce for proofreading the article.

Conflicts of Interest: The authors declare no conflict of interest.

References

1. Bonini, S.A.; Premoli, M.; Tambaro, S.; Kumar, A.; Maccarinelli, G.; Memo, M.; Mastinu, A. Cannabis sativa: A comprehensive ethnopharmacological review of a medicinal plant with a long history. *J. Ethnopharmacol.* **2018**, *227*, 300–315. [CrossRef]
2. Pavlovic, R.; Panseri, S.; Giupponi, L.; Leoni, V.; Citti, C.; Cattaneo, C.; Cavaletto, M.; Giorgi, A. Phytochemical and Ecological Analysis of Two Varieties of Hemp (*Cannabis sativa* L.) Grown in a Mountain Environment of Italian Alps. *Front. Plant Sci.* **2019**, *10*, 1265. [CrossRef] [PubMed]
3. Tremlová, B.; Mikulášková, H.K.; Hajduchová, K.; Jancikova, S.; Kaczorová, D.; Ćavar Zeljković, S.; Dordevic, D. Influence of Technological Maturity on the Secondary Metabolites of Hemp Concentrate (*Cannabis sativa* L.). *Foods* **2021**, *10*, 1418. [CrossRef] [PubMed]
4. Cattaneo, C.; Givonetti, A.; Leoni, V.; Guerrieri, N.; Manfredi, M.; Giorgi, A.; Cavaletto, M. Biochemical aspects of seeds from *Cannabis sativa* L. plants grown in a mountain environment. *Sci. Rep.* **2021**, *11*, 3927. [CrossRef] [PubMed]
5. Farinon, B.; Molinari, R.; Costantini, L.; Merendino, N. The seed of industrial hemp (*Cannabis sativa* L.): Nutritional Quality and Potential Functionality for Human Health and Nutrition. *Nutrients* **2020**, *12*, 1935. [CrossRef] [PubMed]
6. Callaway, J.C. Hempseed as a nutritional resource: An overview. *Euphytica* **2004**, *140*, 65–72. [CrossRef]
7. Shewry, P.R.; Napier, J.A.; Tatham, A.S. Seed storage proteins: Structure and biosynthesis. *Plant Cell* **1995**, *7*, 945–956. [CrossRef] [PubMed]
8. Osborne, T.B. *The Vegetable Proteins*; Longmans: London, UK, 1924.
9. Shewry, P.R. The Protein Chemistry of Dicotyledonous Grains. In *Encyclopedia of Grain Science*; Walker, C., Wrigley, C., Corke, H., Eds.; Elsevier Academic Press: Amsterdam, The Netherlands, 2004; pp. 466–472.
10. Wang, X.S.; Tang, C.H.; Yang, X.Q.; Gao, W.R. Characterization, amino acid composition and in vitro digestibility of hemp (*Cannabis sativa* L.) proteins. *Food Chem.* **2008**, *107*, 11–18. [CrossRef]
11. Tang, C.H.; Ten, Z.; Wang, X.S.; Yang, X.Q. Physicochemical and functional properties of hemp (*Cannabis sativa* L.) protein isolate. *J. Agric. Food Chem.* **2006**, *54*, 8945–8950. [CrossRef] [PubMed]
12. Arbach, C.T.; Alves, I.A.; Serafini, M.R.; Stephani, R.; Perrone, Í.T.; de Carvalho da Costa, J. Recent patent applications in beverages enriched with plant proteins. *NPJ Sci. Food* **2021**, *5*, 28. [CrossRef] [PubMed]
13. Park, S.K.; Seo, J.B.; Lee, M.Y. Proteomic profiling of hempseed proteins from Cheungsam. *Biochim. Biophys. Acta* **2012**, *1824*, 374–382. [CrossRef] [PubMed]
14. Aiello, G.; Fasoli, E.; Boschin, G.; Lammi, C.; Zanoni, C.; Citterio, A.; Arnoldi, A. Proteomic characterization of hempseed (*Cannabis sativa* L.). *J. Proteom.* **2016**, *147*, 187–196. [CrossRef] [PubMed]
15. Dai, H.; Zhang, X.Q.; Harasymow, S.; Roumeliotis, S.; Broughton, S.; Eglinton, J.; Wu, F.; Li, C. MALDI-TOF mass spectrometry provides an efficient approach to monitoring protein modification in the malting process. *Int. J. Mass Spectrom.* **2014**, *371*, 8–16. [CrossRef]
16. Méchin, V.; Damerval, C.; Zivy, M. Total protein extraction with TCA-acetone. *Methods Mol. Biol.* **2007**, *355*, 1–8. [CrossRef] [PubMed]
17. Salem, M.; Bernach, M.; Bajdzienko, K.; Giavalisco, P. A Simple Fractionated Extraction Method for the Comprehensive Analysis of Metabolites, Lipids, and Proteins from a Single Sample. *J. Vis. Exp.* **2017**, *124*, 55802. [CrossRef] [PubMed]
18. Bradford, M. A rapid and sensitive method for the quantitation of microgram quantities of protein utilizing the principle of protein-dye binding. *Anal. Biochem.* **1976**, *72*, 248–254. [CrossRef]
19. Mamone, G.; Picariello, G.; Ramondo, A.; Nicolai, M.A.; Ferranti, P. Production, digestibility and allergenicity of hemp (*Cannabis sativa* L.) protein isolates. *Food Res. Int.* **2019**, *115*, 562–571. [CrossRef] [PubMed]
20. Potin, F.; Lubbers, S.; Husson, F.; Saurel, R. Hemp (*Cannabis sativa* L.) Protein Extraction Conditions Affect Extraction Yield and Protein Quality. *J. Food Sci.* **2019**, *84*, 3682–3690. [CrossRef] [PubMed]

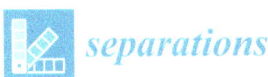

separations

Article

Immunomodulatory Activity of *Phyllanthus maderaspatensis* in LPS-Stimulated Mouse Macrophage RAW 264.7 Cells

Uoorakkottil Ilyas [1], Deepshikha P. Katare [2], Punnoth Poonkuzhi Naseef [3,*], Mohamed Saheer Kuruniyan [4], Muhammed Elayadeth-Meethal [5] and Vidhu Aeri [6,*]

[1] Department of Pharmacognosy and Phytochemistry, Moulana College of Pharmacy, Perinthalmanna 679321, Kerala, India; ukhamdard@gmail.com
[2] Department of Pharmaceutical Biotechnology, Faculty of Pharmacy, Amity University, Noida 201301, India; ukponkkala@gmail.com
[3] Department of Pharmaceutics, Moulana College of Pharmacy, Perinthalmanna 679321, Kerala, India
[4] Department of Dental Technology, College of Applied Medical Sciences, King Khalid University, Abha 61421, Saudi Arabia; mkurunian@kku.edu.sa
[5] Department of Animal Breeding and Genetics, College of Veterinary and Animal Sciences, Kerala Veterinary and Animal Sciences University, Pookode, Wayanad 673576, Kerala, India; muhammed@kvasu.ac.in
[6] Department of Pharmacognosy and Phytochemistry, Faculty of Pharmacy, Jamia Hamdard University, New Delhi 110062, India
* Correspondence: drnaseefpp@gmail.com (P.P.N.); aerividhu@yahoo.com (V.A.)

Citation: Ilyas, U.; Katare, D.P.; Naseef, P.P.; Kuruniyan, M.S.; Elayadeth-Meethal, M.; Aeri, V. Immunomodulatory Activity of *Phyllanthus maderaspatensis* in LPS-Stimulated Mouse Macrophage RAW 264.7 Cells. *Separations* **2021**, *8*, 129. https://doi.org/10.3390/separations8090129

Academic Editor: Ernesto Reverchon

Received: 2 August 2021
Accepted: 17 August 2021
Published: 24 August 2021

Publisher's Note: MDPI stays neutral with regard to jurisdictional claims in published maps and institutional affiliations.

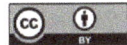
Abstract: *Phyllanthus* species (Family Euphorbiaceae) has been used in traditional medicine of several countries as a cure for numerous diseases, including jaundice and hepatitis. This study is an attempt to evaluate the immunomodulatory activity of various fractions, column eluents of ethyl acetate fraction, and their polyphenols. *Phyllanthus maderaspatensis* were standardized using high-performance liquid chromatography to identify and quantify polyphenols, and purification of polyphenols was carried out using vacuum liquid chromatography. Subsequently, we tested various fractions, column eluents of ethyl acetate fraction, and polyphenols in vitro to assess their impact on nitric oxide (NO) production in LPS-stimulated mouse macrophage RAW 264.7 cells. The ethyl acetate fraction (100 µg mL^{-1}) had a more significant stimulatory effect on LPS-stimulated NO production by the RAW 264.7 cells. We found that the ethyl acetate fraction contains a high amount of catechin, quercetin, ellagic acid kaempferol, and rutin, which are responsible for immunomodulation. The ethyl acetate fraction at concentrations of 25 and 50 µg mL^{-1} had a significant inhibitory effect and 100 µg mL^{-1} had a more significant stimulatory effect when compared with the LPS control. The percentage of inhibition by LPS control ranged from zero percentage, kaempferol ranged from 45.4% at 50 µg mL^{-1} to 41.88% at 100 µg mL^{-1}, catechin ranged from 50% at 50 µg mL^{-1} to 35.28% at 100 µg mL^{-1}, rutin ranged from 36.2% at 50 µg mL^{-1} to 47.44% at 100 µg mL^{-1}, gallic acid ranged from 28.4% at 50 µg mL^{-1} to 50.9% at 100 µg mL^{-1}, ellagic acid ranged from 45.12% at 50 µg mL^{-1} to 38.64% at 100 µg mL^{-1}, and purified quercetin ranged from 26.2% at 50 µg mL^{-1} to 45.48% at 100 µg mL^{-1}. As NO plays an important role in the immune function, polyphenols' treatment could modulate several aspects of host defense mechanisms owing to the stimulation of the inducible nitric oxide synthase.

Keywords: extraction; fractionation; active principles; *Phyllanthus maderaspatensis*; polyphenols; vacuum liquid chromatography; HPTLC; LPS; immunomodulation

1. Introduction

Phyllanthus maderaspatensis, belonging to the genus *Phyllanthus* (Euphorbiaceae), is widely distributed in Sri Lanka, South Africa, China, and southern India. In India, the whole plant is used against kidney and urinary tract infections, digestive disorders, hepatitis, and diabetes. In Tanzania, the whole plant is used as a topical application for scabies.

A root decoction has been indicated to cure constipation, gastrointestinal disorders, menstrual problems, intestinal pain and diarrhea, lack of appetite, testicular swelling, chest complaints, and snakebites. Leaves are mixed with lemon juice and applied to the skin for the treatment of rheumatics. The plant is used for a variety of ailments including smallpox, syphilis, asthma, and bleeding gums, as well as in various biological activities such as chronic hepatitis B infection [1], antihepatotoxic and choleretic activities [2], adulticidal and larvicidal efficacy [3], antidiabetic activity [4], hepatoprotective and antioxidant activity [5], anti-Epstein–Barr virus [6], antiretroviral reverse transcriptase [7], and antiherpes simplex virus type 1 and type [8]. Compounds with immunomodulatory activities like flavonoids, fatty acids, triterpenes, and polysaccharides are found in many plants [9]. *Phyllanthus* genus was found to be rich in polyphenols, lignans, flavonoids, triterpenes, hydrolysable tannins, sterol, and alkaloids [10]. Nowadays, HPTLC is used instead of HPLC owing to the easiness, specificity, speed, and low cost [11].

Chronic inflammation has been concerned with various steps involved in tumorigenesis, including metastasis, cellular transformation, promotion, survival, invasion proliferation, and angiogenesis. Only a minority of all tumors are caused by germline mutation, whereas approximately 90% are linked to environmental and somatic mutation factors. Many environmental causes of tumors and risk factors are associated with some form of chronic inflammation [12]. Throughout, chronic inflammation acts as an associate accommodative multitude resistance against illness or injury and is primarily a self-limiting methodology; inadequate resolution of inflammatory responses typically ends up in numerous chronic ailments such as AIDS and cancer [13,14]. At the time of infection, the immune system goes under the attack of a large number of viruses, bacteria, and fungi [15]. The immune system is a part of the body that detects the pathogen using a specific receptor to produce an immediate response by the activation of immune components' cells, chemokines, and cytokines, as well as release inflammatory mediators [16,17]. The immune system can be manipulated by the use of immunomodulators in disease conditions by achieving immunostimulation (as in the treatment of coronavirus, cancer, and AIDS) or immunosuppression (suppression of normal or excessive immune function (e.g., the treatment of graft rejection or autoimmune disease)) [18,19]. Nitric oxide (NO) is a highly reactive and diffusible gas molecule that exerts many biological effects, which include iron homeostasis, smooth muscle relaxation, platelet reactivity, neurotransmission, and cytotoxic defense mechanism against pathogens [20]. NO is also involved in the pathogenesis of many human pathological conditions such as inflammatory disease, cancer, and neurodegenerative disorders [21]. Nitric oxide acts through the stimulation of the soluble guanyl cyclase; is expressed in the cytoplasm of almost all mammalian cells; and mediates a wide range of important physiological functions such as immunomodulation, inhibition of platelet aggregation, vasodilation, and neuronal signal transduction. Nitric oxide is also generated by phagocytes (neutrophils, monocyte, and macrophages) as part of the human immune response [22]. Phagocytes are formed with inducible nitric oxide synthase (iNOS), which is activated by interferon-gamma (IFN-γ) as a single signal or by tumor necrosis factor (TNF) along with a second signal. In this way, the immune system may regulate the armamentarium of phagocytes that play a role in inflammation and immune responses [23]. Lipopolysaccharide (LPS) is widely reported as a major inducer for the production of inflammatory cytokines, which in turn stimulate iNOS induction during the inflammatory process in RAW 264.7 cells macrophages [24]. These cytokines can be formed from macrophages in response to bacterial LPS, inflammatory stimulation, and infection. They also play an important role in the immune system by aiding cytostatic and cytotoxic effects on malignant or infected cells [25].

2. Materials and Methods

2.1. Reagents and Apparatus

We purchased reference standards for quercetin rutin, ellagic acid, catechin, and kaempferol from Natural Remedies Pvt. Ltd. (Bangalore, India). All chemicals used were of analytical grade, including mouse macrophage RAW 264.7 cells (National Centre for Cell Science (NCCS), Pune, India, Dulbecco's modified Eagle's medium (DMEM), fetal bovine serum (FBS) and MTT assay kit, trypsin EDTA, penicillin and streptomycin and DMSO (Sigma-Aldrich Co. LLC, St. Louis, MO, USA), Trypan blue solution, galactosamine, and absolute ethanol (Himedia Lab Pvt. Ltd., Mumbai, India). Tissue culture flasks, 96- and 24-well micro-culture plates, Eppendorf tube, inverted microscope, serological pipette, heamocytometer (Himedia Lab Pvt. Ltd., Mumbai, India), laminar flow hoods (Khera instrument, New Delhi, India), CO_2 incubator (NuAire, Plymouth, MA, USA), water bath, deep freezer ($-20\,^{\circ}C$) were used.

2.2. Collection of Plant Material

The fresh whole plant was collected from the Kanyakumari district of Tamil Nadu state in India. Dr. R.P Pandey, Plant taxonomist of Tropical Botanical Garden and Research Institute (TBGRI), Trivandrum, India, identified and authenticated the specimen. A voucher specimen was placed at the herbarium of TBGRI (TBGRI 65616 dated 24 December 2010) for future reference.

2.3. Extraction of Plant Materials
2.3.1. Preparation of Aqueous Ethanolic Extract

We extracted dried powdered plant material using aqueous ethanolic solvent (50%, for 6 h at 37 $^{\circ}C$), then pooled the hydroalcoholic extract, and it dried under reduced pressure at 40 $^{\circ}C$ with a rotator evaporator. For hydroalcoholic extracts, the percentage yields of the crude extracts were 15.58% w/w.

2.3.2. Standardization of Polyphenols in *P. maderaspatensis* by HPTLC

Standard solutions of ellagic acid, gallic acid, catechin, quercetin, rutin, and kaempferol were applied in triplicate on silica gel 60 F_{254} plates, using a CAMMAG Linomat-5 Automatic Sample Spotter. The plates were developed in a solvent system, toluene/ethyl acetate/formic acid/methanol (3:3:0.8:0.2 v/v) in a CAMAG glass twin trough chamber (20 × 10 cm) up to a distance of 8 cm, dried in the air, and scanned at 254 nm. The developed plates were dried in the air and scanned at 254 nm using CAMAG TLC scanner 3 and win CATS 4 software. The peak areas were recorded. Calibration curves of ellagic acid, gallic acid, catechin, quercetin, rutin, and kaempferol were obtained by plotting peak areas versus applied crude extracts, and the concentration of ellagic acid, gallic acid, catechin, quercetin rutin, and kaempferol was calculated, respectively.

2.3.3. Estimation of Different Markers

Each sample solution (10 µL) was applied in triplicate on silica gel 60 F_{254} plates with CAMAG Linomat-5 Automatic Sample Spotter and the peak areas and absorption spectra were recorded. We calculated the number of bioactive compounds in *P. maderaspatensis* using the peak areas and the absorption spectra were recorded. The number of bioactive compounds in *P. maderaspatensis* was calculated using the respective standard calibration curves of ellagic acid, gallic acid, catechin, quercetin, rutin, and kaempferol.

2.3.4. Fractionation of Potent Aqueous Ethanolic (50% v/v) Extracts of *P. maderaspatensis*

The aqueous ethanolic extract of *P. maderaspatensis* was dissolved in 10% distilled water and was successively fractionated thrice with hexane (3 × 600 mL), chloroform (3 × 600 mL), ethyl acetate (3 × 500 mL), and water-soluble fractions. The combined fractions of *P. maderaspatensis* were evaporated to dryness under reduced pressure at 40 $^{\circ}C$ in a rotary evaporator.

2.3.5. Nitric Oxide Estimation of Various Fractions of *P. maderaspatensis*

Nitric oxide was measured as nitrite released from mouse macrophage cells, RAW 264.7. Cells were suspended in DMEM (Sigma) supplemented with 10% FCS, seeded in a

96-well culture dish at a density of 1×10^6 cells/well, and incubated for 48 h at 37 °C in an atmospheric of 5% CO_2 and 95% humidity. After incubation, 100 µL of the medium was transferred from the surface of the cultures of each well and replenished with the same amount of fresh medium. Further incubation for 24 h was done with concentrations of 25, 50, and 100 µg mL^{-1} of alcoholic and aqueous-alcoholic (50% v/v) extracts/metabolites (100 and 200 µg mL^{-1}) of *P. maderaspatensis* in the presence or absence of the indicated amount of LPS (10 µg mL^{-1}). Nitric oxide production was estimated in terms of the amount of nitrite. After incubation, 100 µL from the surface of the cultures was transferred into a new plate and the equivalent amount of Griess reagent was added (1% sulfanilamide in 5% phosphoric acid, 0.1% N-(1-naphthyl)-ethylenediamine dihydrochloride in 5% phosphoric acid). This plate was incubated for 10 min at room temperature and measured by an ELISA reader at 570nm. NO concentration was determined using a standard curve plotted using a known quantity of sodium nitrite. The outcome is obtainable in µM concentration obtained from the mean OD of triplicate wells of each group.

The percentage of NO inhibition/stimulation by the extracts was calculated as follows:

$$\% \text{ inhibition} = 100 \times [([NO_2^-] \text{ control} - [NO_2^-] \text{ sample})/[NO_2^-] \text{ control}]$$

2.3.6. Isolation and Purification of Potent Fractions by Vacuum Liquid Chromatography

The air-dried whole plant of *P. maderaspatensis* was coarsely powdered, defatted with extraction procedure thrice. Using a rotary evaporator, the aqueous ethanolic extracts were pooled and dried at 40 °C under reduced pressure. The crude extracts of *P. maderaspatensis* were successively fractionated thrice with chloroform, ethyl acetate, and water. Ethyl acetate fraction was found to have significant immunomodulatory and hepatoprotective activity compared with other fractions. Hence, this fraction was subjected to vacuum liquid chromatography to separate various components present in the fraction. An amount of 16 gm of ethyl acetate fraction was mixed with a small amount of Silica gel G (Merck) to form a dry slurry, which was then loaded onto a sintered glass funnel filled with silica gel gas stationary phase. The column was eluted stepwise under vacuum with solvents of accelerating polarity, starting from pure toluene, and ethyl acetate mixture, to pure ethyl acetate. To elaborate, after initially eluting with 5% ethyl acetate in toluene, the ethyl acetate portion was increased by 5% increments up to 50% and then in 10% increments up to 100% ethyl acetate with a concomitant decrease in the toluene levels. After elution with ethyl acetate, elution with 5% methanol in ethyl acetate, the methanol portion was increased by 5% increments up to 100% methanol. The solvents were eluted until they ran clear of the funnel. The flow rate of solvent was monitored constantly (100 mL/min) throughout the experiment. Various fractions were collected individually and monitored by TLC to match homogeneity. Similar fractions having the same R_f values were combined and crystallized.

2.3.7. Statistical Analysis

Statistical analysis was performed using Dunnett's multiple comparison tests and one-way analysis of variance (ANOVA) using Graphpad prism 5.0 (Graphpad Software, Inc., San Diego, CA, USA). The level of significance was set at $p < 0.05$.

2.3.8. Maintenance of Cell Lines

HepG2 cell lines were grown in 25 cm^2 tissue culture flasks containing minimum essential medium (MEM) supplemented with 10% FBS and 1% penicillin/streptomycin at 37 °C in a CO_2 incubator in an atmosphere of humidified 5% CO_2 and 95% air. The cells were maintained by routine sub-culturing in 25 cm^2 tissue culture flasks.

2.3.9. Method for Passaging the Cells

All the reagents were brought to room temperature before use. Media was removed from the 80–90% confluent flasks by a 10 mL serological pipette. Cells in the T-75 flask were washed with 10 mL of PBS. Two milliliters of 0.1% trypsin EDTA was added to the flask.

The flask was kept at 37 °C in the CO_2 incubator for 2–3 min and was observed under a microscope for detachment. Six milliliters of growth medium were added to the flask for inhibition of trypsin action and re-suspended properly by pipetting. The cell suspension was collected in a 15 mL falcon tube and then centrifuged at 1200 rpm for 3 min. The supernatant was discarded and the pellet was resuspended in 3 mL of complete medium. Cells were counted, and then 0.2–0.4 million cells were kept in a T-25 flask for growing. The flasks were incubated in a CO_2 incubator at 37 °C and the cells were periodically monitored for any morphological changes and contamination. After the formation of an 80–90% confluent monolayer, the cells were further utilized.

2.3.10. Calibration Curves for Standard Markers

Standard solutions of kaempferol, rutin, ellagic acid, catechin, and quercetin were applied in triplicate on silica gel 60 F_{254} plates, using a CAMMAG Linomat-5 Automatic Sample Spotter. The plates were developed in a solvent system, toluene/ethyl acetate/formic acid/methanol (3:3:0.8:0.2 *v/v*) in a CAMAG glass twin trough chamber (20 × 10 cm) up to a space of 8 cm. Further, the developed plates were dried and scanned at 254 nm using CAMAG TLC scanner 3 and win CATS 4 software. The peak areas were recorded. The quantification of polyphenols was carried out based on peak area with a linear calibration curve at concentration ranges of 40–200, 100–1600, 20–200, 200–1400, and 10–160 ng/band of kaempferol, rutin, ellagic acid, catechin, and quercetin, respectively. Calibration curves of polyphenols were obtained by plotting peak areas versus applied crude extracts, and the concentrations of kaempferol, rutin, ellagic acid, catechin, and quercetin were calculated, respectively.

3. Results

3.1. Percentage Yield of the Different Crude Extracts of P. maderaspatensis

We found that the yield of aqueous extract, crude ethanolic extract, and aqueous ethanolic extract was 13.7 ± 1.9% *w/w*, 15.18 ± 0.19% *w/w*, and 15.58 ± 0.45% *w/w*, respectively.

3.2. HPTLC Fingerprint Profile of Aqueous Ethanolic Extracts of P. maderaspatensis
Development of Optimum Mobile Phase

Chromatographic separation studies were carried out on the working standard solution of polyphenols' compounds (1 mg mL^{-1}) in methanol. Initially, various trials were carried out with different solvent systems. Finally, toluene/ethyl acetate/formic acid/methanol (3:3:0.8:0.2) was used for simultaneous determination of ellagic acid, gallic acid, catechin, rutin, kaempferol, and quercetin, showing a sharp and well-defined peak. At room temperature, we obtained well-defined bands upon saturating the chamber with the mobile phase for 30 min. The standard band of ellagic acid, gallic acid, catechin, quercetin, rutin, and kaempferol, along with ethanolic, aqueous ethanolic, and aqueous extracts of *P. maderaspatensis* separated on HPTLC plate, were scanned at 254 nm (Figure 1).

3.3. Fractionation of Aqueous Ethanolic Extract of P. maderaspatensis

Fractionation of the most potent aqueous ethanolic extract into hexane soluble, ethyl acetate sediment, ethyl acetate soluble, chloroform sediment, chloroform soluble, methanol, and water-soluble fractions was carried out. These fractions were studied for their TLC pattern using the above-mentioned solvent systems. The data regarding the number of spots and their resolution are given in Table 1.

The solvent system no.7 indicated the best separation of polyphenols in the ethyl acetate fraction. Except for the ethyl acetate fraction, none of the other fractions indicated the presence of selected polyphenols. Other fractions were discarded. The ethyl acetate fraction was selected for vacuum liquid chromatography.

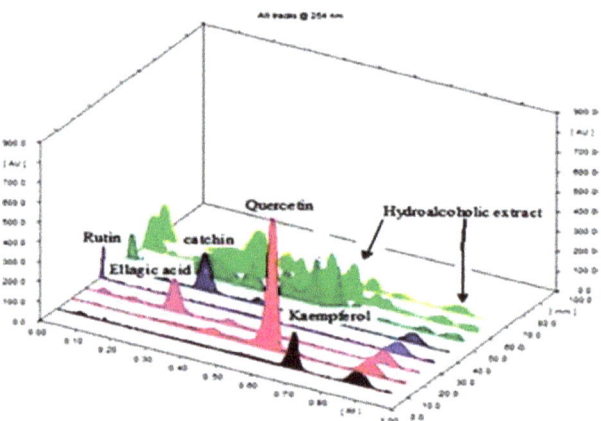

Figure 1. Simultaneous HPTLC profile of hydroethanolic extracts of *P. maderaspatensis* with different markers in the solvent system: toluene/ethyl acetate/formic acid/methanol (3:3:0.08:0.02) (*v/v*) at 254 nm.

Table 1. TLC analysis of ethyl acetate fraction using different solvent systems and visualising agents.

Sl. No.	Solvent System	Visualizing Agents	Inference
01	Hexane/ethyl acetate (7:3)	Anisaldehyde sulphuric acid	Poor separation
02	Ethyl acetate/chloroform (40:60)	Anisaldehyde sulphuric acid	Poor separation
03	Ethyl acetate/methanol/water (100:13.5:10)	Anisaldehyde sulphuric acid	Poor separation
04	Ethyl acetate/formic acid/acetic acid/water (100:11:11:27)	Anisaldehyde sulphuric acid	Tailing
05	n-propanol/ethyl acetate/water (40:40:30)	Anisaldehyde sulphuric acid	Tailing
06	Toluene/ethyl acetate/formic acid (5:4:1)	NP reagents	Good separation
07	Toluene/ethyl acetate/formic acid/methanol (3:3:0.8:0.02)	NP reagents	Best separation

3.4. Stimulation of Inducible NO Synthesis by the Different Fractions of P. maderaspatensis

Ethyl acetate, chloroform, hexane, and water soluble fractions, along with sediment of chloroform and ethyl acetate, were then screened at different concentrations (25, 50, and 100 µg mL^{-1}) for invitro immunomodulatory activity using the nitric oxide assay method. Hexane, chloroform, and sediment between chloroform and water-soluble fractions had no significant effect on LPS-stimulated NO production by the RAW 264.7 cells, while chloroform sediment (25 µg mL^{-1}) and ethyl acetate fraction at concentrations of 25 and 50 µg mL^{-1} had a significant inhibitory effect on LPS-stimulated NO production when compared with LPS control. The ethyl acetate fraction and chloroform fraction (100 µg mL^{-1}) had a more significant stimulatory effect on LPS-stimulated NO production by the RAW 264.7 cells, as represented in Table 2 and Figure 2.

Table 2. Effect of *P. maderaspatensis* fractions on NO production in LPS-stimulated RAW 264.7cells.

Dose	Control	LPS	Hexane	Chloroform	Chloroform Std.	Ethyl Acetate	Std b/w chl3: aq.
-	1.3 ± 0.6	25.77 ± 1.4					
LPS + 25 µg mL^{-1}	-	-	25.9 ± 0.6	27.03 ± 1.4	15.96 ± 2.5	10.97 ± 2.1	22.99 ± 2.6
LPS + 50 µg mL^{-1}	-	-	25.56 ± 1.4	25.43 ± 1.3	33.45 ± 2.34	15.76 ± 2.9	26.62 ± 1.9
LPS + 100 µg mL^{-1}	-	-	25.19 ± 1.6	23.33 ± 2.0	35.92 ± 1.6	37.17 ± 1.3	29.25 ± 1.74

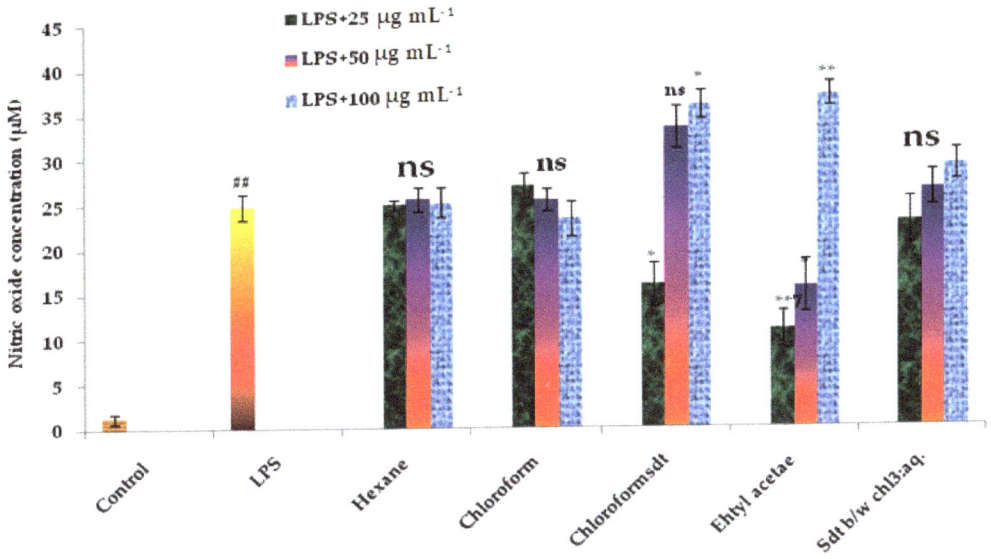

Figure 2. Effect of various fractions based on polarity on LPS-stimulated RAW 264.7 cells. Cells in 96-well plates (1×106 cells/well) were first incubated with and without specified concentrations of crude extracts for 2 h, and then incubated with LPS ($10 \, \mu g \, mL^{-1}$) for 20 h. ## LPS treated. Untreated is the negative control without LPS treatment. Each value was expressed as mean $\pm$ SEM in the triplicate experiment. ns: non-significant, $n = 3$, data $\pm$ S.E.M. Groups 3–7 were compared against group II using Dunnett's post-hoc test (* significant at < 0.01; ** significant at < 0.001).

3.5. Vacuum Liquid Chromatography and Selected Activity of Column Eluents of Ethyl Acetate Fraction

Fourteen column eluents were obtained from the column chromatography of the ethyl acetate fraction of *P. maderaspatensis*. These column eluents were subjected to the HPTLC profile. Different components present in the eluents were identified by spraying with NP reagent and subsequently matching the R_f value with the standards (1–6). The detailed HPTLC profile of each fraction is represented in Table 3.

The standards (1–6) were identified as follows: ellagic acid (R_f value: 0.55) standard was matched with track no. 19 (100% ethyl acetate elutes), eupalitin(R_f value: 0.23) standard was not matched with any track, kaempferol (R_f value: 0.81) standard was matched with track no. 8 (25% ethyl acetate in toluene elutes), rutin (R_f value: 0.08) standard was matched with track no. 13 (50% ethyl acetate in toluene 3rd elutes), epicatechin (R_f value: 0.50) standard was matched with track no. 28 (75% ethyl acetate in toluene elutes), epicatechin (R_f value: 0.50) standard was matched with track no. 15 (75% ethyl acetate in toluene elutes), and catechin (R_f value: 0.54) standard was matched with track no. 15 (75% ethyl acetate in toluene elutes).

3.6. Effect of Column Eluents of Ethyl Acetate Fraction on LPS-Stimulated NO Production in RAW 264.7 Cells

The effect of nine column eluents of ethyl acetate fractions on NO production was determined by treating the RAW cell of LPS stimulation/inhibition by pre-incubating the cells with or without the elutes. LPS significantly increased NO production in RAW 264.7 cells. The levels of NO production induced by LPS-stimulated were significant (** $p < 0.01$) in a dose-dependent manner when treated with concentrations of 25 and 50 $\mu g \, mL^{-1}$ of each elute and significantly stimulated by column eluents of ethyl acetate fractions. NO production was 25 and 50 $\mu g \, mL^{-1}$ of column eluents of ethyl acetate fractions of *P. maderaspatensis* compared with LPS treatment alone. In this study, a comparison of column elutes of ethyl acetate fractions was carried out in mouse monocyte cell lines RAW 264.7 cells, as shown in Figure 3.

Table 3. HPTLC analyses of column eluent of ethyl acetate fractions of *P. maderaspatensis* using VLC.

Tracks	Solvent Combination	Rf Values	Tracks	Solvent Combination	Rf Values
01	Ellagic acid	0.55	11	Toluene + 50% ethyl acetate-1	0.48, 0.48, 0.52, 0.72, 0.78
02	eupalitin	0.23	12	Toluene + 50% ethyl acetate-2	0.27, 0.48
03	Rutin	0.08	13	Toluene + 50% ethyl acetate-3	0.08, 0.12, 0.18, 0.26, 0.36, 0.42, 0.51, 0.60, 0.67
04	Kaempferol	0.81	14	Toluene + 50% ethyl acetate-4	0.08, 0.16, 0.26, 0.56, 0.62, 0.70, 0.87
05	Epicatechin	0.50	15	Toluene + 75% ethyl acetate-1	0.17, 0.27, 0.34, 0.50, 0.54, 0.75
06	Catechin	0.54	16	Toluene + 75% ethyl acetate-2	0.17, 0.27, 0.35, 0.46, 0.54
07	Toluene + 25% ethyl acetate-1	0.76, 0.81	17	Toluene + 75% ethyl acetate-3	0.17, 0.27, 0.35, 0.46, 0.55, 0.68, 0.75
08	Toluene + 25% ethyl acetate-2	0.25, 0.34, 0.48, 0.59, 0.64, 0.7, 0.81, 0.90	18	Toluene + 75% ethyl acetate-4	0.05, 0.17, 0.27, 0.35, 0.46, 0.55
09	Toluene + 25% ethyl acetate-3	0.58, 0.68, 0.72	19	100% ethyl acetate	0.08, 0.55
10	Toluene + 25% ethyl acetate-4	0.48	20	50% ethyl acetate remain	0.25, 0.08

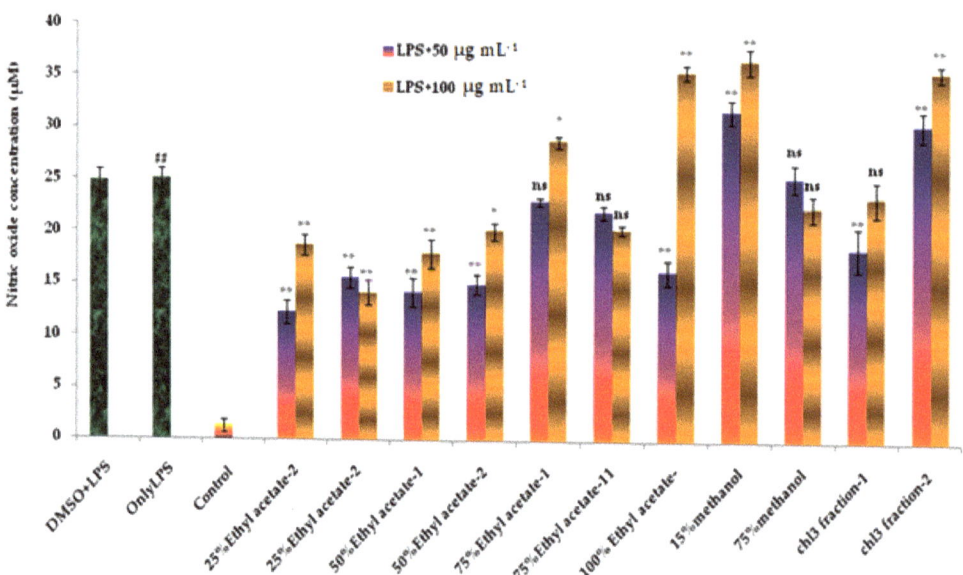

Figure 3. Effect of column eluents of ethyl acetate fractions on NO levels in LPS-stimulated RAW 264.7 cells. Cells (1×106 cells/well) in 96-well plates were first incubated with and without specified concentrations of column eluents for 2 h, and then incubated with LPS (10 µg/mL) for 20 h. ## LPS treated. Untreated is the negative control without LPS treatments. Values are expressed as mean ±SEM. ns: non-significant, $n = 3$, data ± S.E.M. Groups 3–7 were compared against group II using Dunnett's post-hoc test (* significant at < 0.01; ** significant at < 0.001).

3.7. Stimulation of Inducible NO Synthesis by Compounds

The significant suppressive effect by concentration at 50 µg mL^{-1} and 100 µg mL^{-1} of rutin, kaempferol, gallic acid, and ursolic acid; the minimum concentration of ellagic acid (50 µg mL^{-1}); and the more significant stimulatory effect of oleanolic acid, ellagic acid, and quercetin in LPS stimulated NO production by the RAW 264.7 cells were observed (Figure 4).

The compounds indicated significant invitro immunomodulation: ellagic acid > quercetin > oleanolic acid and immunosuppressive effect: kaempferol > catechin > rutin > gallic acid > ellagic acid (50 µg mL^{-1}), when compared with LPS.

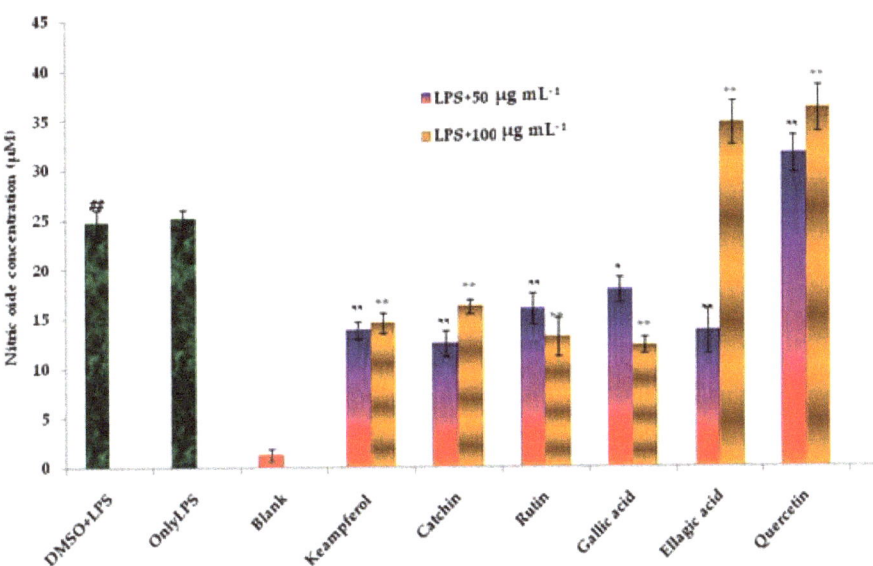

Figure 4. Effect of polyphenols on NO levels in LPS-stimulated RAW 264.7 cells. Cells (2×10^4 cells /well) in 96-well plates were first incubated with and without indicated concentrations of polyphenols for 2 h and then incubated with LPS (10 µg mL^{-1}) for 20 h. ## LPS treated. Untreated is the negative control without LPS treatments. Values are expressed as mean ± SEM. ns: non-significant, $n = 3$, data ± S.E.M. Groups 3–7 were compared against group II using Dunnett's post-hoc test (* significant at < 0.01; ** significant at < 0.001).

4. Discussion

A single solvent system (toluene/ethyl acetate/formic acid/methanol (3:3:0.8:0.2 *v/v*) was developed for densitometric quantification of polyphenols by HPTLC in aqueous-alcoholic extracts with reference to respective marker compounds such asrutin, kaempferol, quercetin, catechin, ellagic acid, gallic acid, and quercetin present in *P. maderaspatensis*. Ethyl acetate supernatant fractions showed significant immunomodulatory activity compared with other fractions, and we subsequently separated ethyl acetate fraction by vacuum liquid chromatography. Using ethyl acetate fraction in *P. maderaspatensis*, we performed isolation, purification, and characterization of rutin, kaempferol, ellagic acid, gallic acid, and catechin. Ellagic acid showed more significant immunomodulatory activity, while quercetin exhibited significant immunomodulation when compared with the crude. Specifically, ethyl acetate (100%) column eluents indicated that ellagic acid exhibited significant immunomodulation, followed by 15% methanol elutes, followed by chloroform second sediment fraction (oleanolic acid and ursolic acid), followed by 75% ethyl acetate(catechin, epicatechin) and 50% ethyl acetate elutes showed highly significant suppression (rutin, gallic acid), followed by 25% ethyl acetate (kaempferol and quercetin) and 75% methanol indicated non-significant active fraction, followed by 75% ethyl acetate second elutes and chloroform first fraction when compared with LPS.

Synthetic agents, natural adjuvant, and antibody reagents are used as immunosuppressive and immunostimulants. However, there is a major limitation to the general use of these agents, that is, the increased risk of infection and generalized effect throughout the immune system [26]. Many therapeutic effects of plant extracts have been claimed to be thanks to their influence on the immune system of the human body [27]. Many herbal preparations such as *Panax ginseng, Picrorhiza scrophulariiflora, Centella asiatica, Tinospora cordifolia, Phyllanthus debilis, Trigonella foenum graecum,* and *Pouteria cambodiana* have been shown to alter the immune function and report a wide array of immunomodulatory effects [28–34]. Most research concerning the immunomodulatory activities of the plant has been carried out using crude extracts [35,36]. In some, combinations of various herbs or herbs in combination with minerals have been used, taking into consideration Unani, Ayurvedic, or Chinese traditional formulation. Although it may be rational to use a single plant or its single constituents, it has been a general experience that the single constituent shows more efficacy compared with the total plant extract. *Phyllanthus* genus was found to be rich in polyphenols, lignins, flavonoids, triterpenes, hydrolysable tannins, sterol, and alkaloids [37].

5. Conclusions

We evaluated the immunomodulatory activity of various fractions, column eluents of ethyl acetate fraction, and their polyphenols present in *P. maderaspatensis* obtained from the Maruthmallai region of Kanyakumari district, Tamilnadu, India. Rutin, gallic acid, kaempferol, and catechin, each 200 µg mL^{-1}, as well as ellagic acid (100 µg mL^{-1}), showed a significant immunosuppressive effect owing to the inhibition of NO production compared with the LPS-stimulated RAW 264.7 cells group, and the most significant immunostimulatory effect was produced by ellagic acid and quercetin, each 200 µg mL^{-1}, when compared with the LPS control group.

Author Contributions: Conceptualization, U.I., D.P.K. and V.A.; methodology, U.I., D.P.K. and V.A.; investigation, U.I.; data curation, U.I., D.P.K., V.A., P.P.N. and M.E.-M.; writing—original draft preparation, U.I., D.P.K., V.A. and P.P.N.; writing—review and editing, U.I., D.P.K., V.A., P.P.N., M.E.-M. and M.S.K.; visualization, U.I.; supervision, V.A.; funding acquisition, U.I., D.P.K., V.A., P.P.N., M.E.-M. and M.S.K. All authors have read and agreed to the published version of the manuscript.

Funding: The authors extend their appreciation to the Deanship of scientific research at king Khalid University, Grant No: RGP2/191/42 Saudi Arabia for financial assistance.

Institutional Review Board Statement: Not applicable.

Informed Consent Statement: Not applicable.

Acknowledgments: The authors would like to thank the National Medicinal Plant Board, Department of AYUH, Delhi, India.

Conflicts of Interest: The authors declare no conflict of interest. The funders had no role in the design of the study; in the collection, analyses, or interpretation of data; in the writing of the manuscript; or in the decision to publish the results.

References

1. Munshi, A.; Mehrotra, R.; Ramesh, R.; Panda, S.K. Evaluation of anti-hepadnavirus activity of *Phyllanthus amarus* and *Phyllanthus maderaspatensis* in duck hepatitis B virus carrier Pekin ducks. *J. Med. Virol.* **1993**, *41*, 275–281. [CrossRef]
2. Asha, V.V.; Akhila, S.; Wills, P.J.; Subramoniam, A. Further studies on the antihepatotoxic activity of *Phyllanthus maderaspatensis* Linn. *J. Ethnopharmacol.* **2004**, *92*, 67–70. [CrossRef]
3. Bagavan, A.; Kamaraj, C.; Elango, G.; Abduz Zahir, A.; Abdul Rahuman, A. Adulticidal and larvicidal efficacy of some medicinal plant extracts against tick, fluke and mosquitoes. *Vet. Parasitol.* **2009**, *166*, 286–292. [CrossRef]
4. Prashanth, D.; Padmaja, R.; Samiulla, D.S. Effect of certain plant extracts on alpha-amylase activity. *Fitoterapia* **2001**, *72*, 179–181. [CrossRef]
5. Srirama, R.; Deepak, H.B.; Senthilkumar, U.; Ravikanth, G.; Gurumurthy, B.R.; Shivanna, M.B.; Chandrasekaran, C.V.; Agarwal, A.; Shaanker, R.U. Hepatoprotective activity of Indian *Phyllanthus. Pharm. Biol.* **2012**, *50*, 948–953. [CrossRef] [PubMed]
6. Zhang, X.; Xia, Q.; Yang, G.; Zhu, D.; Shao, Y.; Zhang, J.; Cui, Y.; Wang, R.; Zhang, L. The anti-HIV-1 activity of polyphenols from *Phyllanthus urinaria* and the pharmacokinetics and tissue distribution of its marker compound, gallic acid. *J. Tradit. Chin. Med. Sci.* **2017**, *4*, 158–166. [CrossRef]
7. Tan, W.C.; Jaganath, I.B.; Manikam, R.; Sekaran, S.D. Evaluation of antiviral activities of four local Malaysian *Phyllanthus* species against herpes simplex viruses and possible antiviral target. *Int. J. Med. Sci.* **2013**, *10*, 1817–1829. [CrossRef]

8. Yang, C.M.; Cheng, H.Y.; Lin, T.C.; Chiang, L.C.; Lin, C.C. Acetone, ethanol and methanol extracts of *Phyllanthus urinaria* inhibit HSV-2 infection in vitro. *Antiviral. Res.* **2005**, *67*, 24–30. [CrossRef]

9. Kumar, D.; Arya, V.; Kaur, R.; Bhat, Z.A.; Gupta, V.K.; Kumar, V. A review of immunomodulators in the Indian traditional health care system. *J. Microbiol. Immunol. Infect.* **2012**, *45*, 165–184. [CrossRef]

10. Patel, J.R.; Tripathi, P.; Sharma, V.; Chauhan, N.S.; Dixit, V.K. *Phyllanthus amarus*: Ethnomedicinal uses, phytochemistry and pharmacology: A review. *J. Ethnopharmacol.* **2011**, *18*, 286–313. [CrossRef] [PubMed]

11. Srivastava, A.; Misra, H.; Verma, R.K.; Gupta, M.M. Chemical fingerprinting of *Andrographis paniculata* using HPLC, HPTLC and densitometry. *Phytochem. Anal.* **2004**, *15*, 280–285. [CrossRef]

12. Singh, N.; Baby, D.; Rajuguru, J.P.; Patil, P.B.; Thakkannavar, S.S.; Pujari, V.B. Inflammation and cancer. *Ann. Afr. Med.* **2019**, *18*, 121–126. [CrossRef]

13. Schottenfeld, D.; Beebe-Dimmer, J. Chronic inflammation: A common and important factor in the pathogenesis of neoplasia. Ca. *Cancer J. Clin.* **2006**, *56*, 69–83. [CrossRef]

14. Ilyas, U.; Katare, D.P.; Aeri, V.; Naseef, P.P. A Review on hepatoprotective and immunomodulatory herbal plants. *Pharmacogn. Rev.* **2016**, *10*, 66–70.

15. Tomar, N.; De, R.K. A brief outline of the immune system. In *Immunoinformatics*; Humana Press: New York, NY, USA, 2014; pp. 3–12.

16. Chaplin, D.D. Overview of the immune response. *J. Allergy Clin. Immunol.* **2010**, *125*, 3–23. [CrossRef] [PubMed]

17. Chandra, R.K. Nutrition and the immune system: An introduction. *Am. J. Clin. Nutr.* **1997**, *66*, 460S–463S. [CrossRef] [PubMed]

18. Catanzaro, M.; Corsini, E.; Racchi, M.; Lanni, C. Immunomodulatory inspired by nature: A review on curcumin and echinacea. *Molecules* **2018**, *23*, 2778. [CrossRef] [PubMed]

19. Sattler, S. The role of the immune system beyond the fight against infection. *Adv. Exp. Med. Biol.* **2017**, *1003*, 3–14.

20. Schaller, M. The behavioral immune system and the psychology of human sociality. *Philos. Trans. R Soc. Lond. B Boil. Sci.* **2011**, *366*, 3418–3426. [CrossRef]

21. Calabrese, V.; Cornelius, C.; Dinkova-Kostova, A.T.; Calabrese, E.J.; Mattson, M.P. Cellular stress responses, the hormesis paradigm, and vitagenes: Novel targets for therapeutic intervention in neurodegenerative disorder. *Antioxid. Redox Signal.* **2010**, *13*, 1763–1811. [CrossRef]

22. Hsieh, H.L.; Yang, C.M. Role of redox signaling in neuroinflammation and neurodegenerative diseases. *BioMed. Res. Int.* **2013**, *2013*, 484613. [CrossRef]

23. Green, S.J.; Mellouk, S.; Hoffman, S.L.; Meltzer, M.S.; Nacy, C.A. Cellular mechanisms of nonspecific immunity to intracellular infection: Cytokine-induced synthesis of toxic nitrogen oxides from L-arginine by macrophages and hepatocytes. *Immunol. Lett.* **1990**, *25*, 15–19. [CrossRef]

24. Yue, G.G.L.; Lau, C.B.S.; Leung, P.C. Medicinal Plants and Mushrooms with Immunomodulatory and Anticancer Properties—A Review on Hong Kong's Experience. *Molecules* **2021**, *26*, 2173. [CrossRef] [PubMed]

25. Sanjeewa, K.K.A.; Nagahawatta, D.P.; Yang, H.W.; Oh, J.Y.; Jayawardena, T.U.; Jeon, Y.J.; De Zoysa, M.; Whang, I.; Ryu, B. Octominin inhibits LPS-induced chemokine and pro-inflammatory cytokine secretion from RAW 264.7 macrophages via blocking TLRs/NF-κB signal transduction. *Biomolecules* **2020**, *10*, 511. [CrossRef]

26. Arango, D.G.; Descoteaux, A. Macrophage cytokines: Involvement in immunity and infectious diseases. *Front. Immunol.* **2014**, *5*, 491. [CrossRef]

27. Shivaprasad, H.N.; Kharya, M.D.; Rana, A.C.; Mohan, S. Preliminary immunomodulatory activities of the aqueous extract of *Terminalia chebula*. *Pharm. Biol.* **2016**, *44*, 32–34. [CrossRef]

28. Bayan, L.; Koulivand, P.H.; Gorji, A. A review of potential therapeutic effects. *Avicenna J. Phytomed.* **2014**, *4*, 1–14.

29. Muhammad, R.; Najm, U.-R.; Muhammad, Z.-U.-H.; Hawa, Z.E.J.; Rosana, M. Ginseng: A dietary supplement as immune-modulator in various diseases. *Trends Food Sci. Tech.* **2019**, *83*, 12–30.

30. Smit, H.F.; Kroes, B.H.; van den Berg, A.J.; Van der Wal, D.; Van den Worm, E.; Beukelman, C.J.; Van Dij, K.H.; Labadie, R.P. Immunomodulatory and anti-inflammatory activity of *Picrorhiza scrophulariiflora*. *J. Ethnopharmacol.* **2000**, *73*, 101–109. [CrossRef]

31. Punturee, K.; Wild, C.P.; Kasinrerk, W.; Vinitketkumnuen, U. Immunomodulatory activities of *Centella asiatica* and *Rhinacanthus-nasutus* extracts. *Asian Pac. J. Cancer Prev.* **2005**, *6*, 396–400.

32. Sharma, U.; Bala, M.; Kumar, N.; Singh, B.; Munshi, R.K.; Bhalerao, S. Immunomodulatory active compounds from *Tinospora cordifolia*. *J. Ethnopharmacol.* **2012**, *14*, 918–926. [CrossRef]

33. Jantan, I.; Haque, M.A.; Ilangkovan, M.; Arshad, L. An insight in to the modulatory effects and mechanisms of action of *Phyllanthus* species and their bioactive metabolites on the immune system. *Front. Pharmacol.* **2019**, *10*, 878. [CrossRef] [PubMed]

34. Bin-Hafeez, B.; Haque, R.; Parvez, S.; Pandey, S.; Sayeed, I.; Raisuddin, S. Immunomodulatory effects of fenugreek (*Trigonella foenum graecum* L.) extract in mice. *Int. Immunopharmacol.* **2003**, *3*, 257–265. [CrossRef]

35. Sudam, V.S.; Potnuri, A.G.; Subhashini, N.J.P. Syk—GTP RAC-1 mediated immune-stimulatory effect of *Cuscutaepithymum*, *Ipomoea batata* and *Euphorbia hirta* plant extracts. *Biomed. Pharmacother.* **2017**, *96*, 742–749. [CrossRef] [PubMed]

36. Ramesh, K.V.; Padmavathi, K. Assessment of immunomodulatory activity of *Euphorbia hirta* L. *Indian J. Pharm. Sci.* **2010**, *72*, 621–625. [PubMed]

37. Zhou, Y.; Tang, Q.; Du, H.; Tu, Y.; Wu, S.; Wang, W.; Xu, M. Antiviral effect of ovotransferrin in mouse peritoneal macrophages by up-regulating type I interferon expression. *Food Agric. Immunol.* **2018**, *29*, 600–614. [CrossRef]

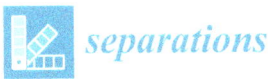

separations

Article

An Evaluation of the Antioxidant Activity of a Methanolic Extract of *Cucumis melo* L. Fruit (F1 Hybrid)

R. S. Rajasree [1,*], Sibi P. Ittiyavirah [2], Punnoth Poonkuzhi Naseef [3,*], Mohamed Saheer Kuruniyan [4], G. S. Anisree [5] and Muhammed Elayadeth-Meethal [6]

[1] College of Pharmaceutical Sciences, Government Thirumala Devaswom Medical College, Alappuzha 688005, India
[2] Department of Pharmaceutical Sciences, Centre for Professional and Advanced Sciences Cheruvandoor, Kottayam 686631, India; sibitho@gmail.com
[3] Department of Pharmaceutics, Moulana College of Pharmacy, Perinthalmanna 679321, India
[4] Department of Dental Technology, College of Applied Medical Sciences, King Khalid University, Abha 61421, Saudi Arabia; mkurunian@kku.edu.sa
[5] AES College of Pharmacy, Alappuzha 688561, India; anisreegs@gmail.com
[6] Department of Animal Breeding and Genetics, College of Veterinary and Animal Sciences, Kerala Veterinary and Animal Sciences University, Pookode, Wayanad 675621, India; muhammed@kvasu.ac.in
* Correspondence: rajasreejkrishnan@gmail.com (R.S.R.); drnaseefpp@gmail.com (P.P.N.)

Citation: Rajasree, R.S.; Ittiyavirah, S.P.; Naseef, P.P.; Kuruniyan, M.S.; Anisree, G.S.; Elayadeth-Meethal, M. An Evaluation of the Antioxidant Activity of a Methanolic Extract of *Cucumis melo* L. Fruit (F1 Hybrid). *Separations* 2021, 8, 123. https://doi.org/10.3390/separations8080123

Academic Editor: Didier Thiébaut

Received: 27 July 2021
Accepted: 13 August 2021
Published: 18 August 2021

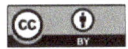
Abstract: *Cucumis melo* L. (*C. melo*) is a fruit with many medicinal properties and is consumed in various countries. It is utilised for chronic eczema and to treat minor burns and scrapes. The present study was conducted to evaluate the antioxidant activity of a methanolic extract of *Cucumis melo* Linn (MECM). A coarse powder prepared from the fruit and seeds was extracted with methanol (absolute) by a hot continuous percolation process in accordance with the standard protocols. All the extracts were estimated for potential antioxidant activities with tests such as an estimation of total antioxidant activity, hydroxyl radical and nitric oxide scavenging activity and reducing power ability. The qualitative analysis of the methanolic extract of *C. melo* fruit showed the presence of various phytochemical constituents such as carbohydrates, alkaloids, sterols, phenolic compounds, terpenes and flavonoids. The total antioxidant activity of concentrations of 50, 100 and 200 μg were tested and observed to be 3.3 ± 0.1732, 6.867 ± 0.5457 and 13.63 ± 0.8295 μg of ascorbic acid, respectively. The results also showed significant nitric oxide and DPPH scavenging activities as well as a reducing power activity of MECM. Thus, our results suggest that MECM may serve as a putative source of natural antioxidants for therapeutic and nutraceutical applications.

Keywords: antioxidants; methanolic extract; DPPH; *Cucumis melo*

1. Introduction

Traditional medicines composed of plants and their extracts used to cure various infections and ailments are being modified and refined to modern formulations in order to play a significant role in the treatment of various diseases such as diabetes, ischemic heart diseases, atherosclerosis and the initiation of carcinogenesis or liver diseases [1,2]. The physiological response imparted by the phytochemicals induces the desired therapeutic action [3,4]. The most essential of these bioactive constituents are phenolic compounds, alkaloids, saponins, tannins and flavonoids. *Cucurbits* form an important and large fruit crop set, cultivated extensively in subtropical and tropical countries, and contains a terpenoid substance known as Cucurbitacin [5]. The whole fruit of *Cucumis melo* L. (*C. melo* or muskmelon) is indicated for chronic eczema and to treat light burns and scrapes [6].

Dose-dependent cytotoxic activities exhibited by an aqueous fruit extract of *C. melo* in human prostate carcinoma PC 3 cell lines is evidence of its anti-cancer property [7]. High superoxide dismutase activity (SOD) is responsible for the in vitro and in vivo antioxidant and anti-inflammatory properties of their extract [8]. The in vitro evaluation of the antioxidant properties of *C. melo* leaves and fruit extracts reported concentration-dependent scavenging activity. 1,1-diphenyl-2-picrylhydrazyl (DPPH) was employed as the free radical in the evaluation of the reducing substances [9]. Previous investigations suggested that *C. melo* is a potential source of natural antioxidants and can act as a therapeutic agent in preventing oxidative stress-related disorders [10–12]. Advanced techniques using supercritical and subcritical CO_2 are also recommended to improve the bioavailability of the active ingredients [13]. In the present study, the antioxidant activity of a methanolic extract of *C. melo* fruit (F1 hybrid) was evaluated using standard procedures.

2. Materials and Methods

2.1. Chemicals

The chemicals and drugs were of pharmacopoeia/AnalaR or HPLC grade as required by the nature of the experiment and extraction. They were purchased from the licensed distributors of the Central Drug House (New Delhi, India), Himedia Labs (Mumbai, India) and Sigma-Aldrich chemicals (Bangalore, India).

2.2. Procurement of the Research Raw Materials

C. melo (family: Cucurbitaceae) fruit (Figure 1) were purchased from Vadanerkunam (Tindivanam T.K., Villupuram District, Tamilnadu, India) and identified and authenticated by experts of the Department of Botany, St. Berchmans College, Changanacherry, Kottayam-686101, India.

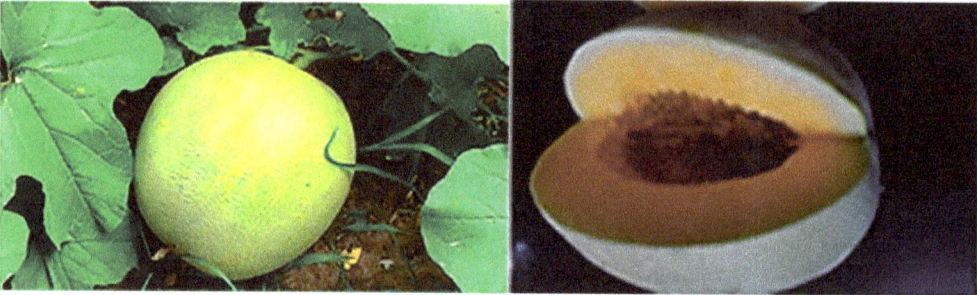

Figure 1. Muskmelon is a member of the Cucurbitaceae family, genus *Cucumis*, which comprises about 118 genera and 825 species. The fruit has been cultivated in China since 2000 BC. Diverse fruit forms have evolved around the world and are widely spread in subtropical and tropical regions. China and the USA are the highest producers of muskmelons.

2.3. Fruit Extract Preparation

The fruit of *C. melo* were cut into pieces with a stainless-steel knife. The mean dimensions were 1.8 cm diameter × 3.5 to 4.0 cm cylinders [14] and weighed approximately 100 g (including the seeds). These were dried in an oven at 60 °C. The dried fruit were then comminuted to a coarse powder and then passed through a No.10 sieve.

2.4. Preparation of MECM

The coarse powder was extracted with methanol (absolute) by a hot continuous percolation process. A total of 100 g of the dry powder was packed in a filter paper thimble each time and extracted in a Soxhlet extractor (five cycles/day for three consecutive days). The marc was then further extracted until it was colourless with 95% methanol. The process was repeated with fresh powder and the entire alcoholic extractives were mixed. Excess solvent was recovered by distillation under a reduced pressure and evaporated under a vacuum to form a soft extract, which was then weighed, re-heated (ensuring it was free of alcohol) and again weighed. The yield was calculated as the percentage weight per weight (w/w) of powder.

Product yield = (the total weight of extract obtained ÷ the total weight of the dry material used for extraction) × 100.

2.5. Phytochemical Screening

The following chemical tests were performed on the methanol extracts of *C. melo* (MECM) [15].

2.5.1. Tests for Carbohydrates

MECM (1 g) was boiled with 10 mL of distilled water for 10 min. It was cooled and filtered. The filtrate was used to conduct the following tests:

a. Molisch's test: Filtrate (2 mL) was added with two drops of alcoholic solution of α-naphthol. The mixture was shaken well and 1 mL of concentrated sulphuric acid was added slowly along the sides of the test tube. It was allowed to stand for a few seconds. The colour of the mixture was noted.

b. Iodine test: Filtrate (2 mL) was added with a few drops of dilute iodine solution and observed for the formation of a blue, orange or red colour.

c. Fehling's test: Filtrate (1 mL) was boiled in a water bath with 2 mL of a mixed Fehling's solution (1 mL each of Fehling's solutions A and B). The change in the colour of the solution was noted.

d. Benedict's test: Filtrate (0.5 mL) was added with 0.5 mL of Benedict's reagent and heated. The mixture was kept on a boiling water bath for 2 min. The change in the colour of the solution was noted.

e. Barfoed's test: Filtrate (1 mL) was added with 1 mL of Barfoed's reagent. It was heated in a boiling water bath for 2 min. The change in the colour of the solution was noted.

2.5.2. Tests for Glycosides

MECM was hydrolysed (50 mg) by heating with concentrated hydrochloric acid for 2 h on a water bath. It was filtered and, in the hydrolysate obtained, the following tests were conducted:

a. Borntrager's test: Filtered hydrolysate (2 mL) was added with 3 mL chloroform and shaken. The chloroform layer was separated and a 10% ammonia solution was added to it. The change in the colour of the solution was noted.

b. Legal's test: MECM (50 mg) was dissolved in pyridine. A sodium nitroprusside solution was added and made alkaline by using a 10% sodium hydroxide solution. The change in the colour of the solution was noted.

2.5.3. Tests for Alkaloids

MECM (2 g) was shaken with an ammonia solution for 20 min and then filtered. The mixture was extracted with petroleum ether and the ethereal extract was acidified with dilute HCl and extracted with 10 mL of water. The aqueous extract was again made ammoniacal and re-extracted with petroleum ether. The ethereal extract was evaporated to dryness and the residue was stirred with 10 mL of dilute hydrochloric acid and filtered. The filtrate was tested carefully with various reagents for the detection of alkaloids as follows:

a. Mayer's test: Filtrate (2 mL) was taken in a test tube. Two drops of Mayer's reagent were added along the sides and the change in the colour was noted.

b. Dragendorff's test: Filtrate (2 mL) was added with 1 mL of Dragendorff's reagent and the colour change and formation of any precipitate were noted.

c. Hager's test: Filtrate (2 mL) was added with 1 mL of Hager's reagent and the change in the colour of the solution was noted.

d.	Wagner's test: Filtrate (2 mL) was added with 1 mL of Wagner's reagent and the change in the colour of the solution was noted.

2.5.4. Tests for Amino acids

A total of 500 mg of MECM was shaken vigorously with 10 mL distilled water and filtered through a Whatman No.1 filter paper. The filtrate was used to tests for proteins and amino acids as follows:

a.	Biuret test: Filtrate (2 mL) was treated with one drop of a 2% copper sulphate solution. A total of 1 mL of (95%) ethanol was added to the solution followed by an excess of potassium hydroxide pellets and the change in the colour was observed.

b.	Ninhydrin test: Ninhydrin solution of 1% was added (2 drops) to the aqueous filtrate (2 mL). The mixture was heated and the change in the colour was observed.

c.	Million's test: A few drops of Million's reagent were added to the filtrate (2 mL) and the colour change was noted.

d.	Xanthoprotein test: The filtrate (3 mL) was added with 1 mL of concentrated nitric acid. The solution was cooled and made alkaline with 10% sodium hydroxide. The change in the colour of the solution was noted.

2.5.5. Tests for Sterols/Steroids

a.	Liebermann's sterol test: MECM (500 mg) was mixed with 2 mL of glacial acetic acid and one drop of concentrated sulphuric acid was added. The change in the colour of the solution was noted.

b.	Liebermann–Burchard test: MECM (500 mg) was mixed with 5 mL chloroform and a few mL of acetic anhydride was added. The mixture was added with one drop of concentrated sulphuric acid. This was then shaken well and the change in the colour was observed.

c.	Salkowski's test: MECM (500 mg) was shaken vigorously with 3 mL of chloroform and concentrated sulphuric acid was added through the sides of the test tube. The colour change of the solution was observed.

2.5.6. Tests for Fixed Oils and Fats

a.	Grease spot test: MECM (a small quantity) was pressed between two filter papers.

b.	Saponification test: MECM (a small quantity) was added with a few drops of a 0.5 N alcoholic potassium hydroxide solution along with a drop of phenolphthalein and the mixture was heated on a water bath for 2 h. The solution was observed for the formation of soap or any colour change indicating the neutralisation of potassium hydroxide on saponification.

2.5.7. Tests for Phenolic Compounds and Tannins

a.	Ferric chloride test: MECM (50 mg) was boiled with 5 mL distilled water and filtered. A few drops of a neutral, freshly prepared 5% ferric chloride solution were added to the filtrate and the colour change was noted (brownish green or blue-black colouration indicated the presence of tannins and phenolic compounds).

b.	Test for phlobatannins: MECM (1 g) was boiled with 1% HCl in a boiling tube and observed for the deposition of a red precipitate.

c.	Lead acetate test: MECM (50 mg) was boiled with distilled water and filtered. The filtrate was added with 3 mL of a 10% lead acetate solution. The formation of any precipitate was observed.

d.	Gelatine test: MECM (50 mg) was boiled with distilled water and 2 mL of a 1% solution of gelatine was added containing 10% sodium chloride. The solution was observed for the formation of a precipitate.

2.5.8. Tests for Terpenes/Terpenoids

a.   Tin and Thionyl chloride test: MECM (1 g) was boiled with 5 mL distilled water and filtered and the filtrate was treated with tin and thionyl chloride. Any change in the colour that occurred in the solution was noted.

2.5.9. Tests for Saponins

a.   Foam test: MECM (50 mg) was dissolved in distilled water and was diluted to 20 mL. The suspension was shaken vigorously in a graduated cylinder for 15 min. It was observed for the formation of foam.

b.   MECM (1 g) was boiled with 20 mL distilled water for 5 min and then cooled and filtered. The filtrate (10 mL) was shaken vigorously after adding 5 mL of distilled water. The frothing solution was mixed with a few drops of arachis oil and again shaken vigorously and observed for the formation of an emulsion.

2.5.10. Tests for Gums and Mucilage

a.   Precipitation test: MECM (100 mg) was shaken vigorously with 10 mL of distilled water and 25 mL of absolute alcohol was then added with constant stirring.

b.   Ruthenium red test: MECM (50 mg) was allowed to swell in water and then a few drops of Ruthenium red were added.

2.5.11. Tests for Flavones and Flavonoids

a.   Aqueous sodium hydroxide: An MECM solution of 2 mL was added with an aqueous solution of sodium hydroxide and mixed well. The change in the colour was observed.

b.   Concentrated sulphuric acid: An MECM solution (50 mg dissolved in 10 mL of water) was added with a concentrated sulphuric acid solution.

c.   Shinoda test: MECM (50 mg) was dissolved in alcohol. A few magnesium turnings and concentrated hydrochloric acid (dropwise) were added and the change in the colour was noted.

2.6. HPTLC Analysis

HPTLC was used for the detection of the phenolic compounds. HPTLC is a highly efficient, reliable and cost-efficient separation technique that is ideally applicable for the analysis of herbal drugs as well as botanicals. A Camag HPTLC instrument with a Linomat V automatic spotter fitted with a 100 µL syringe connected to a nitrogen cylinder and a Scanner-III were used. The developing chamber used was a twin trough and the viewing cabinet was equipped with dual-wavelength UV lamps (Camag, Muttenz, Switzerland). The precoated HPTLC plates used were aluminium backed with silica gel 60 F254 and the thickness was 0.2 mm. The HPTLC plates were cleaned by predevelopment with methanol before the analysis and activated at 110 °C for 5 min for the removal of solvents. Specific mobile phases were used for the separation of a particular group of phytochemicals.

Sample Application

A total of 10 µL of the sample was spotted using Linomat V on a precoated TLC plate as a narrow bandwidth (8 mm) 10 mm from the bottom and 15 mm from left and right edges of the plates. The samples were applied under a continuous dry stream of nitrogen gas.

THF (toluene, formic acid and water with a ratio of 16:8:2:1) was used as mobile phase for the development of the plates spotted with the samples for the detection of the phenolic compounds. The method of development was linear ascending and it was carried out in a 10 × 10 cm twin trough glass chamber that was equilibrated with the mobile phase. It was saturated for 20 min at 25 ± 2 °C with a relative humidity of 60 ± 5%. The volume of the mobile phase used for the development was 10 mL (5 mL in a trough containing the plate and 5 mL in another trough). It was allowed to migrate up to a distance of 85 mm from the point of the sample application. The TLC plate was dried after the development and the chromatogram was viewed in a UV chamber at 254 nm and 366 nm to visualise the phenolic compounds. Fast blue salt B was used to detect the phenolic compounds.

2.7. Total Antioxidant Activity Estimation

Test solutions containing 50, 100 and 200 µg/mL of MECM in methanol were prepared and 0.3 mL of the solution was mixed with a reagent solution (3 mL) containing 0.6 mL H_2SO_4, 28 mM sodium phosphate and 4 mM ammonium molybdate. The tubes containing the reaction solutions were incubated at 95 °C for 90 min and then cooled to room temperature. The absorbance of the resulting solution was measured at 695 nm against a blank. The solution of methanol (0.3 mL) was the control

The antioxidant activity was expressed as the number of grams equivalent to ascorbic acid. The antioxidant activity values were portrayed in standard graphs plotted with an OD of the standard against the various concentrations of ascorbic acid (10, 25, 50, 100, 250 and 500 µg/mL) treated similarly.

2.8. DPPH Radical Scavenging Assay

The free radical scavenging property of the extracts was estimated by a DPPH radical scavenging assay [16–19]. The hydrogen atom-donating capability of the plant extractives was determined by the decolourisation of the methanol solution of the DPPH (2,2-diphenyl-1-picrylhydrasyl) that produces a violet/purple colour in the methanol solution and fades to shades of yellow in the presence of antioxidants. A solution of 0.1 mM DPPH in methanol was prepared and 2.4 mL of this solution was mixed with 1.6 mL of the methanol extract at different concentrations (12.5–150 µg/mL). The reaction mixture was vortexed thoroughly and left in the dark at RT for 30 min. The absorbance of the mixture was measured spectrophotometrically at 517 nm. The percentage DPPH radical scavenging activity was calculated by the following equation:

$$\% \text{ DPPH radical scavenging activity} = \{(A_0 - A_1)/A_0\} \times 100$$

where A_0 was the absorbance of the control and A_1 was the absorbance of the extractives/standard. The % of inhibition was then plotted against the concentration and, from the graph, the IC_{50} was calculated. The experiment was repeated three times at each concentration [20–24].

2.9. Hydroxyl Radical Scavenging Activity

The assay principle was based on the competition estimation between the MECM and 2-deoxyribose for the hydroxyl radical that was formed by the Fenton's reaction [24,25]. The underlying mechanism is the oxidation of ferrous ion to ferric ion by hydrogen peroxide and hydroxyl free radicals and hydroxide ions are also formed. The Fe^{3+} form is reduced back to the Fe^{2+} form by reacting with another molecule of H_2O_2, forming a superoxide radical and an H^+. This reaction is essential in biological systems because transition metals such as iron and copper can donate or accept free electrons through various reactions taking place within the cells and can generate free radicals. The hydroxyl ion formed in the Fenton's reaction can react with barbituric acid and convert it into alloxan [26].

$$Fe^{2+} + H_2O_2 \rightarrow Fe^{3+} + OH. + OH^-.$$

$$Fe^{3+} + H_2O_2 \rightarrow Fe^{2+} + HOO. + H^+.$$

2.10. Nitric Oxide Generation and the Assay of Nitric Oxide Scavenging

Nitric oxide (NO) was generated from sodium nitroprusside and measured by the Greiss reaction as described previously. Sodium nitroprusside in an aqueous solution at a physiological pH spontaneously generates NO, which interacts with oxygen to produce nitrite ions that can be estimated by the Greiss reagent [27,28]. Scavengers of NO compete with oxygen, leading to a reduced production of NO. Sodium nitroprusside (5 mM) in phosphate-buffered saline was mixed with different concentrations of various plant extracts dissolved in suitable solvent systems and incubated at 258 °C for 150 min and reacted with the Greiss reagent (1% sulphanilamide, 2% H_3PO_4 and 0.1% naphthylethylenediamine dihydrochloride). The absorbance of the chromophore formed during the diazotisation of the nitrite with sulphanilamide and the subsequent coupling was noted.

2.11. Evaluation of the Reducing Power Activity

Concentrations of 50, 100 and 200 µg/mL of MECM and standard ascorbic acid of 50, 100 and 200 µg/mL each were mixed with 2.5 mL of phosphate buffer (pH 6.6). To the resultant solution, 1% potassium ferricyanide (2.5 mL) was added and boiled for 20 min at 50 °C. To that mixture, TCA (2.5 mL) was added and centrifuged for 10 min at 2000 rpm. The supernatant was collected and distilled water (1 mL) and 0.1% ferric chloride (250 µL) were added. The absorbance of the solution was then measured at 700 nm. The reducing power activity was indicated by the increase in the optical density [29,30].

3. Results

3.1. Qualitative Screening Tests of the Methanolic Extract of Muskmelon

The qualitative analysis of the methanolic extract of *C. melo* fruit showed the presence of various phytochemical constituents such as carbohydrates, alkaloids, sterols, phenolic compounds, terpenes and flavonoids (Table 1). The Rf value obtained from HPTLC analysis of the MECM for phenolic compounds were 0.80, 0.83 and 0.86 (Figure 2).

Table 1. Qualitative chemical tests of the methanolic extract of muskmelons.

Sl No	Phytochemicals	Test/Reagent Used	Result
01	Carbohydrates	Molisch's test	+
		Iodine test	−
		Fehling's test	−
		Benedict's test	−
		Barfoed's test	−
		Million's test	−
02	Proteins	Biuret test	−
		Xanthoproteic test	−
		Ninhydrin test	−
03	Fats/oil	Grease spot test	−
		Saponification test	−
04	Alkaloids	Bontrager's test	−
		Hager's test	+
		Dragendorff's test	+
05	Sterols/steroids	Liebermann's sterol test	+
		Liebermann–Burchard test	+
		Salkowski's test	+
06	Phenolics	Ferric chloride test	+
		Lead acetate test	+
		Gelatine test	−
07	Terpenes/terpenoids	Tin and thionyl chloride test	+
08	Saponin glycosides	Form test	−
		Haemolysis test	−
09	Gums/mucilage	Precipitation test	−
		Ruthenium red test	−
10	Flavones/flavonoids	Alkali (aqueous NaOH)	+
		Conc. H_2SO_4	+
		Shinoda test	+

+ Present, − Absent.

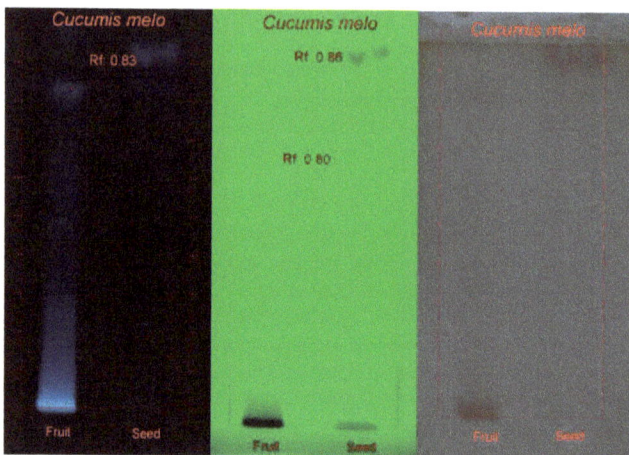

Figure 2. HPTLC of the phenolic compounds: UV 366 nm, UV 254 nm and derivatised under visible light using a fast blue salt B reagent.

3.2. Estimation of the Total Antioxidant Activity

The antioxidant activity of MECM in concentrations of 50, 100 and 200 µg were equated to the antioxidant activity of 3.3 ± 0.1732, 6.867 ± 0.5457 and 13.63 ± 0.8295 µg of ascorbic acid, respectively (Figure 3).

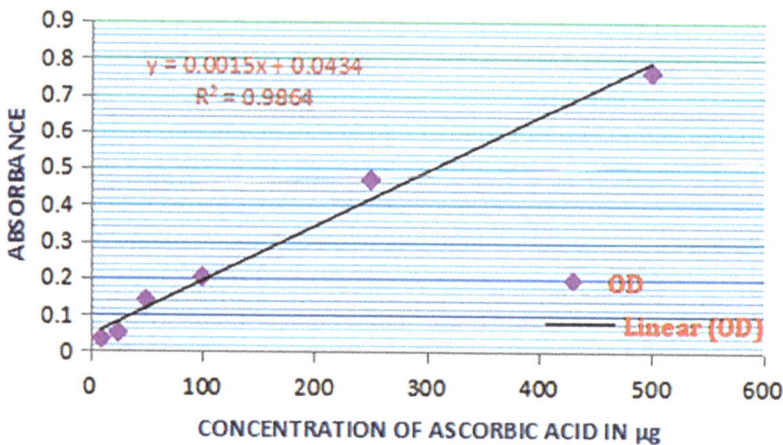

Figure 3. Evaluation of the total antioxidant activity: a standard curve of ascorbic acid.

3.3. DPPH Scavenging Activity

DPPH, 2,2-Diphenyl-1-picrylhydrasyl, is a dark-coloured compound composed of stable free radical molecules. The purple colour of DPPH decays in the presence of antioxidants. The change in absorbance at 517 nm in the presence of antioxidants can be equated with the antioxidant potential of the compound.

The % scavenging activity = $100 \times$ [(OD control − OD test)/OD control].

The standard employed was ascorbic acid. Both the extract and the ascorbic acid were tested in concentrations of 100, 250 and 500 µg. It was observed that the calculated percentage scavenging activity of ascorbic acid at these concentrations was 29.24 ± 0.8712,

36.76 ± 1.3 and 52.06 ± 0.7963, respectively (mean ± SEM). The percentage inhibition for MECM calculated at similar concentrations was 11.79 ± 0.5469, 16.50 ± 1.065 and 22.45 ± 1.131; when compared with the control, these values were significant ($p < 0.001$). The results are summarised in Table 2 and Figure 4.

Table 2. DPPH scavenging activity.

Sl No.	Concentrations Exposed (μg/mL)	% Scavenging		
		Control	MECM	Ascorbic Acid
1	100		11.79 ± 0.5469 ***	29.24 ± 0.8712 ***
2	250	0.00	16.50 ± 1.065 ***	36.76 ± 1.3 ***
3	500		22.45 ± 1.131 ***	52.06 ± 0.7963 ***

*** Significant, $p < 0.001$, ANOVA, Dunnett's multiple comparison with control, F = 356.3.

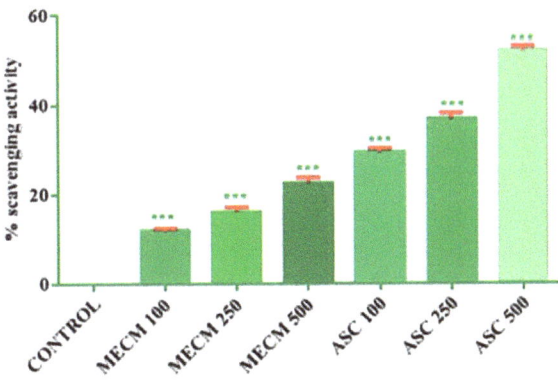

Groups and concentrations exposed

Figure 4. The DPPH scavenging activity of MECM using ascorbic acid as a standard. Compared with ascorbic acid in its pure form, MECM showed a significant DPPH scavenging activity (*** Significant, $p < 0.001$).

The ability of MECM to scavenge hydroxyl radicals generated by Fenton's reaction was tested in this study. The test depends upon the formation of the coloured product by the reaction of hydroxyl radicals with thiobarbituric acid and the measurement of its optical density by a colorimetric assay. A reduction in the OD correlated with the ability of MECM to scavenge the hydroxyl radicals from the reaction mixture.

The standard employed was ascorbic acid. Both the extracts and the ascorbic acid were tested in concentrations of 50, 100 and 200 μg. It was observed that the calculated percentage inhibition by ascorbic acid at these concentrations was 36.09 ± 0.296, 52.4 ± 0.387 and 65.98 ± 0.589, respectively (mean ± SEM). The percentage inhibition for MECM calculated at similar concentrations was 19.56 ± 0.194, 24.92 ± 0.194 and 33.3 ± 0.194; when compared with the control, these values were significant ($p < 0.001$). The results are summarised in Table 3 and Figure 5.

The IC_{50} calculated for the ascorbic acid was 108.95 μg whereas that of MECM was 385 μg. A comparison of the inhibitory activities of ascorbic acid and MECM is shown in Figure 4.

Table 3. Evaluation of the hydroxyl radical scavenging activity of MECM.

Group Treated	Concentration Exposed (µg)	% Inhibition (Mean ± SEM)	Groups Compared and Significance
Control (A)	–	00	–
Standard (B) ascorbic acid	50 (B1)	36.09 ± 0.296	A and B1 ***
	100 (B2)	52.4 ± 0.387	A and B2 ***
	200 (B3)	65.98 ± 0.589	A and B3 ***
Test (C) MECM	50 (C1)	19.56 ± 0.194	A and C1 ***
	100 (C2)	24.92 ± 0.194	A and C2 ***
	200 (C3)	33.3 ± 0.194	A and C3 ***

*** Significant, 0.001, ANOVA, post-hoc test by Dunnett's multiple comparisons, all groups with control, F = 470.

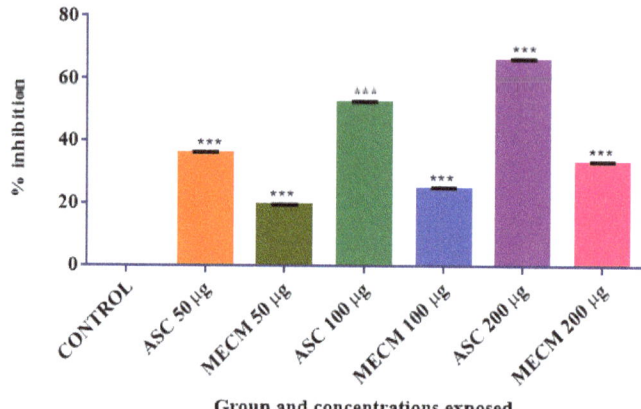

Figure 5. Comparison of the hydroxyl radical scavenging activity of MECM and ascorbic acid. Compared with ascorbic acid in its pure form, MECM showed a significant hydroxyl radical scavenging activity (*** Significant, $p < 0.001$).

3.4. Nitric Oxide Scavenging Activity

We evaluated the nitric oxide scavenging activity of MECM. The standard used for the comparison was gallic acid. The increased concentration of nitric oxide generated was indicated by the increase in the optical density. Thus, the decrease in the optical density evaluated the nitric oxide scavenging activity (Table 4).

Table 4. Nitric oxide scavenging activity of MECM.

Sl No	Group	% Inhibition (Mean ± SEM)			Level of Significance and Groups Compared
		50 µg (A)	100 µg (B)	200 µg (C)	
1	Control (I)	00.00	00.00	00.00	—
2	Std (II) (Gallic acid)	51.8 ± 0.744	68.8 ± 0.562	85.7 ± 0.342	I(A) and II(A), II(B), II(C) ***
3	MECM (III)	10.1 ± 1.39	20.13 ± 0.281	36.5 ± 1.55	I(A) and III(A), III(B), III(C) ***

*** Significant, ANOVA and Dunnett's multiple comparison against control, F = 1026, N = 3.

The observed mean OD of the control group was 0.201 ± 0.007, which corresponded with a zero % inhibition. As the exposed concentrations of gallic acid were increased from 50, 100 and 250 µg/mL, there was a significant reduction in the OD ($p < 0.05$). Hence, the inhibitory effect on the nitric oxide generation had to be considered inhibited in a corresponding gradation. The percentage inhibition calculated (with reference to the control OD) for the optical density values of 0.099, 0.064 and 0.029 was 51.8 ± 0.744, 68.83 ± 0.562 and $85.7 \pm 0.342\%$ for the gallic acid standard. These values were statistically significant at 0.05 levels.

The OD values of MECM for concentrations of 50, 100 and 200 µg/mL were 0.184 ± 0.004, 0.163 ± 0.003 and 0.130 ± 0.002, respectively. These values corresponded with the percentage inhibition of 10.1 ± 1.39, 20.13 ± 0.281 and 36.5 ± 1.55. When compared with the inhibition produced by gallic acid at the same concentrations, these values were significantly low ($p < 0.05$). Moreover, although the decrease in the OD was significant at 100 and 200 µg/mL concentrations, the effect of 50 µg was found to be insignificant at $p < 0.05$.

The IC_{50} for gallic acid was calculated to be 30.74 µg and that for MECM was 275.29 µg (Figure 6).

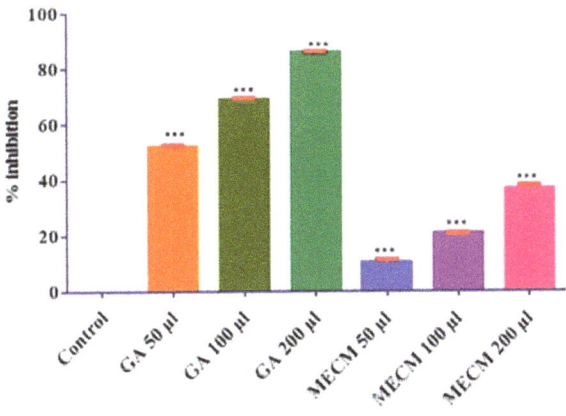

Figure 6. Evaluation of the nitric oxide scavenging activity of MECM: a comparison with gallic acid (*** Significant, $p < 0.001$).

3.5. Evaluation of the Reducing Power Activity

The evaluation of the reducing power activity was conducted by a simple colorimetric method. The change in the absorbance of a reaction system containing trichloroacetic acid, ferric chloride and potassium ferricyanide was extrapolated to calculate the reducing power activity of a compound.

The percentage increase in the absorbance with respect to the control was taken as the percentage reducing power. The result of the study is tabulated in Table 5.

The reducing power of ascorbic acid at concentrations of 50, 100 and 200 µg was found to be (mean $\pm$ SEM) 40.42 ± 1.35, 53.98 ± 0.2405 and 69.14 ± 0.2309 whereas that of MECM in similar concentrations was 11.8 ± 0.6132, 19.37 ± 0.8192 and 24.78 ± 0.8110 (Figure 7).

Table 5. Evaluation of the reducing power of MECM.

Sl NO	Concentration (µg /mL)	Reducing Power as % (Mean ± SEM)			Statistics
		Control (A)	MECM (B)	Ascorbic Acid (C)	
1	50 (i)	0.0	11.8 ± 0.6132	40.42 ± 1.35.	Bi and Ci *** Bi and A *** Ci and A ***
2	100 (ii)		19.37 ± 0.8192	53.98 ± 0.2405	Bii and Cii ** Bii and A *** Cii and A ***
3	200 (iii)		24.78 ± 0.8110	69.14 ± 0.2309	Biii and Ciii *** Biii and A *** Ciii and A ***

*** Significant, $p < 0.001$, ANOVA and Tukey's multiple comparison (comparison of all pairs of columns) $N = 7$, F: 1108.

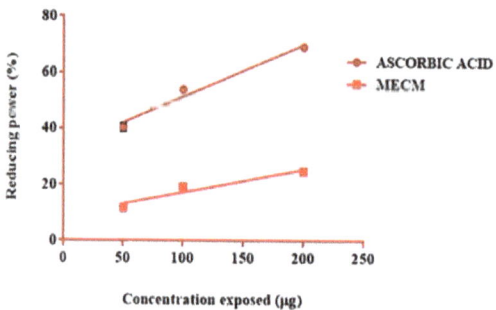

Figure 7. A comparison of the reducing power of MECM with that of ascorbic acid at concentrations of 50,100 and 200 micrograms. The x-axis shows the concentrations exposed and the y-axis shows the percentage reducing activity. Compared with ascorbic acid in its pure form, MECM showed a significant reducing power.

4. Discussion

Oxidative stress plays an important role in the development and pathophysiology of many diseases [1]. The *C. melo* extract showed good activities in hydroxyl, nitric oxide radical and DPPH radical scavenging activity [11]. Moreover, the antioxidant potency of MECM was evaluated by estimating the total antioxidant activity and reducing power activity [12]. Our finding indicates that MECM is a good source of antioxidant constituents, which may be due to the presence of a series of components acting synergistically by different mechanisms. Natural antioxidants are considered better than synthetic compounds due to minimum adverse effects and *C. melo* fruit could be a dietary supplement that could be recommended to prevent oxidative stress.

The phytochemical analysis revealed the presence of a series of phytochemicals in MECM and the HPTLC analysis revealed the presence of polyphenolic compounds. The study mainly aimed to evaluate the antioxidant activity of MECM. Hence, by comparing the antioxidant activity with the standard ascorbic acid in its pure form, we demonstrated that MECM had an antioxidant activity. Ascorbic acid was used in its pure form and is a standard and potent antioxidant. Specifically, the study proved that MECM had an activity compared with the control, with a significance level of a *p*-value less than 0.05.

4.1. DPPH Radical Scavenging Activity of MECM

This method is one of the most popular procedures to test the antioxidant potential of a plant extract. DPPH is a relatively stable radical that acts as an antioxidant or free radical scavenger by donating hydrogen ions to the compounds in the oxidised state [31]. The estimation of the free radical scavenging activity in food and plant-based drugs is extensively performed utilising this assay and the fruit extract had an excellent activity [32,33].

4.2. Hydroxyl Radical Scavenging Potential of MECM

The neutral form of a hydroxide ion (OH^-) is a hydroxyl radical and is highly reactive. Therefore, it exists only for a short period. Several biological membranes including DNA can be damaged by hydroxyl radicals. To neutralise this radical, no endogenous enzymatic scavenging pathways are present inside the body and most often it is neutralised by several endogenous molecules such as glutathione, melatonin and antioxidants supplemented through diet [34]. MECM showed a statistically significant hydroxyl radical scavenging potential and the fruit could act as an excellent dietary source to produce this activity.

4.3. Nitric Oxide Scavenging Potential of MECM

Nitric oxide (NO), which is an important bioactive molecule, possesses several physiological functions [35]. It assists in maintaining vascular homeostasis, fights against pathological microorganisms and it is known to have an anti-cancer activity. NO can also act on the blood vessels, producing vasodilatation, altering the vascular endothelial permeability and acting as a neurotransmitter. When combined with a superoxide radical, it generates a peroxynitrite anion and becomes highly reactive and causes severe damage to intracellular components. The substances that scavenge nitric oxide could have a cytoprotecting property [35].

The methanolic extract of the F1 Hybrid variety of *C. melo* was tested for its ability to scavenge nitric oxide using gallic acid as a standard. In the in vitro study, the significant capacity of MECM to reduce the formation of NO in the reaction system was established. It can act as a potent scavenger of free radicals, thus inferring its cytoprotective effect [36–38].

5. Conclusions

Cucumis melo Linn. (*C. melo*) is an important horticultural crop cultivated worldwide. In the present study, we evaluated the antioxidant activity of a methanolic extract of *Cucumis melo Linn* (MECM) quantitatively and qualitatively using standard protocols. The qualitative analysis showed that MECM contained carbohydrates, alkaloids, sterols, phenolic compounds, terpenes and flavonoids. The total antioxidant activity of the concentrations of 50, 100 and 200 µg was 3.3 ± 0.1732, 6.867 ± 0.5457 and 13.63 ± 0.8295 µg of ascorbic acid, respectively. Significant nitric oxide and DPPH scavenging activities as well as a reducing power activity were also observed.

Author Contributions: Conceptualization, S.P.I., R.S.R.; methodology, R.S.R., S.P.I.; investigation, R.S.R.; data curation, P.P.N., M.E.-M.; writing—original draft preparation, R.S.R.; writing—review and editing, R.S.R., P.P.N., M.E.-M., M.S.K., G.S.A.; visualization, R.S.R.; supervision, S.P.I.; funding acquisition, R.S.R., P.P.N., M.E.-M., M.S.K. All authors have read and agreed to the published version of the manuscript.

Funding: This research received no external funding.

Institutional Review Board Statement: Not applicable.

Informed Consent Statement: Not applicable.

Acknowledgments: The authors extend their appreciation to the Deanship of Scientific Research at King Khalid University, Saudi Arabia for funding this work through the Research Group Program under Grant No: RGP 2/191/42.

Conflicts of Interest: There is no conflict of interest.

References

1. Adwas, A.A.; Elsayed, A.S.I.; Azab, A.E. Oxidative stress and antioxidant mechanisms in human body. *J. Appl. Biotechnol. Bioeng.* **2019**, *6*, 43–47. [CrossRef]
2. Kasole, R.; Martin, H.D.; Kimiywe, J. Traditional medicine and its role in the management of diabetes mellitus: "patients' and herbalists' perspectives. *Evid.-Based Complement. Altern. Med.* **2019**, *2019*, 2835691. [CrossRef] [PubMed]
3. Contardi, M.; Lenzuni, M.; Fiorentini, F.; Summa, M.; Bertorelli, R.; Suarato, G.; Athanassiou, A. Hydroxycinnamic acids and derivatives formulations for skin damages and disorders: A review. *Pharmaceutics* **2021**, *13*, 999. [CrossRef] [PubMed]
4. Nuzzo, D.; Contardi, M.; Kossyvaki, D.; Picone, P.; Cristaldi, L.; Galizzi, G.; Bosco, G.; Scoglio, S.; Athanassiou, A.; Di Carlo, M. Heat-resistant *Aphanizomenon flos-aquae* (AFA) Extract (Klamin®) as a functional ingredient in food strategy for prevention of oxidative stress. *Oxid. Med. Cell. Longev.* **2019**, *2019*, 9481390. [CrossRef] [PubMed]
5. Mujeeb, F.; Bajpai, P.; Pathak, N. Phytochemical evaluation, antimicrobial activity, and determination of bioactive components from leaves of *Aegle marmelos*. *Biomed Res. Int.* **2014**, *2014*, 497606. [CrossRef] [PubMed]
6. Tungmunnithum, D.; Thongboonyou, A.; Pholboon, A.; Yangsabai, A. Flavonoids and other phenolic compounds from medicinal plants for pharmaceutical and medical aspects: An overview. *Medicines* **2018**, *5*, 93. [CrossRef]
7. Larayetan, R.; Ololade, Z.S.; Ogunmola, O.O.; Ladokun, A. Phytochemical constituents, antioxidant, cytotoxicity, antimicrobial, antitrypanosomal, and antimalarial potentials of the crude extracts of *Callistemon citrinus*. *Evid.-Based Complement. Altern. Med.* **2019**, *2019*, 5410923. [CrossRef]
8. Rajasree, R.S.; Sibi, P.I.; Francis, F.; William, H. Phytochemicals of Cucurbitaceae family—A review. *Int. J. Pharmacogn. Phytochem. Res.* **2016**, *8*, 113–123.
9. Marwat, S.K.; Rehman, F.U. Medicinal folk recipes used as traditional phytotherapies in district Dera Ismail Khan, KPK, Pakistan. *Pak. J. Bot.* **2011**, *43*, 1453–1462.
10. Ittiyavirah, S.P.; George, A.; Santhosh, A.M.; Kurian, S.T.; Pappachan, P.; Jacob, G. Studies of cytotoxic potential of *Cucumis-melo*. Linn fruit aqueous extract in prostate cancer cell lines PC-3 using MTT and neutral red assay. *Iran. J. Pharmacol. Ther.* **2013**, *12*, 24–30.
11. Mallek-Ayadi, S.; Bahloul, N.; Kechaou, N. Characterization, phenolic compounds and functional properties of *Cucumis melo* L. peels. *Food Chem.* **2017**, *221*, 1691–1697. [CrossRef]
12. Ismail, H.I.; Chan, K.W.; Mariod, A.A.; Ismail, M. Phenolic content and antioxidant activity of cantaloupe (*Cucumis melo*) methanolic extracts. *Food Chem.* **2010**, *119*, 643–647. [CrossRef]
13. Baldino, L.; Scognamiglio, M.; Reverchon, E. Supercritical fluid technologies applied to the extraction of compounds of industrial interest from *Cannabis sativa* L. and to their pharmaceutical formulations: A review. *J. Supercrit. Fluids* **2020**, *165*, 104960. [CrossRef]
14. Portela, S.I.; Cantwell, M.I. Cutting blade sharpness affects appearance and other quality attributes of fresh-cut cantaloupe melon. *J. Food Sci.* **2001**, *66*, 1265–1270. [CrossRef]
15. Gokhale, S.B.; Kokate, C.K.; Purohit, A.P. *A Textbook of Pharmacognosy*, 28th ed.; Niraliprakashan: New Delhi, India, 2007; pp. 1–20.
16. Becket, A.H.; Stenlake, J.B. *Practical Pharmaceutical Chemistry*, 2nd ed.; C.B.S. Publishers and Distributors: New Delhi, India, 1986; pp. 333–337.
17. Vouldoukis, I.; Lacan, D.; Kamate, C.; Coste, P.; Calenda, A.; Mazier, D.; Conti, M.; Dugas, B. Antioxidant and anti-inflammatory properties of a *Cucumis melo* LC. extract rich in superoxide dismutase activity. *J. Ethnopharmacol.* **2004**, *94*, 67–75. [CrossRef]
18. Reddy, G.M.; Muralikrishna, A.; Padmavathi, V.; Padmaja, A.; Tilak, T.K.; Rao, C.A. Synthesis and antioxidant activity of styryl sulfonyl methyl 1, 3, 4-oxadiazoles, pyrazolyl/isoxazolyl-1, 3, 4-oxadiazoles. *Chem. Pharm. Bull.* **2013**, *61*, 1291–1297. [CrossRef] [PubMed]
19. Chandran, P.R.; Jothi, T.A. Multisource five level inverter using an improved PWM scheme. *Int. J. Sci. Res.* **2013**, *2*, 279–282.
20. Nishikimi, M.; Rao, N.A.; Yagi, K. The occurrence of superoxide anion in the reaction of reduced phenazine methosulfate and molecular oxygen. *Biochem. Biophys. Res. Commun.* **1972**, *46*, 849–854. [CrossRef]
21. McCord, J.M.; Fridovich, I. The utility of superoxide dismutase in studying free radical reactions: I. Radicals generated by the interaction of sulfite, dimethyl sulfoxide, and oxygen. *J. Biol. Chem.* **1969**, *244*, 6056–6063. [CrossRef]
22. Umamaheswari, M.; Chatterjee, T.K. In vitro antioxidant activities of the fractions of *Coccinia grandis* L. leaf extract. *Afr. J. Tradit. Complement. Altern. Med.* **2008**, *5*, 61–73. [CrossRef]
23. Blois, M.S. Antioxidant determinations by the use of a stable free radical. *Nature* **1958**, *181*, 1199–1200. [CrossRef]
24. Brand-Williams, W.; Cuvelier, M.E.; Berset, C.L. Use of a free radical method to evaluate antioxidant activity. *LWT-Food Sci Technol.* **1995**, *28*, 25–30. [CrossRef]
25. Elizebeth, K.; Rao, M.W.A. Oxygen radical scavenging activity of Curcumin. *Int. J. Pharm.* **1991**, *58*, 237–240.
26. Enrol, D.; Mechmet, U.; Ferda, C.; Dimitra, D.; Gulhan, V.U.; Mosschos, P.; Atalay, S. Antimicrobial and antioxidant activities of essential oils and methanol extract of *Saliva cryptantha* (Montbret et AucherexBenth) and *Saliva multicaulis* (Vahl). *J. Food Chem.* **2013**, *84*, 519–525.
27. Kumaran, A.; Karunakaran, R.J. Nitric oxide radical scavenging active components from *Phyllanthus emblica* L. *Plant Foods Hum. Nutr.* **2006**, *61*, 1. [CrossRef] [PubMed]
28. Yen, G.C.; Duh, P.D.; Tsai, C.L. Relationship between antioxidant activity and maturity of peanut hulls. *J. Agric. Food Chem.* **1993**, *41*, 67–70. [CrossRef]

29. Lu, Y.; Foo, L.Y. Antioxidant activities of polyphenols from sage (*Salvia officinalis*). *Food Chem.* **2001**, *75*, 197–202. [CrossRef]

30. Da Porto, C.; Calligaris, S.; Celotti, E.; Nicoli, M.C. Antiradical properties of commercial cognacs assessed by the DPPH test. *J. Agric. Food Chem.* **2000**, *48*, 4241–4245. [CrossRef]

31. Soare, J.R.; Dinis, T.C.; Cunha, A.P.; Almeida, L. Antioxidant activities of some extracts of *Thymus Zygis*. *Free Radic. Res.* **1997**, *26*, 469–478. [CrossRef]

32. Badarinath, A.V.; Rao, K.M.; Chetty, C.M.; Ramkanth, S.T.; Rajan, T.V.; Gnanaprakash, K. A review on *in-vitro* antioxidant methods: Comparisons, correlations and considerations. *Int. J. Pharmtech. Res.* **2010**, *2*, 1276–1285.

33. Pham-Huy, L.A.; He, H.; Pham-Huy, C. Free radicals, antioxidants in disease and health. *Int. J. Biomed. Sci.* **2008**, *4*, 89–96.

34. Garratt, D.C. *The Quantitative Analysis of Drugs, Japan*; Chapman and Hall: Tokyo, Japan, 1964; Volume 3, pp. 456–458.

35. Marcocci, L.; Maguire, J.J.; Droylefaix, M.T.; Packer, L. The nitric oxide-scavenging properties of *Ginkgo biloba* extract EGb 761. *Biochem. Biophys. Res. Commun.* **1994**, *201*, 748–755. [CrossRef] [PubMed]

36. Tamir, S.; Tannenbaum, S.R. The role of nitric oxide (NO) in the carcinogenic process. *Biochim. Biophys. Acta Rev. Cancer* **1996**, *1288*, 31–36. [CrossRef]

37. Sreejayan, N.; Rao, M.N.; Priyadarsini, K.I.; Devasagayam, T.P. Inhibition of radiation-induced lipid peroxidation by curcumin. *Int. J. Pharm.* **1997**, *151*, 127–130. [CrossRef]

38. Kala, M.; Shaikh, M.V.; Nivsarkar, M. Equilibrium between anti-oxidants and reactive oxygen species: A requisite for oocyte development and maturation. *Reprod. Med. Biol.* **2017**, *16*, 28–35. [CrossRef]

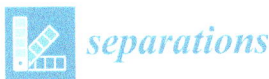

Review

Advanced Analytical Approaches for the Analysis of Polyphenols in Plants Matrices—A Review

Elena Roxana Chiriac [1],*, Carmen Lidia Chiţescu [2],*, Elisabeta-Irina Geană [3], Cerasela Elena Gird [1], Radu Petre Socoteanu [4] and Rica Boscencu [1]

[1] Faculty of Pharmacy, "Carol Davila" University of Medicine and Pharmacy, 6 Traian Vuia St., 020956 Bucharest, Romania; cerasela.gird@umfcd.ro (C.E.G.); rica.boscencu@umfcd.ro (R.B.)

[2] Faculty of Medicine and Pharmacy, "Dunarea de Jos", University of Galaţi, 35 A.I. Cuza Str., 800010 Galaţi, Romania

[3] National Research &Development Institute for Cryogenics and Isotopic Technologies (ICSI Rm. Vâlcea), 4th Uzinei Street, 240050 Râmnicu Vâlcea, Romania; irina.geana@icsi.ro

[4] "Ilie Murgulescu" Institute of Physical Chemistry, Romanian Academy, 202 Splaiul Independentei, 060021 Bucharest, Romania; s.radu@hotmail.com

* Correspondence: roxana.elena.chiriac@gmail.com (E.R.C.); carmen.chitescu@ugal.ro (C.L.C.)

Abstract: Phenolic compounds are plants' bioactive metabolites that have been studied for their ability to confer extensive benefits to human health. As currently there is an increased interest in natural compounds identification and characterization, new analytical methods based on advanced technologies have been developed. This paper summarizes current advances in the state of the art for polyphenols identification and quantification. Analytical techniques ranging from high-pressure liquid chromatography to hyphenated spectrometric methods are discussed. The topic of high-resolution mass spectrometry, from targeted quantification to untargeted comprehensive chemical profiling, is particularly addressed. Structure elucidation is one of the important steps for natural products research. Mass spectral data handling approaches, including acquisition mode selection, accurate mass measurements, elemental composition, mass spectral library search algorithms and structure confirmation through mass fragmentation pathways, are discussed.

Keywords: extraction; high-resolution mass spectrometry; fragmentation pathway; non-targeted analysis; chemical profiling

Citation: Chiriac, E.R.; Chiţescu, C.L.; Geană, E.-I.; Gird, C.E.; Socoteanu, R.P.; Boscencu, R. Advanced Approaches for the Analysis of Polyphenols in Plants Matrices—A Review. *Separations* **2021**, *8*, 65. https://doi.org/10.3390/separations8050065

Academic Editor: Ernesto Reverchon

Received: 6 April 2021
Accepted: 10 May 2021
Published: 12 May 2021

Publisher's Note: MDPI stays neutral with regard to jurisdictional claims in published maps and institutional affiliations.

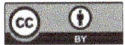
1. Introduction

Plants have been used for centuries as remedies in several forms: unprocessed, as complex mixtures of different species as in Traditional Chinese Medicine [1], or, more recently, in commercial products as phyto-pharmaceuticals and dietary supplements [2–4]. The bioactivity of those natural products is generally high [4–6], supporting the high use of those products as a primary form of healthcare for a large part of the population [7]. Furthermore, about 80% of all synthetic drugs are directly or indirectly derived from them [8,9]. The pharmaceutical industry is currently showing an increasing interest in the development of new formulations with integrated vegetal extracts as a source of bioactive compounds [9]. Therefore, the assessment of the chemical components of herbs, spices or functional foods has become an essential part of our understanding.

Polyphenols are secondary plant metabolites, and comprise a wide range of compounds that strongly differ in their structure, physicochemical and nutritional properties. Dietary polyphenols are one of the most important groups of natural antioxidants and chemopreventive agents in human diets, playing a vital role in supporting the functioning of biological systems [6,10]. Epidemiological, clinical and nutritional studies strongly support the suggestion that polyphenolic compounds enhance human health by lowering risk and preventing several diseases and disorders [5,10]. It has been reported that polyphenolic compounds exhibit anticarcinogenic, anti-inflammatory, antimicrobial, antiviral, antidiabetic and hepatoprotective activities, as well as estrogen-like activities [11–13].

In the last few decades, different studies have intensely investigated the antioxidative, antimicrobial, antiproliferative or enzyme-inhibition effects of polyphenols [6,12,14]. Studies using in vitro and in vivo approaches together with LC-MS analytical techniques have led to a better understanding of the bioavailability and bioactivity of polyphenols. However, the theory that the beneficial effects of polyphenols are direct consequences of antioxidant activity in vivo is obsolete. Their protective activity was firstly attributed to their antioxidant, free radical-scavenging, and metal chelator properties, and then to their ability to inhibit different enzymes [12]. New research supports the hypothesis according to which polyphenols' interaction with signal transduction pathways and cell receptors induce adaptive responses that drive antioxidant, antiplatelet, vasodilatory or anti-inflammatory effects [6,11,15]. Thus, the current research places more emphasis on the individual identification/quantification of each compound rather than on the in vitro assay of bioactive properties [16].

The occurrence of polyphenols in herbs or food and their chemistry have been intensively debated, and as such, they are not the subject of this study. This review aims to provide updated information on the advances in the analytical approaches currently used in sample preparation and subsequent analyses for the determination of the polyphenolic profiles in plant samples. Recent literature (2015–2020) was reviewed for a comparative overview of the advanced analytical techniques.

2. Extraction

The extraction of bioactive compounds from plant material is a key step in the development of various analytical methods. The extraction methods should be simple, safe, reproducible, less expensive, and also suitable for industrial applications in phyto-chemistry.

2.1. Conventional Methods

Conventional methods provided by European Pharmacopoeia, [17] such as infusion, decoction, percolation or maceration, as well as extraction under reflux and Soxhlet extraction, are still currently used. Methanol, ethanol, acetonitrile, acetone, or their mixtures with water are the most used solvents.

2.2. Advanced Methods

The current tendency is to develop and apply new fast, efficient and selective techniques, which are able to meet the special extraction requirements of bioactive compounds and are environmentally clean.

2.2.1. Ultrasound-Assisted Extraction (UAE)

Among the new extraction methods, ultrasound-assisted extraction (UAE) is a modern technique that offers a high yield of active compounds with simple manipulation, energy efficiency and high reproducibility [18]. Commonly used for solid/liquid systems, UAE lead to a disruption of the cellular walls of the plant material, and enhances mass transfer across cell membranes, thus increasing the solvent access to the analytes [18,19]. Several factors, such as solvent composition, solvent-to-sample ratio, ultrasound amplitude and cycle, solvent pH, and temperature, can impact the extraction efficiency [19]. The selection of solvents and temperature were shown to be the most important factors influencing the efficiency of UAE [18,19]. It has been observed that, in the case of highly polar phenolic compounds, extraction with pure organic solvents has low efficiency [19,20]. Ethanol/methanol mixtures with water in various proportions (e.g., 80:20, 60:40, 70:30) are widely used as extraction solvents [19], sometimes with the addition of acids for the adjustment of pH, e.g., ethanol 70% and acetic acid 2% at 60 °C was used for flavonoids extraction in *Dendranthema indicum* [21], and 80% aqueous MeOH with 1% formic acid was successfully used for the extraction of flavonoids from culinary herbs and spices [22].

The extraction of polyphenols is also affected by the duration of contact between phases, and the liquid–solid or liquid–liquid ratio. Bajkacz et al. [23] studied the influence of extraction duration (2 and 5 h) on the extraction efficiency from plant material. An increase in polyphenol content with the extraction duration was observed. However, the potential production of free radicals with prolonged sonication (>40 min) in frequencies above 20 kHz was reported as a disadvantage of the method [24]. The possible degradation of some active principles in plant matrices can also occurs due to oxidative pyrolysis caused by hydroxyl (OH) radicals during the cavitation phenomenon [25].

2.2.2. Microwave-Assisted Extraction (MAE)

In recent years, due to the tendency to reduce the quantity of organic solvents used in the extractions, microwave-assisted extraction (MAE) has been developed and optimized. With the main benefits of extraction time reduction, low cost and sustainability, this technique was found to be suitable for the extraction of phenolic acids, flavones, flavonols and isoflavones from blackberry (*Rubus Fruticosus* L.) [26], myrtle (*Myrtus communis* L.) leaves [27], blackthorn (*Prunus spinosa* L.) flowers [28], basil (*Oscium basilicum*) [29], chilean superfruits (*Aristotelia chilensis*) [30] and pistachio green (*Pistacia vera* L.) [31].

Microwaves consist of electric and magnetic fields that oscillate perpendicularly to each other in a high-frequency range from 0.3 to 300 GHz [24,32]. This condition produces localized heating and causes the destruction of the plant matrix leading, to the easier diffusion of the compounds of interest into the solvent [28,32]. A microwave power between 300 and 900 W and extraction temperatures ranging from 50 to 100 °C are generally used [19].

The main challenge of this extraction technique is to obtain the maximum extraction yield via the destruction of the cellular tissue without affecting the chemical structure of the natural compounds. A special piece of equipment was developed in 2017 by a Romanian research team using a slot end coaxial antenna with a microwave applicator, provided with a cooling system [33]. Consequently, a high specific absorption rate (SAR) was achieved at low temperatures. Polyphenols were extracted from sea buckthorn leaves, showing higher polyphenols contents and higher antioxidant capacities than extracts obtained via conventional methods performed with the same temperature profile [33].

2.2.3. Accelerated Solvent Extraction (ASE)

As an alternative to the extraction and fractionation of nutraceutical compounds from different natural products, accelerated solvent extraction (ASE), also known as pressurized liquid extraction (PLE), allows faster extraction and, by adjusting the process parameters, enhances the extraction selectivity for particular groups of compounds [19]. Due to the high pressure, solvents remain in the liquid state even at high temperatures, allowing high-temperature extraction. These conditions enhance the solubility of target compounds in the solvent and the desorption kinetics of plant matrices. Furthermore, as it is performed in a closed system, the occurrence of oxidation reactions during ASE is limited [19]. Thus, the method has been successfully used to extract thermally sensible phytochemicals from such plants as purple sweet potatoes [34], passion fruit rinds [35], citrus [36], and olive leaves [37].

Regarding the extraction conditions, studies have shown that ASE is more efficient when mixtures of solvents are used, such as methanol or ethanol in water, instead of pure solvents [19], for the reasons of polarity compatibility. Working pressures ranging from 4 to 20 MPa affect the diffusion of the solvent into the pores of the raw material matrix, enhancing the contact of the target compounds with the solvent [32,38]. Temperature is also an important parameter of ASE extraction. Various works have shown that from 40 to 120 °C, there is an increase in the phenolics extraction efficiency [32].

ASE was evaluated by Garcia-Mendoza et al. [38] at different working pressures using several solvents, including ethanol, water, an acidified mixture of ethanol + water and acidified water, for the extraction of polyphenols and anthocyanin from juçara (*Euterpe edulis Mart.*). ASE was compared to different low-pressure extraction methods (Soxlet and UAE) and to supercritical fluids extraction (SFE). The antioxidant activity determined through DPPH was significantly higher in the Soxhlet extracts, suggesting differences in the chemical composition of the extracts, probably due to the long interactions between raw material and solvent. The total polyphenols content obtained in SFE was lower than in ASE and low-pressure extractions, while a significant improvement in the extraction of anthocyanins by SFE compared with ASE was observed [38].

Study results showed that high-pressure methods are, in general, more effective and selective for phenolic compound extraction than low-pressure techniques [37,38]. However, lower recovery rates of thermosensitive polyphenols at high temperatures and incomplete extraction due to limited solvent volume were reported as disadvantages [32,39].

2.2.4. Supercritical Fluids Extraction (SFE)

Besides ASE, supercritical fluids extraction (SFE) is a green extraction technology based on the properties of fluids in a supercritical state (their thermodynamic parameters, pressure and temperature being critical values) to extract bioactive components from vegetal materials [32,40]. Supercritical carbon dioxide (SC-CO_2) is currently considered as an ideal solvent for selectively extracting soluble compounds from vegetable materials [40,41]. For both the food and the pharmaceutical industry, the main advantages of extracts obtained by SFE are the absence of residual organic solvent and the controlled selectivity of the extract's composition, SFE being recognized as safe by the European Food Safety Authority (EFSA) and the Food and Drug Administration (FDA) of the United States of America [32,42].

However, this approach has some limitation. SC-CO_2 is a non-polar solvent that has affinity to non-polar or low-polar compounds. On the other hand, polyphenols have a low degree of solubility in SC-CO_2, which leads to low extraction yields [40]. To overcome this limitation, the addition of chemical modifiers or cosolvents, such as water, methanol, ethanol, acetone, acetonitrile or an acidified ethanol + water mixture, to change the non-polar nature of supercritical CO_2, was tested [42].

2.2.5. Enzyme-Assisted Extraction

Enzymatic hydrolysis is an effective and nontoxic extraction procedure, widely used in various food processes. The enzymatic activity of cellulases, pectinases and hemicellulases leads to cell wall disruption and enhances the extraction of valuable compounds from plants [43]. Furthermore, due to the enzymatic activity of lyases and hydrolases on the glycosidic fractions of natural polyphenols, their biological properties are improved in terms of bioactivity and bioavailability [44]. A mixture of hesperidinase and β-galactosidase was used in a very recent study for the extraction of flavonoids from *Matricaria chamomilla* [44]. Flavonoids, as well as non-flavonoid polyphenols, were significantly structurally modified by the enzymatic treatment, which resulted in the increased bioactivity of the metabolites as inhibitors of pancreatic lipase activity [44].

Mixtures of enzymes, including pectinases, endo- and exo-glucanases, β-glucosidases, β-galactosidase and cellobiases, are used to obtain an overall synergistic effect [45,46]. Enzymatic hydrolysis using cellulose and peptinase was employed for achieving the release of polymeric polyphenols, which are theoretically "non-extractable", from the plant matrix [46].

Extraction parameters such as temperature and pH influence the catalytic activity and the rheological properties of the raw material, as well as the solubilization of bioactive compounds. Although temperature increase enhances the mass transfer rates and solubility of the extracted compounds, it may lead to enzymatic denaturation; therefore, temperatures below 60 °C are usually used [47]. Environment pH values ranging between 4.0 and 6.5 are used for the optimal activity of enzymatic system [43,45]. After incubation for 30 to 90 min, the vegetal mass is subjected to extraction and centrifuged [43].

2.2.6. Extraction with Ionic Liquids (ILs)

Recent studies have focused on the extraction of bioactive components from herbal medicines or other vegetal sources using ionic liquids (ILs) and deep eutectic solvents (DESs) as alternative solvents, showing their potential to substitute organic solvents [48]. ILs are a group of organic salts that are presented in a liquid form below 100 °C and consist of an organic cation (e.g., imidazolium, pyrrolidinium, pyridinium tetraalkyl ammonium, tetraalkyl phosphonium) and an inorganic or organic anion (e.g., tetrafluoroborate, hexafluorophosphate and bromide).

The polarity, hydrophobicity, viscosity and miscibility of the solvent can be selected by choosing the cationic or anionic constituent. The wide variety of possible combinations of cations and anions implies a wide variety of physico-chemical properties that depend on both the nature and the size of the cation, but especially the anion. Depending on their nature, the resulting ionic liquids may have a hydrophobic or a hydrophilic character, higher or lower viscosity and miscibility with water or other different organic phases, as well as specific electrochemical properties [49].

Due to these properties, the use of ionic liquids has been considered a success in stabilizing, pre-concentrating or extracting bioactive analytes. Imidazolium-based ionic liquids have been successfully applied for the extraction of isoflavones by UAE from soy (daidzeinm genistein, and glycosides) [50] and from *Iris tectorum Maxim* (tectoridin, iristectorin B, and iristectorin A) [51]. Choline-chloride based DESs have been used for the extraction of polyphenols from *Ficus carica* L. leaves [52].

2.3. Modeling the Extraction Process by Response Surface Methodology (SRM)

Extraction optimization can be a time-consuming process, as many combinations of different solvents mixtures, with different pH values and temperatures, can be used. In order to save time, solvents and resources, empirical models were created and applied to test the functional relationship between a response of interest and a number of associated inputs [18,53–55].

Response surface methodology (RSM) is based on mathematical and statistical techniques for the modeling and optimization of complex chemical and physical processes [55,56]. In a recent study, for the optimization of the extraction of bioactive components from *Medicago sativa* L., Fumic et al. [54] used the Box–Behnken design (BBD), a spherical three-level–three-factor design, employed to determine the best combination of independent extraction variables (solvents' concentration in water, temperature and pH) for the selected dependent variables (extraction yield, radical scavenging activity, the content of phenolic compounds). The conclusions of the study showed ethanol concentrations as the key variable for the achievement of high total phenol and flavonoid contents, while temperature was the most important variable for the extraction of phenolic acids and the antioxidant activity of the extracts [54].

Improvements in UAE yield and the content of phenolic compounds in apple pomace extracts were obtained by Skrypnik and Novikova [55] using nonionic emulsifiers (Tween 20, Tween 80), compared to 70% ethanol/water. pH value, extraction time, and emulsifiers concentration and volume were subjected to RSM.

Considering the complexity of the influence of the extraction conditions, a very careful analysis of the extraction settings is required according to the desired results, which demonstrates the usefulness of these modeling techniques.

3. Extract Hydrolysis and Purification

The hydrolysis can be performed before, during or after extraction, using different procedures—acidic, alkaline or enzymatic hydrolysis—in order release bound polyphenols and increase the extraction yield of their aglycone form [46,56,57]. While acidic hydrolysis breaks glycosidic bonds, alkaline hydrolysis breaks ester bonds and removes acetyl- or malonyl- groups from glucosides, allowing only β-glucosides and native aglycone forms to remain in the extract [56]. Enzymatic hydrolysis produces aglycone forms, similar to acid hydrolysis [56]. The official AOAC method 2001.10 for isoflavones in soy and in various foods containing soy uses alkaline hydrolysis [57]. For enzymatic hydrolysis, β-glucosidase, β-galactosidase, β-glucuronidase or mixtures of these are usually used [45].

The purification, fractionation and concentration of the extract are of great importance, both for the analysis of polyphenols and for the subsequent use of the extracts in various fields, including pharmaceuticals.

The extract, hydrolyzed or not, may be subjected to clean-up techniques allowing the accurate identification and quantification of the target analytes. The extraction in the solid phase (SPE) is the most-employed technique in clean-up procedures [58]. In SPE, the target compounds are retained in a specific sorbent and then eluted with an adequate solvent, such as methanol, ethanol, and ethyl acetate. The SPE process allows for the purification and concentration of polyphenols at the same time. SPE columns type C18 [23], HLB [58] or Oasis MCX [59] were used as stationary phases. An alternative to traditional SPE is the matrix solid-phase dispersion extraction (MSPD) method, with the advantage of less solvent consumption [60]. Dispersive solid-phase extraction (d-SPE), another alternative to SPE, was recently evaluated for the determination of phenolic compounds in *Myrciaria cauliflora* peel [61], proving its efficiency in removing the interfering compounds without significant retention of polyphenols.

QuEChERS (quick, easy, cheap, effective, rugged, and safe) is an alternative method of polyphenol extraction and purification that reduces solvent amount and procedure duration. Initially developed for the determination of pesticide residues in food matrices, due to its versatility, QuEChERS has been progressively applied for the extraction of other compounds in different matrices, resulting in the good recovery of the target analytes and lower interference [62]. The technique involves liquid–liquid partitioning with organic solvents and purification of the extract using solid-phase dispersive extraction (d-SPE) with sorbents and buffers [62,63].

QuEChERS assisted by ultrasound extraction was recently optimized for the isolation of polyphenols from several fruit and vegetable samples [62]. Acetonitrile, methanol, ethanol, and a combination of them were tested, methanol being selected in the subsequent experiments. An ultra-sonification time of 5 min was also selected as optimum. A mixture of buffered salts, including disodium hydrogen citrate sesquihydrate, trisodium citrate dihydrate sodium chloride, and MgSO4, was used [62].

However, due to the development of advanced, sensitive spectrometric methods, sample preparation has become simplified, often consisting of the filtration and convenient dilution of the extract.

4. Analytical Detection Techniques

Due to polyphenols' structural diversity and low concentrations, and the plant matrix complexity, their analysis remains challenging. Currently, there is a requirement for sensitive and accurate methods for the analysis of polyphenols, as knowledge of their identity and dosage are prerequisites in evaluating health benefits [64]. Novel techniques have been employed in the past few decades, ranging from high-pressure liquid chromatography (HPLC) to mass spectrometry (MS) and spectroscopic methods. Recent (2015–2020) developments, and the application of analytical methods in qualitative and quantitative studies of polyphenols following extraction, were reviewed in the present work. High-resolution mass spectrometry is particularly addressed due to its applicability in the targeted/untargeted metabolomic analysis of polyphenols.

4.1. Liquid Chromatography with Ultraviolet/Visible (UV/Vis)-Based Detection: HPLC Fingerprint with Chemometric Analysis

High-performance liquid chromatography (HPLC) is still one of the most widely used analytical tools for the identification and quantification of polyphenols [65]. The quality consistency of herbal medicines reflects variations in their chemical composition from batch to batch, depending on several factors, such as botanical species, chemotypes, morphological parts of the plant, geographical area, time of harvest, and storage conditions. With the continuous development of HPLC technology, chromatographic fingerprint analysis has been recognized as an innovative, rapid, and comprehensive method for the identification and qualification of herbal medicines [66]. The fingerprint profiles show variations in a given herb in an integrated manner, and can identify a particular herb, distinguishing it from closely related species [66,67]. The chromatographic fingerprint of the herbal profile can be defined as the characteristic signal of selected plant that allows unambiguous identification via the evaluation of the chemical similarities and differences in the obtained chromatograms of studied samples [66]. Fingerprint analysis has been internationally accepted as a method for the evaluation and quality control of herbal medicines and preparations, and is currently applied in combination with other chemometric modeling methods, namely, similarity analysis (SA), hierarchical clustering analysis (HCA), principal component analysis (PCA), and partial least square regression [68–70].

For a reliable investigation of a matrix as complex as is found vegetal extracts, the fingerprint method should display good precision, repeatability, and stability, evaluated based on the relative standard deviations (RSD) of the relative retention times (RRT < 3%), and the relative peak areas (RPA < 3%) of the characteristic peaks compared with the reference peak. Similarity values above 0.98 are accepted [69].

The chromatographic fingerprint method can also distinguish authentic materials from substitutes and adulterants, suggesting new applications for food products and pharmaceuticals. Recently, several methods were developed for the fingerprint analysis of different species, such as Flos Carthami (*Carthamus tinctorius* L.), [71], Aurantii Fructus (*Citrus aurantium* L.) [66], chamomile (*Matricaria chamomilla* L.) [72], licorice (*Glycyrrhiza glabra* L.) [67], and selected lavender species (*Lavandulae* spp.) [73] (Table 1). An HPLC-UV polyphenolic fingerprint method was applied on pure cranberry extracts and cranberry-based extracts adulterated with grape at different percentages [2].

For assessing the chromatographic condition, the C18 or C8 reversed-phase LC (packed with particles of silica bonded with alkyl chains) columns are preferred for the separation. C12 columns have also been investigated in herbal drug standardization [74].

Table 1. Some examples of the recent applications of HPLC fingerprinting methods in natural polyphenols analysis.

Plant Material	Extraction	HPLC Condition	Characteristic Fingerprint Peaks	Chemometric Analysis Approach	Ref.
Cranberry (*Vaccinium macrocarpon*)-based products (fresh and dried fruits, juice)	Lyophilized samples were extracted with an acetone-water-hydrochloric acid (70:29.9:0.1 *v/v*) solution by UAE for 10 min	Kinetex C18 (100 4.6 mm i.d., 2.6 μm particle size) column; mobile phase: 0.1% formic acid in water (*v/v*) and MeOH; flow rate of 1 mL/min; monitoring wavelength range: 190–550 nm	gallic acid, homogentisic acid, protocatechuic acid, protocatechualdehyde, (+) catechin hydrate, gentic acid, *p*-salicilic acid, chlorogenic acid, vanillic acid, (−) epicatechin, syringic acid, syringaldehyde, ethyl gallate, *p*-coumaric acid, ferulic acid, resveratrol and quercitrin	Partial least square regression and PCA	[2]
27 *Salvia* L. Species, leaf and root	Maceration in MeOH (2 × 10 mL for 24 h) followed by solvents removal on rotary evaporator under vacuum at 40 °C to dryness	RP C18 Eurospher-100 column, (5 μm particle, 125 mm × 4 mm); mobile phase: 0.2% (*v/v*) glacial acetic acid in water and ACN; flow rate of 1 mL/min; monitoring wavelength: 280 nm	rosmarinic acid, carnosic acid, caffeic acid, salvianolic acids A and B	PCA	[65]
Aurantii Fructus, dried mature and immature fruits of *Citrus aurantium* L. (medicinal herbs in TCM);	UAE (200 W) with MEOH for 45 min	Symmetry C18 column (250 × 4.6 mm, 5 μm); mobile phase: ACN and 0.1% aqueous phosphoric acid; flow rate of 1 mL/min; monitoring wavelength range: 285–324 nm	eriocitrin, neoeriocitrin, narirutin, naringin, hesperidin, neohesperidin, meranzin, poncirin, naringenin, nobiletin, tangeretin and auraptene	Quantitative analysis of multiple components by single marker (QAMS); similarity analysis; standard method difference; HCA	[66]
Licorice root (*Liquiritiae radix*) –*Glycyrrhiza glabra* L.	UAE with 80% MeOH-water, 120 W, 40 KHZ, 20 min	Cosmosil column (5C18-MS-II, 5 μm, 4.6 × 250 mm), at 35 °C; mobile phase: 5 mmol/L sodium heptane sulfonate solution phosphoric acid (499:1, *v/v*) and ACN-MeOH (9:1, *v/v*); flow rate of 1 mL/min; monitoring wavelengths: 203 nm, 220 nm, 250 nm, 280 nm and 344 nm	glycyrrhizic acid, liquiritigenin, isoliquiritigenin, isoliquiritin, liquiritin apioside, isoliquiritin apioside and glabridin	Geometric linear quantified fingerprint method (GLQFM) and PCA	[67]
Flos Carthami, the dried flower of *Carthamus tinctorius* L.; (medicinal herbs in TCM)	UAE with 50% MeOH, 270 W, 30 min	C18 column (4.6 mm × 250 mm, 5 μm); mobile phase: 0.1% formic acid in water and ACN	guanosine, hydroxysafflor yellow A, anhydrosafflor yellow B, kaempferol 3-O-β-rutinoside, rutin, quercetin, kaempferol	Similarity Evaluation System for Chromatographic Fingerprint of Traditional Chinese Medicine (Version 2004 A)	[71]
Chamomile—*Matricaria chamomilla* L., commercial samples	UAE with MeOH-water mixture (80:20, *v/v*) at 35 °C for 30 min, three times repeated	Hypersil Gold C18 column (250 × 4.6 mm; 5 μm); mobile phase: 0.05% TFA in ACN and 0.05% TFA in water; flow rate of 1 mL/min; monitoring wavelength: 254 nm	gallic acid, caffeic acid, syringic acid, *p*-coumaric acid, ferulic acid, rutin, myricetin, quercetin and kaempferol	ANOVA, PCA, hierarchical cluster analysis (HCA)	[72]
Seven species of *Lavandulae flos*	UAE with xylen (1:30) under reflux for 4 h followed by solvents removal on a rotary evaporator under vacuum to dryness	Kinetex RP18 column (5 μm, 150 × 4.6 mm); mobile phase: MeOH-water–0.1% formic acid (gradient 5–100% (*v/v*) of MEOH) at 30 °C; flow rate of 1 mL/min; monitoring wavelength: 280 nm	apigenin, myricetin, luteolin, luteolin 7-glucoside, chlorogenic acid, caffeic acid, ferulic acid	Cluster analysis using SpecAlign program (Pearson correlation coefficient, r, and Euclidean) and PCA	[73]
Pomegranate (*Punica granatum* L.), dried peel	UAE of the dried samples with 60% ethanol, 26 min	Zorbax SB-C18 column (5 μm, 4.6 mm × 250 mm); mobile phase: glacial acetic acid (99:1, *v/v*; pH 3.0) and MeOH flow rate of 1 mL/min; monitoring wavelength: 280 nm	gallic acid, punicalagin, catechin, chlorogenic acid, caffeic acid, epicatechin, rutin, and ellagic acid	Similarity Evaluation System for Chromatographic Fingerprint of Traditional Chinese Medicine (Version 2004A) software	[75]

Table 1. *Cont.*

Plant Material	Extraction	HPLC Condition	Characteristic Fingerprint Peaks	Chemometric Analysis Approach	Ref.
Sedi linearis Herba, dried whole herb	UAE of the dried samples with 70% methanol, 60 min	BDS Hypersil C18 column (4.6 m × 250 mm, 5 μm), 30 °C; Mobile phase: ACN and 0.1% acetic acid solution; flow rate of 1 mL/min; monitoring wavelength: 265 nm	hyperoside, isoquercetin and astragalin	-	[76]
Black tea samples	Enzymatic extraction using immobilized polyphenol oxidase followed by fractionating using a Mitsubishi SP-207 resin chromatography with an elution gradient of 20%, 30%, 40%, 50% and 70% aqueous ethanol	C18 column; mobile phase: water: ACN: glacial acetic acid (73.5/26/0.5, v/v/v); flow rate of 5 mL/min	caffeine, (−) epigallocatechin gallate, (−) epigallocatechin, (+) epicatechin gallate, (−) epicatechin, (+) gallocatechin gallate, (+) gallocatechin, (+) catechin gallate, (+) catechin, theaflavin, theaflavin 3-monogallate, theaflavin 3'-monogallate and theaflavin 3,3'-digallate	-	[77]
Raw elderberry (*Sambucus nigra* L.)	UAE of the dried samples with 80% methanol, 45 min	C18 column, 35 °C, mobile phase: MeOH and acetic acid in water (1.0%, v/v); flow rate of 1 mL/min; monitoring wavelength: 285 nm	gallic acid, chlorogenic acid, caffeic acid, syringic acid, p-coumaric acid, ferulic acid, rutin, myricetin, quercetin kaempferol and quercetin 3-glucoside	HCA and PCA	[78]
Phyllanthus emblica, dried fruits	Fruit powder was extracted in 70% ethanol (1:8) at 50 °C using a magnetic stirrer	DiKMA C18 column (250 mm × 4.6 mm × 5 μm); mobile phase: 0.2% formic acid in water and methanol; flow rate of 1 mL/min; Monitoring wavelength: 273 nm	gallic acid, corilagin, ellagic acid, quercetin	Similarity Evaluation System for Chromatographic Fingerprints of Traditional Chinese Medicine (Version, 2004A) and HCA	[79]
Medicago spp. in different phenologic stages: vegetative elongation, late bud and late flower; dried leaves	MSPD extraction using C18 column. Elution with methanol: H₂O (9:1, v/v)	Luna 5 U C18 column (5 μm, 150 × 4.60 mm) at 40 °C; mobile phase: acetonitrile and acetic acid in water (1.0%, v/v); flow rate of 1 mL/min; monitoring wavelength: 254 nm	puerarin, daidzin, genistin, daidzein, glyciterin, genistein, pratensein, formononetin, irilone, prunetin and bio-chanin A	generalized linear model (GLM) and linear discriminant analysis (LDA)	[80]
Tithonia diversifolia, dried leaves	Maceration in 80% acetone for 72 h; evaporate to dryness at 40 °C	C18 column (5 μm, 4.6 mm × 250 mm); mobile phase: water/acetic acid, 98.2% v/v and methanol/water/acetic acid, 70:28:2% v/v; flow rate 0.6 mL/min; monitoring wavelengths: 254, 327, 366	gallic acid, chlorogenic acid, caffeic acid and p-coumaric acid, and apigenin	analysis of variance model and Tukey's test	[81]
lyophilized leaves of ten mango varieties	UAE with 70% ethanol, 320 W for 30 min; evaporate to dryness by vacuum rotary evaporator at 30 °C	C18 column (250 mm × 4.6 mm, 5 μm); mobile phase: 0.1% (v/v) formic acid in water and 0.1% (v/v) formic acid in acetonitrile; flow rate: 0.8 mL/min; all wavelengths scanning detection from 200 to 600 nm	neomangiferin, gallic acid, 5-caffeoylquinic acid, 3-chlorogenic acid, mangiferin, 4-hydroxybenzoic acid, sinpic acid, isoquercetin, quercetin	similarity analysis, PCA, HCA, discriminant analysis	[82]

A mixture of water with organic solvents (i.e., methanol, acetonitrile) is usually used as the mobile phase. The development of LC methods for polyphenols analysis is almost always based on a slow solvent gradient (duration between 45 and 80 min) with the advantage of sharper peaks because of the compression effects induced by the gradient, as well as minimizing the LC column contamination due to the increased solvent strength. A gradient based on a combination of acetonitrile/water/methanol is often applied on a C18 column for the separation polyphenols [66,74]. Acetic acid, trimethylamine, phosphoric acid or trifuloroacetic acid (TFA) are usually used as mobile phase additives for enhancing the chromatographic separation [66,73–75,78] (Table 1).

However, conventional HPLC suffers the disadvantages of long analysis time, low resolution and large solvent consumption. UPLC and multi-dimensional separation techniques have emerged as alternatives to HPLC, presenting superior separation capabilities and high levels of system stability, providing technical support for further pharmacological and pharmaceutical research [77,83].

4.2. Liquid Chromatography–Mass Spectrometry Analytical Methods

Although many studies had been published concerning the phenolic profiles of various plant species through RP-HPLC, mass spectrometric techniques have recently gained a considerable advancement in the analysis of complex biological matrices, and thus in evaluating the bioactivity and nutraceutical potential of plants [20,23,84,85].

Due to noise reduction, and improved detection sensitivities and method specificities, these techniques require minimal sample preparation by dilution. Thus, the limitations of LC-UV methods, such as the presence of interferences in complex samples and the high levels of detection and quantification limits, have been overcome [23,84]. Mass spectrometry is currently the most sensitive method of structural analysis, consisting in the ionization of the investigated chemical substances followed by the separation of the ions according to the mass to charge ratio. The mass spectrum represents the plot of the ions' relative abundances versus their mass to charge ratio, and is a characteristic of each compound [20].

4.2.1. Liquid Chromatography (LC) Tandem Low-Resolution Mass Spectrometry

Liquid chromatography (LC) coupled with single–quadruple low-resolution mass spectrometry, or more often, with tandem mass spectrometry (MS-MS) using ion trap spectrometers (IT) [84] or triple quadrupole (QQQ) [23,86-88], is common in targeted screening and quantification methods for polyphenols. The comparative study of the theoretical mass and fragmentation patterns of the reference standards vs. target compounds is used to unequivocally confirm the identity of polyphenolic compounds in "targeted" analysis. However, due to the limited availability of analytical standards, a limited number of compounds can be identified and quantified using this approach.

Four MS scan approaches are possible, and all can generate valuable information: (i) Full scan (FS) and (ii) selective ion monitoring (SIM) represent the most common data acquisition modes in methods without fragmentation. Confirmatory analysis uses the monitoring of the fragment ions through (iii) product reaction monitoring (PRM) or (iv) multiple reactions monitoring (MRM), which monitor all ion fragments resulting from a single selected precursor ion (MS^2 spectra) [86].

The most common ionization source in the LC-MS analysis of polyphenols is electrospray ionization (ESI) in the negative mode, providing the deprotonated molecule $[M-H]^-$ [86]. ESI in the positive ionization mode has also been proposed in various applications [89].

For the chromatographic separation of polyphenols, prior to spectrometric analysis, reverse phase chromatography (RP-LC) using the stationary phases C18 and C8 is the most commonly used in LC-MS. Short columns (e.g., 150 mm for HPLC and 100 mm for UHPLC) with small particle diameters (e.g., 5 μm for HPLC or between 1.8 and 2.6 μm for UHPLC) are generally preferred [23,87,90]. Mixtures of ultrapure water acidified with formic acid or acetic acid 0.05–0.5% and methanol or acetonitrile as organic solvents (often acidified with formic acid or acetic acid) are usually used as mobile phases [20,23]. The addition of 0.1% trifluoroacetic acid can result in improved peak separation, tailing reduction and superior peak symmetry [20].

For adequate detection of the analytes, the parameters of the ESI ion source (nebulizing gas flow, their temperature, voltage and source temperature, declustering potential, etc.) as well as the different parameters of the MS instrument (e.g., collision energy) are optimized by injection of analytical standards.

Liquid chromatography (LC) tandem low-resolution mass spectrometry has recently been used in various targeted analyses of polyphenols in alfalfa (*Medicago sativa* L.), lavender (*Lavandula spica* L.), buckwheat (*Fagopyrum esculentum*), phacelia (*Phacelia tanacetifolia* Benth.) and licorice (*Glycyrrhiza glabra*) root extract [23], Chinese rose (*Dalbergia odorifera*) used in traditional Chinese medicine [88], red clover (*Trifolium pratense* L.) extract [87], and green, black and oolong tea (*Camellia sinensis*) [89] (Table 2).

4.2.2. Non-Targeted High-Resolution Mass Spectrometry Use in "Chemical Profiling"

Although low-resolution mass spectrometry is still used for the identification and quantification of polyphenols in different vegetal matrices, particularly food, high-resolution mass spectrometry (HRMS), represented by quadrupole–flight time spectrometry (Q-TOF) and quadrupole–Orbitrap technologies, have recently gained popularity due to their ability to provide complete information on the exact molecular mass, elemental composition and chemical structure of a given compound [91,92].

The exact mass provided by high-resolution mass spectrometry with a mass error ≤ 2 ppm is currently the ideal tool for the structural characterization of the compounds in various applications, including polyphenols identification [91]. In the MS/MS tandem analysis, the quasi-molecular ion [M-H]− or [M-H]+ fragmentation model can be studied by the retro-Diels–Alder reaction (rDA) or other fragmentation models [91,92].

For polyphenols' analysis, the negative ionization mode provides more characteristic fragments than positive ionization [93–95]. A fragmentation pattern characterized by loss of the carboxylic fraction (CO_2, 44 Da) is observed for phenolic acids. The remaining skeleton showed the ion [MH]− at m/z 137.02 ($C_7H_5O_3$), and in the MS/MS spectra, the fragment [MH-COOH]− at m/z 93.03 (C_6H_5O) is generated [91]. The loss of a hydroxyl radical leads to the fragment m/z 107.01, visible in several such compounds [91].

For O-glycosylated flavonoids, the cleavage to the neutral glycosidic residue is characteristic in both positive and negative ionization modes, resulting in fragments such as 162 Da (glucose), 132 Da (pentose), 146 Da (deoxyhexose), 146 Da (rhamnosis), 180 Da (glucopyranose) and 308 Da (rutinoside) [92]. In aglycones flavonoids, two characteristic fragmentation pathways can be distinguished: ring heterocyclization and gradual degradation of the molecule [92].

Thus, for negatively ionized flavones, isoflavones, flavonols and flavanones, the MS-MS ion spectra show fragmentation following the retro-Diels–Alder reaction path to the C ring, leading to = molecule cleavage at bonds 1 and 3 (Figure 1). Two product ions containing intact A and B rings result [91–93].

On the other hand, small radical losses such as CO and CO_2, H_2O, CH_2-CO, and CH_4O were observed [91,92,95]. The fragments resulting from the rDA reaction are particularly useful for elucidating the structure, because they allow not only the positioning of the OH-group, but also for the identification of the position of glycosidic bonds. March et al. [94] proposed an intermediate structure of the C ring, which successfully explained the mechanism of CO_2 removal at the C ring in the negative ionization of isoflavone-glycoside. Fabre et al. [95] found a loss in ketene moiety (C_2H_2O) in flavones and flavanones at the C ring following fragmentation due to the low probability of rearrangement, whereas Kang et al. [86] showed that the loss of ketene occurs at ring A for isoflavones.

Table 2. Examples of the target screening methods used for the identification/quantification of the selected polyphenols.

Plant Material	Extraction	Hyphenated Technique Used	Instrumental Methodology (HPLC Condition, Ionization, Acquisition Mode)	Selected Polyphenols	Ref.
Flowers, leaves, and stalks of alfalfa (*Medicago sativa* L.) and goldenrod (*Solidago virgaurea* L.); flowers, leaves, stalks, and roots of phacelia (*Phacelia tanacetifolia* Benth.); buckwheat (*Fagopyrum esculentum*); licorice root (*Glycyrrhiza glabra*); and lavender flower (*Lavandula spica* L.)	solid–liquid extraction (SLE) consecutively using H₂O, mixture H₂O/EtOH (1:1; *v/v*), mixture H₂O/MeOH (1:1; *v/v*), and finally NeOH shaking for 5 h; SPE purification using a C18 column	UHPLC-MS/MS	Zorbax Eclipse XDB-C18 column (50 × 2.1 mm, 1.8 μm); mobile phase: 0.1% *v/v* formic acid in water and ACN; ESI ionization source in negative mode, acquisition in selected reactions monitoring mode, SRM	3-(4-hydroxyphenyl) propionic acid, 4-hydroxybenzoic acid, 3,4-dihydroxybenzoic acid, quercetin, rutin, glabridin, and naringenin	[23]
Edible lotus (*Nelumbo nucifera*) rhizome knot	Enzymatic hydrolysis with cellulose and pectinase, at 62 °C, pH 4, 90 min followed by ultrafiltration	HPLC-QqQ-MS/MS	ZORBAX Eclipse XDB-C18 column (150 mm × 4.6 mm, 5 μm; mobile phase: aqueous 0.4% acetic acid, and acetonitrile; ESI in negative ion mode Acquisition in MRM mode	chlorogenic acid, B-type procyanidin dimer, (+)-catechin, B-type procyanidin dimer, gallate, caffeic acid, (−)-epicatechin-3-gallate, (−)-epicatechin, propyl and rutin	[43]
Trifolium pratense L. (Red Clover), dried leaves	MAE, 300 W, with MeOH at 70 °C	HPLC-ESI-MS/MS	Zorbax Eclipse XDB-C18 50 mm × 4.6 mm × 1.8 μm column; mobile phase: 0.05% aqueous formic acid and MeOH; ESI ionisation source in negative mode, acquisition in SRM	43 phenolic including: genistein, daidzein, p-hydroxy-benzoic acid, caffeic acids, kaempferol 3-O-glucoside, quercetin 3-O-glucoside, hyperoside	[87]
Heartwood samples of *Dalbergia odorifera* (medicinal herbs in TCM);	UAE with 70% methanol (*v/v*) for 45 min	UHPLC-QqQ-MS/MS and UHPLC-Q/TOF-MS/MS	Acquity HSS T3 column (100 mm × 2.1 mm, 1.8 μm); mobile phase: ACN and water containing 0.05% formic acid ESI negative ion mode. Acquisition in MRM mode for QqQ analysis.	17 flavonoids including: daidzein, dalbergin, 30-hydroxydaidein, liquiritigenin, isoliquiritigenin, alpinetin, butein, naringenin, butin, prunetin, eriodictyol, tectorigenin, pinocembrin, formononetin, genistein, sativanone	[88]
Green, black and oolong tea (*Camellia sinensis*)	Extraction at high temperature (80 °C) for 3 min with mild stirring	HPLC-QqQ-MS/MS	Capcell Pak C18 MGIII (2.0 mm × 100 mm, 3 m) column; ESI in positive and negative ion mode. Acquisition in MRM mode.	gallocatechin, epigallocatechin, catechin, epigallocatechin gallate, epicatechin, gallocatechin gallate, epicatechin gallate, catechin gallate, theaflavin, theaflavin-3-gallate, theaflavin-3′-gallate; theaflavin-3,3′-digallate.	[89]
Sour Guava (*Psidium friedrichsthalianum* Nied) lyophilized whole fruits	UAE of lyophilized fruits with acetone:water (7:3). The extract was submitted to successive partitions with ethyl ether, ethyl acetate, and N-butanol.	UPLC-ESI/QqQ-MS/MS	UPLC BEH C18-column (2.1 × 100 mm, 1.7 μm); mobile phase water/formic acid (99.9:0.1, *v/v*) and ACN/formic acid (99.9:0.1, *v/v*) ESI ionization source in negative mode. Acquisition in MRM	22 phenolic compounds including several hydroxybenzoic, phenylacetic, and hydroxycinnamic acid derivatives	[90]
Barks of *Connarus* var. *angustifolius*, and leaves of *Cecropia obtusa*, *Cecropia palmata* and *Mansoa alliacea*; dried samples	UAE in 70% hydroethanolic, butanol/ethyl acetate, 4 h Butanol and ethyl acetate were evaporated at 40 °C	HPLC-ESI/QqQ-MS/MS	SB-C18 Rapid Resolution HD column (2.1 × 50 mm, 1.8 μm; mobile phase 0.1% acetic acid in water and ACN; ESI ionization source in negative mode Acquisition in MRM	gallic acid, catechin, caffeic acid, rutin, ferulic acid, quercitrin and resveratrol	[96]

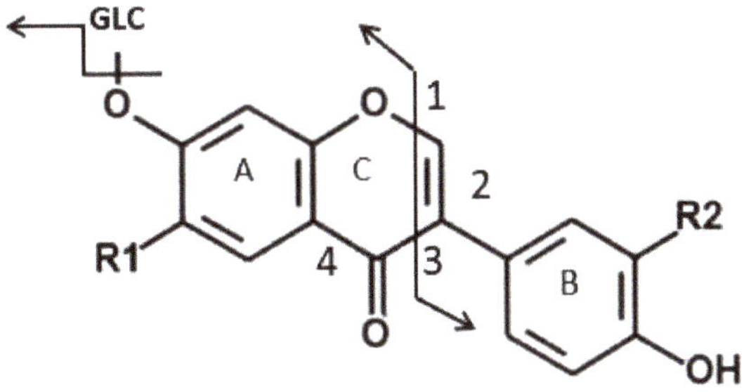

Figure 1. The proposed fragmentation model for flavonoids following the retro-Diels–Alder path to the C ring (after Gao et al. [91]).

In addition, the ion $[MH-C_3O_2]^-$ has shown a relatively high abundance in flavonones fragmentation (luteolin, apigenin, genistein), it being one of the key ions for the differentiation of isobaric compounds apigenin and genistein. The subsequent fragmentation MS^3 of this ion from the apigenin showed the ion $[MH-2C_3O_2]$ resulting from the loss of another C_3O_2 fragment, and in genistein the loss of CO from $[MH-C_3O_2]$ was displayed [97].

For methoxylated flavonoids (biochanin, formononetin, prunetin, calicosin, glycitein), the $[M-H-CH_3]^-$ ion is characteristic of negative ionization [94]. The ionic fragments CH_3, CHO, and CO_2, resulting from successive or simultaneous losses, are attributed to the type of isoflavone [4'-OCH₃], [86,97]. In addition, for isoflavones containing a hydroxyl group or a methoxy- group at the B ring, a relatively highly abundant fragment ion at m/z 132 was detected and assigned to [0.3B-2H]- for prunetin and glycitein, and [0.3B-CH₃-H]- for formononetin and biochanin A [86,97]. The fragment ion at m/z 117 indicates the presence of a hydroxyl group at ring B or in position 3. On the other hand, the fragments $[MH-CH_3-CO]$ are characteristic of methoxilates isoflavones, CO loss being subsequent to radical loss $[CH_3]$. The fragment $[MH-CH_3-CO-B-ring]$ was found to be characteristic of the distinction between glycitein and other isomers as collision energy increases [98]. Thus, the mass spectral decomposition of polyphenols under ESI-HRMSⁿ allows a structural characterization of the corresponding compounds by assigning specific key ions.

Analytical approaches based on HRMS have been successfully applied for polyphenols profiling in herbal remedies from traditional Chinese medicine, such as Dingkun Dan [91] or *Aster tartaricus* risoma [99], rare plants such as *Ophryosporus triangularis* (native to the Acatama Desert, Chile) [100], or common plants, e.g., culinary herbs [22], green tea products [101], leaves of green perilla [102], pomegranates [103] and goji [104] (Table 3).

Table 3. Examples of the non-target screening methods used for chemical profiling of the plant extracts.

Plant Material	Extraction	Hyphenated Technique Used	Instrumental Methodology (LC Condition, Ionization, Acquisition Mode)	Data Processing Approach Used for Tentatively Identification	Ref.
Ground dried culinary herbs and spices: dill (*Anethum graveolens*), marjoram (*Origanum majorana*), turmeric (*Curcuma longa*), caraway (*Carum carvi*), and nutmeg (*Myristica fragans*)	UAE with 5 mL of 50% ethanol in 0.1% formic acid in ultrapure water; 5 min	UHPLC–LTQ Orbitrap MS	Atlantis T3 C18 (100 × 2.1 mm, 3 μm) column; mobile phase; 1% formic acid in water and 0.1% formic acid in ACN. Full scan MS mode at 60,000 FWHM and MS/MS mode with the Orbitrap at 30,000 FWHM DDA scan.	In-house database Comparison with HR-MS data found in literature PCA, HCA	[22]
Dingkun Dan (traditional Chinese medicine prescription)	Ultrasonic extraction with MeOH, 30 min	UHPLC-Q/Orbitrap –HRMS/MS	Acquity T3 (2.1 × 100 mm, 1.8 μm) column; mobile phase: 0.1% formic acid in water (A) and 0.1% formic acid in MeOH. HESI II ionization source in positive and negative mode; collision energy: 25–60 V. Data-dependent acquisition (DDA).	In-house database Searching in Chemspider; Pubchem.	[91]
Aster tataricus rhizoma	UAE with MeOH for 30 min	UHPLC-Q-TOF-MS	Poroshell 120 EC-C18 column (100 mm × 2.1 mm, 2.6 μm); mobile phase: water + 0.1% formic acid and ACN + 0.1% formic acid. ESI source in both positive and negative ion mode. DDA and IDA acquisition methods. Multiple mass defect filter (MMDF) and dynamic background subtraction (DBS) by AB Sciex software	Searching for reported metabolites; in-house database. Searching in Chemspider database using MasterView™ 1.0. Product ions strategy (KPIs). Clog P (calculated by Chemdraw Ultra 12.0 software)—used for distinguishing isomers.	[99]
Ophryosporus triangularis Meyen, dried aerial parts (leaves and stems) and flowers	UAE with MeOH, 30 min	UHPLC-Q-Orbitrap HRMS/MS	Acclaim UHPLC C18 column, (150 mm × 4.6 mm ID, 2.5 μm); mobile phases: 1% formic aqueous solution and ACN; HESI negative ionization mode; full scan at 70,000 FWHM followed by targeted MS/MS at −7,500 FWHM; collision energy (HCD cell)–30 kv	In-house database comparison with HR-MS data found in literature	[100]
Dried leaves of green perilla (*Perilla frutescens*)	Extraction with MeOH by shaking for 8 h at ambient temperature	LC–TOF-MS/MS	Poroshell 120 EC-C18 150 × 2.1 mm, I.D., 4 mm; mobile phase: 0.1% formic acid in water and MeOH; ESI source in negative ion mode; resolution of 2700; collision energy 10 eV.	The analyst TF software (version 1.7); identification of the compounds by comparison with previous studies. Tentatively characterized by fragmentation pathway identification.	[102]
Goji berries (*Lycium barbarum* L.)	Extraction in 1% formic acid in 80:20 methanol/water solution by centrifugation at 25,000 rpm/3 min	UHPLC-ESI-QTOF-MS	Zorbax eclipse plus C 8 column (50 × 2.1 mm, 1.8 μm); mobile phase: water and MeOH ESI ionisation source in positive; full scan MS² (30,000 FWHM); mass accuracy ≤ 5	Profinder B.07 software. Phenol-Explorer 3.6 database	[104]
Stellera chamaejasme extracts	reflux with MeOH for 30 min at 50 °C.	UHPLC-LTQ-Orbitrap MSⁿ	Agilent Zorbax Eclipse Plus C18 column (100 × 3.0 mm, 1.8 μm) at 50 °C; mobile phase water with 0.5% FA and ACN; HESI in positive and negative mode DDA, MSⁿ scan (four scans for MS² and one ion for MS³); resolution of M 32–60,000 and MS³–30,000; collision energy: MS²–30 V and MS³–35 V.	SciFinder database (https://scifinder.cas.org) for chemical formula annotation; comparison with HR-MS data found in literature	[105]

Table 3. *Cont.*

Plant Material	Extraction	Hyphenated Technique Used	Instrumental Methodology (LC Condition, Ionization, Acquisition Mode)	Data Processing Approach Used for Tentatively Identification	Ref.
The male flowers of date palm (*Phoenix dactylifera*)	Soxhlet extraction with 80% MeOH for 6 h at 50 °C, fractionation in a C18 column	HPLC-ESI-ITMS	Symmetry C18 column (5 μm, 2.1 mm × 150 mm; mobile phase: ACN containing 0.03% (v/v) formic acid and water containing 0.03% (v/v) formic acid; ESI ion source in negative ion mode full-scan followed by MS-MS	Density functional theory (DFT) study	[106]
Mentha rotundifolia (L.) Huds, aerial parts	maceration in MeOH for 24 h at room temperature	UHPLC-ESI-Q-Orbitrap-HRMS/MS	Kromasil RP-18 column (250 mm 10 mm); mobile phase: water/ACN 75:25, 0.25% FA and ACN, 0.25% FA; HESI ionization source in negative mode; full MS followed by DDA scan	In-house database, confirmation by NMR approaches	[107]
Baoyuan decoction (traditional Chinese medicine formula)	reflux with water for 1.5 h	UHPLC-Q-TOF-MS/MS	Cortecs UPLC C18 column (1.6 μm, 2.1 × 100 mm; mobile phase: 0.05% aqueous formic acid and ACN containing 0.05% formic acid; ESI ionization in negative mode; DDA	UNIFI software. In-house database	[108]
The bark, twigs, leaves, and fruits of *Alnus japonica*, *Alnus hirsuta* and *Alnus hirsuta var. sibirica*	UAE with MeOH (1:10 g DW/g), 60 °C, 60 min, at 60 kHz	UHPLC-Q-TOF-MS/MS	Acquity BEH C18 (100 × 2.1 mm 1.7 μm) column; mobile phase: H₂O and MeCN, both of which were acidified with 0.1% formic acid; ESI ionization mode in negative ion; DDA (full MS followed by MS/MS scans for the three most intense ion).	Spectral preprocessing using MZmine; in silico annotation with network; annotation propagation GNPS molecular networking; integration of annotation data using MolNetEnhancer	[109]
Medicago sativa L. and *Trifolium pratense* L. dried sprouts	UAE with 70% ethanol (1:10 g DW/g), 60 °C, 60 min, at 60kHz	UHPLC-Q-Orbitrap HRMS/MS	Accucore U-HPLC Column C18 (150 × 2.1 mm, 2.6 μm); mobile phase: water containing 500 μL/L⁻¹ formic acid (pH 2.5) and MeOH; HESI ionization in negative mode; DIA (Full scan 70,000 FWHM, MS/MS 35,000 FWHM). Normalized collision energy: 30, 60 and 80 NCE	Chemspider database; NORMAN MassBank, mzCloude™ Advanced Mass Spectral Database; in silico fragmentation with ACD.Labs MS Fragmenter 2019.2.1 software	[110]
Blackcurrant (*Ribes nigrum* L.) leaves	UAE with ethanol/water (1:1), 20 °C, 60 min	ESI-LTQ-Orbitrap MS	Kinetex Evo C18 5 μm column; mobile phase: water + 0.1% formic acid and ACN + 0.1% formic acid. ESI source in negative ion mode. DDA	MZmine; PCA.	[111]
Persimmon leaves (Chinese traditional medicine)	UAE with methanol/water (80:20, v/v)	LC-ESI-LTQ-Orbitrap-MS	Atlantis T3 column 2.1 × 100 mm, 3 m; mobile phase water/0.1% formic acid and ACN; ESI source in both positive and negative ion mode; DDA approach–full scan at 30,000 FWHM and MS/MS at 15,000 FWHM; Collision energy (HCD cell)–35 kv	Identification by generating the molecular formula using accurate mass (C = 30, H = 100, O = 15), and matching with the isotopic pattern. Searching in polyphenol database: (http://phenol-explorer.eu/). Confirmation by comparison with HR-MS data in literature and databases	[112]
Flowers and leaves of Chilean Mistletoe (Quintral, *Tristerix tetrandus*)	Lyophilized flowers and leaves were defatted thrice with N-hexane (1:10) and then extracted by UAE with 0.1% HCl in MeOH (1:10) for 60 min. Purification with XAD-7 column.	UHPLC-Q/Orbitrap/HRMS/MS	UHPLC C18 Column, Acclaim, 150 mm × 4.6 mm ID, 5 μm. Mobile phase: 0.1% aqueous formic acid and ACN 0.1% formic acid. HESI II ionization source in positive and negative mode. Full scan MS (70,000 FWHM) acquisition followed by targeted MS/MS analysis (17,500 FWHM). Collision energy: 30 kv. Mass accuracy ≤ 5	Trace Finder 3.2 software	[113]

Hybrid mass spectrometers using linear ion capture technology, such as LTQ-Orbitrap, have also become common in this field. LTQ-Orbitrap provides the possibility of the screening, identification and structural characterization of unknown compounds using MS^n fragmentation [111,112]. For example, the UHPLC technique coupled with LTQ-Orbitrap has recently been used for the characterization of components in *Stellera chamaejasme* [105] and in blackcurrant leaves [111].

Regarding the methods' optimization, in the LC-HRMS/MS non-targeted screening analysis, resolution, scan rate and mass acquisition interval are the most critical parameters [99]. In addition to data acquisition modes also common in low-resolution spectrometry (SIM and MRM, PRM), new approaches such as data-dependent acquisition (DDA) and independent data acquisition (DIA) strategies, used so far only in proteomics, have recently been transposed into the analysis of small molecules in HRMS [110,114].

The limitation of the DDA strategy comes from the selection of precursors for MS/MS analysis [99]. Instead, in the recently developed independent data acquisition (DIA) strategy, all molecules within consecutive preselected m/z windows are subject to fragmentation, leading to higher specificity compared to the AIF (all ions fragmentation) approach [99,110]. As a disadvantage, the lack of precursor preselection can lead to impure mass spectra and low sensitivity. In this particular situation, the scan speed is the critical parameter [99,114].

In a recent study, Sun et al. [99] compared the DDA and DIA acquisition mode approaches using UHPLC-Q-TOF-MS technology for chemical characterization of the Aster tataricus rhizome, a traditional Chinese medicinal remedy. The key product ions strategy (KPIs) was used for the first time for searching for and identifying bioactive compounds. A total of 131 compounds, of which 31 were flavonoids, were identified or provisionally characterized. For the DDA setting, a complete scan and the ten most intense ion fragments from each analyte were applied to perform a TOF scan. For flavonoids, the ionic fragment m/z 153.0180 of kaempferol was used as the key ion in positive ionization. Based on the metabolic patterns of apigenin, isorhamnetin and kaempferol, several flavonoids were provisionally characterized: asapigenin-5-ramnoside, isorhamnetin-3-O-neohespeidoside, isorhamnetin-3-O-glucoside and biorobine (kaempferios 3-robin). The DDA strategy allowed the identification of 120 compounds, while 131 was identified by the DIA approach. However, certain glycosides identified in the DDA could not be detected by DIA [99].

The use of the DIA-MS strategy using an HRMS Q-Exactive Orbitrap instrument has recently been reported for the identification of polyphenols in extracts of red clover and alfalfa sprouts [110].

A workflow strategy in chemical profiling and metabolomics using HRMS technologies is shown in Figure 2.

Although HRMS non-target screening offers clear advantages, investigating the enormous amount of data produced by such techniques remains a challenge [110]. The identification of unknown compounds in complex samples always requires MS and MS/MS databases, and the evaluation of the exact mass of the ions obtained by HRMS (molecular ion, ionic fragments, isotopic models) for provisionally assigning the chemical formula based on the rules defined in organic chemistry or using designed software.

Practically, considering polyphenolic compounds, the potential elementary molecular compositions of the compounds are established as C, H and O, then molecular formulas calculated based on mass accuracy are generated with a reasonable degree of measurement error ($\leq$2 ppm). Based on molecular fragments and a "match" factor of 70%, presumptive compounds are selected from a database, such as the Chemspider, (http://www.chemspider.com/), Pub-chem, (https://pubchem.ncbi.nlm.nih.gov/) or SciFinder database (https://scifinder.cas.org) or the polyphenol database (http://phenol-explorer.eu/) [105,110,111].

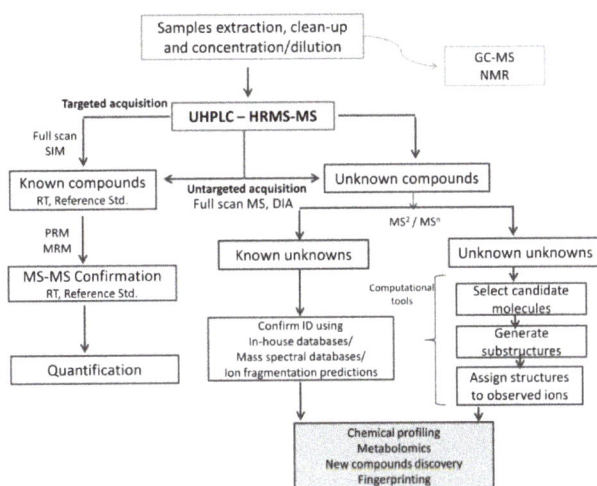

Figure 2. Workflow strategy in chemical profiling and metabolomics using HRMS technologies.

The comparison of the fragmentation patterns in MS-MS databases in the literature led to structure confirmation. There are currently various collections of public and private MS/MS mass spectra, such as NBS/EPA/NIH Mass Spectral Date Base, G.W.A. National Bureau of Standards Washinton; "eight peck index" at the Mass Spectrometry Data Center of Royal Society, Cambrige; Norman MassBank (https://massbank.eu/MassBank/); network clusters such as as mzCloudeTM (https://www.mycloud.com/#/); ReSpect, NIST (The National Institute of Standards and Technology; http://www.nist.gov/srd/nist1a.cfm) and Global Molecular Social Networking (GNPS). These allow users to compare the obtained MS-MS spectra with reference spectra for chemical structure annotation.

Spectrum processing and comparative analysis can be done manually, requiring extensive work and time, or automatically using software such as Compound Discoverer^{TM}, Trace Finder^{TM}, MassHunter, MasterView^{TM}, MZmine, MAGMa software, or MetabolitePilot^{TM}.

In addition, predictors of silico fragmentation, such as as software tools like ACD Labs MS Fragmenter or Mass Frontier^{TM}, are used to extend the primary annotation of presumptively identified molecules to the confirmation of the chemical structure [110].

Peak selection is one of the key steps in any non-target screening, and it can be done using a software algorithm (e.g., UNIFI platform by Waters Corporation). In the "suspect" compounds screening, the selection is made based on theoretical/predicted reference data. In non-target screening, presumptive peak identification can be performed when the signal strength for both the precursor ion and the fragments is sufficient to elucidate the molecular formula. Recently, Xu et al. [115] applied a UPLCQ-TOF-MSE method using data processing in the UNIFI computer platform for the determination of the chemical composition of Gandou decoction, a traditional Chinese medicine (TCM) formula. In total, 96 compounds, including flavonoids and phenolic acid, were identified or provisionally characterized based on retention time, exact mass (mass separation window of 5 ppm) and MS-MS fragmentation patterns [115].

In addition to MS databases, information on the environmental context (samples source, literature) may also be essential for the compounds' identification. As well, combined statistical approaches, including chemometrics and bioinformatics, are currently being used to identify unknown or new compounds [116].

Guo et al. [116] performed a chemical profiling of several Keemun black tea classes via LC-Orbitrap-MS/MS. Data were subsequently analyzed using multivariate metabolomics statistics (PCA and HCA), leading to the identification of tea class markers (theasinensin A, afzelechin galate and kaempferol-glucoside).

The reported studies have highlighted that the digitized analysis of MS/MS data significantly improves the phytochemical analysis. Moreover, it demonstrates that molecules with high complexity can be identified and chemically characterized only with specialized software tools and require highly qualified personnel.

4.3. Analysis of Phenolic Compounds in Plants by GC-MS Using Derivatization Techniques

Although the use of GC coupled with MS and tandem MS-MS has been proven a powerful analytical tool for natural products' characterization [117], there is a limited range of polyphenolic compounds that can be analyzed by GC-MS methods. Phenolic acids, phenolic aldehydes, ketones and phenolic alcohols were recently analyzed by GC-MS in wild plant fruits [117], fruit samples [36,118], *Curcuma caesia Roxb* [119], Kodo millet (*Paspalum scrobiculatum*) [120], and *Scambiosa Columbabria* L. [121]. Although newer two-dimensional GC x GC systems improved the separation performance and resolution [122], currently, the GC-MS technique is less commonly employed mainly because complex sample pre-treatments are required to increase the volatility and stability of the phenolic compounds. In addition to sample extraction and clean-up, a previous chemical derivatization step is needed to convert the hydroxyl groups to ethers, or make esters more volatile and thermostable.

Among the variety of derivation reagents, the most used is the trialkylsilyl, substituting the active hydrogen in alcohols and other polar organic compounds by the trimethylsilyl (TMS) group, $-Si(CH_3)_3$. N,O-bis-(trimethylsilyl)trifluoroacetamide (BSTFA), N,O-bis-(trimethylsilyl)acetamide (BSA), *N*-methyl-*N*-(trimethylsilyl)trifluoroacetamide (MSTFA) and *N*-[dimethyl-(2-methyl-2-propyl)silyl]-2,2,2-trifluoro-*N*-methylacetamide (MTBSTFA) are the most commonly used reagents [118,122]. Regarding the chromatographic conditions, fused silica capillary columns with lengths ranging from 25 to 30 m and inner dimensions from 0.25 to 0.5 mm, coated with 5% phenyl-95% dimethylpolysiloxane, are commonly used. The temperature gradients use initial column temperatures ranging from 40 to 80 °C, and final temperatures between 200 and 370 °C, with increasing rates ranging from 2 to 50 °C/min. High-purity helium is commonly used as a carrier gas at a flow-rate ranging from 0.4 to 3 mL/min, although high-purity hydrogen has also been used. Usually, GC-MS systems use the electron ionization (EI) mode prior to quadrupole MS quadrupole ion trap (QIT) and time-of-flight (TOF) analyzers [118,122].

4.4. Metabolomic Analysis of Polyphenolc Using Nuclear Magnetic Resonance Spectroscopy

Nuclear magnetic resonance (NMR) spectroscopy and high-resolution mass spectrometry (HRMS) are currently the main analytical methods applied in metabolomics studies [123]. Both techniques can enable two approaches for "profiling" studies: a non-targeted approach using chemometric analysis; and a targeted approach for the identification and quantification of known compounds in the plant extract [123,124]. Both techniques have met the requirements of metabolomics by being able to provide information that can lead to molecular structure characterization.

One of the disadvantages of HRMS compared to NMR is the complexity of operations, including elaborate sample preparation, chromatographic separation, molecule fragmentation, and extensive data processing, all of which requiring highly qualified personnel. In addition, because of the complexity and variability of the factors that influence the analysis, analytical protocols are difficult to standardize. Although less sensitive than mass spectrometry, NMR is highly reproducible, allowing the operations' standardization [124]. Due to the distinct advantages of each method, NMR and HRMS are considered complementary techniques for the characterization of plant extracts [123].

Various open databases for the metabolites' identification are currently being developed, such as the Human Metabolism Database (http://www.hmdb.ca), and the Biological Magnetic Resonance Databank (BMB) (http://www.bmrb.wisc.edu/). However, most of these databases contain information on human metabolites and very few resources for the identification of secondary metabolites of plants [74].

In NMR spectroscopy, the intensity of the peaks is directly proportional to the number of atomic nuclei, and hence, in combination with chemometric analysis, NMR is currently used to classify plant samples according to species, origin, processing, age or other quality parameters, based on the NMR profiles [74]. The main approach of metabolomics is to compare two data sets (for example, in the case of plant matrices several species of the same genus) and, through data filtering and multivariate analysis (PCA) techniques, a discrimination between these two data sets is performed. This process highlights any differences between the data and aims to identify the compounds responsible for this differentiation [74].

A typical NMR workflow for the identification of unknown compounds in natural extracts involves the collection of fractions containing the metabolites of interest after chromatographic separation followed by off-line NMR analysis. RMB databases and computational methods, such as the prediction and simulation software PERCH, or StrucEluc from ACD Labs, in combination with complete 1 H NMR iterative full-spin analysis (HiFSA approach), provide an accurate distinction between the natural compounds with almost identical NMR spectra. In addition, computer-assisted structural elucidation (CASE) is a methodology that allows users to enter NMR data and identify clusters by comparison algorithms [123–125].

Using an integrated approach (HPLC-DAD-MS/MS) and nuclear magnetic resonance (NMR) techniques, four derivatives of ellagic acid (ellagic hexoside, ellagic pentoside, methyl ellagic deoxiexoside acid, 4- (alpha-Ramnopyranosyl) ellagic acid (eschweilenol C)) were characterized for the first time in the biomass of Brazil nuts, *Bertholletia excelsa Bonpl.* (*Lecythidaceae*) [123]. A triple-quadrupole negative ionization was used for MS analysis, and NMR analysis was performed after an SPE fractionation of the plant extract.

5. Conclusions

Currently, the complete characterization of the chemical profiles of medicinal plants, functional foods and other nutraceuticals, and the identification of their secondary metabolites, is becoming more and more important for better understanding the biochemical and pharmacological actions, as well as the curative/preventive potential.

Recent instrumental developments have resulted in improved chromatographic resolution and MS detection (higher sensitivity, acquisition speed, resolution and mass accuracy). Due to the differences in the fragmentation mechanisms of the $[M + H]+$ and $[M - H]-$ ions, the fragmentation patterns in the MS-MS analysis reflect the structural properties of the polyphenolic compounds and allow their identification in complex plant matrices.

Due to the high mass accuracy, high-resolution MS-MS spectra are particularly useful for identifying polyphenols in plant extracts, establishing new applications in metabolomics and complex phytochemical analysis.

Thus, current technologies enable targeted and non-targeted analysis, and are able to provide the chemical characterization of unknown compounds, chemical profiling and metabolomics in various plant. Chemometric analysis is also a powerful tool that can be used in the preliminary stages of analytical methods optimization, but is also efficient in data processing.

These new approaches may be the key to the analysis of polyphenols, although there are challenges in identifying and annotating those compounds due to the limited availability of analytical standards and structural diversity.

Author Contributions: Conceptualization, E.R.C. and C.L.C.; methodology, E.R.C.; investigation, E.R.C., C.L.C.; resources, E.R.C., C.E.G., R.P.S.; data curation, E.R.C., C.L.C., E.-I.G.; writing—original draft preparation, E.R.C.; writing—review and editing, E.R.C., C.L.C., E.-I.G., R.B.; visualization, E.-I.G., C.E.G., R.P.S.; supervision, R.B. All authors have read and agreed to the published version of the manuscript.

Funding: This research received no external funding.

Separations **2021**, *8*, 65

Institutional Review Board Statement: Not applicable.

Informed Consent Statement: Not applicable.

Data Availability Statement: Not applicable.

Conflicts of Interest: The authors declare no conflict of interest.

References

1. Sun, Z.; Zuo, L.; Sun, T.; Tang, J.; Ding, D.; Zhou, L.; Kang, J.; Zhang, X. Chemical Profiling and Quantification of XueBiJing Injection, a Systematic Quality Control Strategy Using UHPLC-Q Exactive Hybrid Quadrupole-Orbitrap High-Resolution Mass Spectrometry. *Sci. Rep.* **2017**, *7*, 16921. [CrossRef]
2. Pardo-Mates, N.; Vera, A.; Barbosa, S.; Hidalgo-Serrano, M.; Núñez, O.; Saurina, J.; Hernández-Cassou, S.; Puignou, L. Characterization, Classification and Authentication of Fruit-Based Extracts by Means of HPLC-UV Chromatographic Fingerprints, Polyphenolic Profiles and Chemometric Methods. *Food Chem.* **2017**, *221*, 29–38. [CrossRef]
3. Baranowska, I.; Bajkacz, S. A New UHPLC-MS/MS Method for the Determination of Flavonoids in Supplements and DPPH-UHPLC-UV Method for the Evaluation of the Radical Scavenging Activity of Flavonoids. *Food Chem.* **2018**, *256*, 333–341. [CrossRef]
4. Chen, L.-R.; Ko, N.-Y.; Chen, K.-H. Isoflavone Supplements for Menopausal Women: A Systematic Review. *Nutrients* **2019**, *11*, 2649. [CrossRef]
5. Minatel, I.O.; Borges, C.V.; Ferreira, M.I.; Gomez, H.A.G.; Chen, C.-Y.O.; Lima, G.P.P. Phenolic Compounds: Functional Properties, Impact of Processing and Bioavailability. In *Phenolic Compounds: Biological Activity*; IntechOpen: London, UK, 2017; pp. 1–24. ISBN 978-953-51-2960-8. [CrossRef]
6. Fraga, C.G.; Croft, K.D.; Kennedy, D.O.; Tomás-Barberán, F.A. The Effects of Polyphenols and Other Bioactives on Human Health. *Food Funct.* **2019**, *10*, 514–528. [CrossRef]
7. Šatínský, D.; Jägerová, K.; Havlíková, L.; Solich, P. A New and Fast HPLC Method for Determination of Rutin, Troxerutin, Diosmin and Hesperidin in Food Supplements Using Fused-Core Column Technology. *Food Anal. Methods* **2013**, *6*, 1353–1360. [CrossRef]
8. Bidlack, W.R.; Omaye, S.T.; Meskin, M.S.; Topham, D.K.W. *Phytochemicals as Bioactive Agents*; CRC Press: Boca Raton, FL, USA, 2000; ISBN 978-1-56676-788-0.
9. Veeresham, C. Natural Products Derived from Plants as a Source of Drugs. *J. Adv. Pharm. Technol. Res.* **2012**, *3*, 200–201. Available online: https://www.japtr.org/article.asp?issn=2231-4040;year=2012;volume=3;issue=4;spage=200;epage=201;aulast=Veeresham (accessed on 5 April 2021). [CrossRef] [PubMed]
10. Tomás-Barberán, F.A.; González-Sarrías, A.; García-Villalba, R. *Dietary Polyphenols: Metabolism and Health Effects*; John Wiley & Sons: Hoboken, NJ, USA, 2020; ISBN 978-1-119-56371-6.
11. Kim, H.-S.; Quon, M.J.; Kim, J. New Insights into the Mechanisms of Polyphenols beyond Antioxidant Properties; Lessons from the Green Tea Polyphenol, Epigallocatechin 3-Gallate. *Redox Biol.* **2014**, *2*, 187–195. [CrossRef]
12. Li, A.N.; Li, S.; Zhang, Y.-J.; Xu, X.-R.; Chen, Y.-M.; Li, H.-B. Resources and Biological Activities of Natural Polyphenols. *Nutrients* **2014**, *6*, 6020–6047. [CrossRef]
13. Granado-Lorencio, F.; Hernández-Alvarez, E. Functional Foods and Health Effects: A Nutritional Biochemistry Perspective. *Curr. Med. Chem.* **2016**, *23*, 2929–2957. [CrossRef]
14. Sarian, M.N.; Ahmed, Q.U.; Mat So'ad, S.Z.; Alhassan, A.M.; Murugesu, S.; Perumal, V.; Syed Mohamad, S.N.A.; Khatib, A.; Latip, J. Antioxidant and Antidiabetic Effects of Flavonoids: A Structure-Activity Relationship Based Study. *BioMed Res. Int.* **2017**, *2017*, 8386065. [CrossRef]
15. Goszcz, K.; Duthie, G.G.; Stewart, D.; Leslie, S.J.; Megson, I.L. Bioactive Polyphenols and Cardiovascular Disease: Chemical Antagonists, Pharmacological Agents or Xenobiotics That Drive an Adaptive Response? *Br. J. Pharmacol.* **2017**, *174*, 1209–1225. [CrossRef] [PubMed]
16. Plaza, M.; Domínguez-Rodríguez, G.; Castro-Puyana, M.; Marina, M.L. 6—Polyphenols analysis and related challenges. In *Polyphenols: Properties, Recovery, and Applications*; Galanakis, C.M., Ed.; Woodhead Publishing: Cambridge, UK, 2018; pp. 177–232. ISBN 978-0-12-813572-3.
17. European Pharmacopoeia (Ph. Eur.) 10th Edition | EDQM—European Directorate for the Quality of Medicines. Available online: https://www.edqm.eu/en/european-pharmacopoeia-ph-eur-10th-edition (accessed on 5 April 2021).
18. Vural, N.; Cavuldak, Ö.A.; Anlı, R.E. Multi Response Optimisation of Polyphenol Extraction Conditions from Grape Seeds by Using Ultrasound Assisted Extraction (UAE). *Sep. Sci. Technol.* **2018**, *53*, 1540–1551. [CrossRef]
19. Oreopoulou, A.; Tsimogiannis, D.; Oreopoulou, V. Chapter 15—Extraction of Polyphenols From Aromatic and Medicinal Plants: An Overview of the Methods and the Effect of Extraction Parameters. In *Polyphenols in Plants*, 2nd ed.; Watson, R.R., Ed.; Academic Press: Cambridge, MA, USA, 2019; pp. 243–259, ISBN 978-0-12-813768-0.
20. López-Fernández, O.; Domínguez, R.; Pateiro, M.; Munekata, P.E.S.; Rocchetti, G.; Lorenzo, J.M. Determination of Polyphenols Using Liquid Chromatography–Tandem Mass Spectrometry Technique (LC–MS/MS): A Review. *Antioxidants* **2020**, *9*, 479. [CrossRef]

21. Zhong, L.; Liu, Y.; Xiong, B.; Chen, L.; Zhang, Y.; Li, C. Optimization of Ultrasound-Assisted Extraction of Total Flavonoids from Dendranthema Indicum Var. Aromaticum by Response Surface Methodology. *J. Anal. Methods Chem.* **2019**, *2019*, e1648782. [CrossRef]

22. Vallverdú-Queralt, A.; Regueiro, J.; Alvarenga, J.F.R.; Martinez-Huelamo, M.; Leal, L.N.; Lamuela-Raventos, R.M.; Vallverdú-Queralt, A.; Regueiro, J.; Alvarenga, J.F.R.; Martinez-Huelamo, M.; et al. Characterization of the Phenolic and Antioxidant Profiles of Selected Culinary Herbs and Spices: Caraway, Turmeric, Dill, Marjoram and Nutmeg. *Food Sci. Technol.* **2015**, *35*, 189–195. [CrossRef]

23. Bajkacz, S.; Baranowska, I.; Buszewski, B.; Kowalski, B.; Ligor, M. Determination of Flavonoids and Phenolic Acids in Plant Materials Using SLE-SPE-UHPLC-MS/MS Method. *Food Anal. Methods* **2018**, *11*, 3563–3575. [CrossRef]

24. Phenolics in Foods: Extraction, Analysis and Measurements | IntechOpen. Available online: https://www.intechopen.com/books/phenolic-compounds-natural-sources-importance-and-applications/phenolics-in-foods-extraction-analysis-and-measurements (accessed on 5 April 2021).

25. Ameer, K.; Shahbaz, H.M.; Kwon, J.-H. Green Extraction Methods for Polyphenols from Plant Matrices and Their Byproducts: A Review. *Compr. Rev. Food Sci. Food Saf.* **2017**, *16*, 295–315. [CrossRef]

26. Machado, A.P.D.F.; Pasquel-Reátegui, J.L.; Barbero, G.F.; Martínez, J. Pressurized Liquid Extraction of Bioactive Compounds from Blackberry (*Rubus fruticosus* L.) Residues: A Comparison with Conventional Methods. *Food Res. Int.* **2015**, *77*, 675–683. [CrossRef]

27. Dahmoune, F.; Nayak, B.; Moussi, K.; Remini, H.; Madani, K. Optimization of Microwave-Assisted Extraction of Polyphenols from *Myrtus communis* L. Leaves. *Food Chem.* **2015**, *166*, 585–595. [CrossRef]

28. Lovrić, V.; Putnik, P.; Bursać Kovačević, D.; Jukić, M.; Dragović-Uzelac, V. Effect of Microwave-Assisted Extraction on the Phenolic Compounds and Antioxidant Capacity of Blackthorn Flowers. *Food Technol. Biotechnol.* **2017**, *55*, 243–250. [CrossRef] [PubMed]

29. Filip, S.; Pavlić, B.; Vidović, S.; Vladić, J.; Zeković, Z. Optimization of Microwave-Assisted Extraction of Polyphenolic Compounds from Ocimum Basilicum by Response Surface Methodology. *Food Anal. Methods* **2017**, *10*, 2270–2280. [CrossRef]

30. Vázquez-Espinosa, M.; Espada-Bellido, E.; González de Peredo, A.V.; Ferreiro-González, M.; Carrera, C.; Palma, M.; Barroso, C.G.; Barbero, G.F. Optimization of Microwave-Assisted Extraction for the Recovery of Bioactive Compounds from the Chilean Superfruit (*Aristotelia chilensis* (Mol.) Stuntz. *Agronomy* **2018**, *8*, 240. [CrossRef]

31. Kazemi, M.; Khodaiyan, F.; Labbafi, M.; Saeid Hosseini, S.; Hojjati, M. Pistachio Green Hull Pectin: Optimization of Microwave-Assisted Extraction and Evaluation of Its Physicochemical, Structural and Functional Properties. *Food Chem.* **2019**, *271*, 663–672. [CrossRef] [PubMed]

32. Chaves, J.; Souza, M.; Silva, L.; Lachos Perez, D.; Torres Mayanga, P.; Machado, A.; Forster-Carneiro, T.; Vázquez Espinosa, M.; Velasco González de Peredo, A.; Barbero, G.; et al. Extraction of Flavonoids From Natural Sources Using Modern Techniques. *Front. Chem.* **2020**, *8*, 507887. [CrossRef] [PubMed]

33. Calinescu, I.; Lavric, V.; Asofiei, I.; Gavrila, A.I.; Trifan, A.; Ighigeanu, D.; Martin, D.; Matei, C. Microwave Assisted Extraction of Polyphenols Using a Coaxial Antenna and a Cooling System. *Chem. Eng. Process. Process. Intensif.* **2017**, *122*, 373–379. [CrossRef]

34. Cai, Z.; Qu, Z.; Lan, Y.; Zhao, S.; Ma, X.; Wan, Q.; Jing, P.; Li, P. Conventional, Ultrasound-Assisted, and Accelerated-Solvent Extractions of Anthocyanins from Purple Sweet Potatoes. *Food Chem.* **2016**, *197*, 266–272. [CrossRef]

35. Viganó, J.; Brumer, I.Z.; Braga, P.A.D.C.; da Silva, J.K.; Maróstica Júnior, M.R.; Reyes Reyes, F.G.; Martínez, J. Pressurized Liquids Extraction as an Alternative Process to Readily Obtain Bioactive Compounds from Passion Fruit Rinds. *Food Bioprod. Process.* **2016**, *100*, 382–390. [CrossRef]

36. Barrales, F.M.; Silveira, P.; Barbosa, P.D.P.M.; Ruviaro, A.R.; Paulino, B.N.; Pastore, G.M.; Macedo, G.A.; Martinez, J. Recovery of Phenolic Compounds from Citrus By-Products Using Pressurized Liquids—An Application to Orange Peel. *Food Bioprod. Process.* **2018**, *112*, 9–21. [CrossRef]

37. Dobrinčić, A.; Repajić, M.; Garofulić, I.E.; Tuđen, L.; Dragović-Uzelac, V.; Levaj, B. Comparison of Different Extraction Methods for the Recovery of Olive Leaves Polyphenols. *Processes* **2020**, *8*, 1008. [CrossRef]

38. Garcia-Mendoza, M.D.P.; Espinosa-Pardo, F.A.; Baseggio, A.M.; Barbero, G.F.; Maróstica Junior, M.R.; Rostagno, M.A.; Martínez, J. Extraction of Phenolic Compounds and Anthocyanins from Juçara (*Euterpe edulis* Mart.) Residues Using Pressurized Liquids and Supercritical Fluids. *J. Supercrit. Fluids* **2017**, *119*, 9–16. [CrossRef]

39. Lachos-Perez, D.; Baseggio, A.M.; Torres-Mayanga, P.C.; Ávila, P.F.; Tompsett, G.A.; Marostica, M.; Goldbeck, R.; Timko, M.T.; Rostagno, M.; Martinez, J.; et al. Sequential Subcritical Water Process Applied to Orange Peel for the Recovery Flavanones and Sugars. *J. Supercrit. Fluids* **2020**, *160*, 104789. [CrossRef]

40. Da Silva, R.P.F.F.; Rocha-Santos, T.A.P.; Duarte, A.C. Supercritical Fluid Extraction of Bioactive Compounds. *TrAC Trends Anal. Chem.* **2016**, *76*, 40–51. [CrossRef]

41. King, J.W. Modern Supercritical Fluid Technology for Food Applications. *Annu. Rev. Food Sci. Technol.* **2014**, *5*, 215–238. [CrossRef]

42. Cvjetko Bubalo, M.; Vidović, S.; Radojčić Redovniković, I.; Jokić, S. New Perspective in Extraction of Plant Biologically Active Compounds by Green Solvents. *Food Bioprod. Process.* **2018**, *109*, 52–73. [CrossRef]

43. Zhu, Z.; Li, S.; He, J.; Thirumdas, R.; Montesano, D.; Barba, F.J. Enzyme-Assisted Extraction of Polyphenol from Edible Lotus (*Nelumbo nucifera*) Rhizome Knot: Ultra-Filtration Performance and HPLC-MS2 Profile. *Food Res. Int.* **2018**, *111*, 291–298. [CrossRef] [PubMed]

44. De Franco, E.P.D.; Contesini, F.J.; da Silva, B.L.; Fernandes, A.M.A.P.; Leme, C.W.; Cirino, J.P.G.; Campos, P.R.B.; Carvalho, P.D.O. Enzyme-Assisted Modification of Flavonoids from Matricaria Chamomilla: Antioxidant Activity and Inhibitory Effect on Digestive Enzymes. *J. Enzym. Inhib. Med. Chem.* **2020**, *35*, 42–49. [CrossRef] [PubMed]
45. Gligor, O.; Mocan, A.; Moldovan, C.; Locatelli, M.; Crişan, G.; Ferreira, I.C.F.R. Enzyme-Assisted Extractions of Polyphenols—A Comprehensive Review. *Trends Food Sci. Technol.* **2019**, *88*, 302–315. [CrossRef]
46. Domínguez-Rodríguez, G.; Marina, M.L.; Plaza, M. Strategies for the Extraction and Analysis of Non-Extractable Polyphenols from Plants. *J. Chromatogr. A* **2017**, *1514*, 1–15. [CrossRef]
47. Swer, T.L.; Mukhim, C.; Bashir, K.; Chauhan, K. Optimization of Enzyme Aided Extraction of Anthocyanins from *Prunus nepalensis* L. *LWT* **2018**, *91*, 382–390. [CrossRef]
48. Xiao, J.; Chen, G.; Li, N. Ionic Liquid Solutions as a Green Tool for the Extraction and Isolation of Natural Products. *Molecules* **2018**, *23*, 1765. [CrossRef]
49. Zhang, J.; Zong, A.; Xu, T.; Zhan, P.; Liu, L.; Qiu, B.; Liu, W.; Jia, M.; Du, F.; Tian, H. A Novel Method: Ionic Liquid-Based Ultrasound-Assisted Extraction of Polyphenols from Chinese Purple Yam. *Nat. Prod. Res.* **2018**, *32*, 863–866. [CrossRef]
50. Magiera, S.; Sobik, A. Ionic Liquid-Based Ultrasound-Assisted Extraction Coupled with Liquid Chromatography to Determine Isoflavones in Soy Foods. *J. Food Compos. Anal.* **2017**, *57*, 94–101. [CrossRef]
51. Sun, Y.; Li, W.; Wang, J. Ionic Liquid Based Ultrasonic Assisted Extraction of Isoflavones from Iris Tectorum Maxim and Subsequently Separation and Purification by High-Speed Counter-Current Chromatography. *J. Chromatogr. B* **2011**, *879*, 975–980. [CrossRef] [PubMed]
52. Wang, M.; Wang, J.; Zhou, Y.; Zhang, M.; Xia, Q.; Chen, D.Y. Ecofriendly Mechanochemical Extraction of Bioactive Compounds from Plants with Deep Eutectic Solvents. *ACS Sustain. Chem. Eng.* **2017**, *5*, 6297–6303. [CrossRef]
53. Izadiyan, P.; Hemmateenejad, B. Multi-Response Optimization of Factors Affecting Ultrasonic Assisted Extraction from Iranian Basil Using Central Composite Design. *Food Chem.* **2016**, *190*, 864–870. [CrossRef]
54. Fumic, B.; Jug, M.; Koncic, M.Z. Multi-Response Optimization of Ultrasound-Assisted Extraction of Bioactive Components from *Medicago sativa* L. *Croat. Chem. Acta* **2017**, *90*, 481–492. [CrossRef]
55. Skrypnik, L.; Novikova, A. Response Surface Modeling and Optimization of Polyphenols Extraction from Apple Pomace Based on Nonionic Emulsifiers. *Agronomy* **2020**, *10*, 92. [CrossRef]
56. Rodrigues, S.; Fernandes, F.A.N.; de Brito, E.S.; Sousa, A.D.; Narain, N. Ultrasound Extraction of Phenolics and Anthocyanins from Jabuticaba Peel. *Ind. Crops Prod.* **2015**, *69*, 400–407. [CrossRef]
57. Collison, M.W. Determination of Total Soy Isoflavones in Dietary Supplements, Supplement Ingredients, and Soy Foods by High-Performance Liquid Chromatography with Ultraviolet Detection: Collaborative Study. *J. AOAC Int.* **2008**, *91*, 489–500. [CrossRef]
58. Köseoğlu Yılmaz, P.; Kolak, U. SPE-HPLC Determination of Chlorogenic and Phenolic Acids in Coffee. *J. Chromatogr. Sci.* **2017**, *55*, 712–718. [CrossRef] [PubMed]
59. Ruiz, A.; Sanhueza, M.; Gómez, F.; Tereucán, G.; Valenzuela, T.; García, S.; Cornejo, P.; Hermosín-Gutiérrez, I. Changes in the Content of Anthocyanins, Flavonols, and Antioxidant Activity in Fragaria Ananassa Var. Camarosa Fruits under Traditional and Organic Fertilization. *J. Sci. Food Agric.* **2019**, *99*, 2404–2410. [CrossRef] [PubMed]
60. Ding, M.; Bai, Y.; Li, J.; Yang, X.; Wang, H.; Gao, X.; Chang, Y. A Diol-Based-Matrix Solid-Phase Dispersion Method for the Simultaneous Extraction and Determination of 13 Compounds From Angelicae Pubescentis Radix by Ultra High-Performance Liquid Chromatography. *Front. Pharmacol.* **2019**, *10*, 227. [CrossRef]
61. Senes, C.E.R.; Nicácio, A.E.; Rodrigues, C.A.; Manin, L.P.; Maldaner, L.; Visentainer, J.V. Evaluation of Dispersive Solid-Phase Extraction (d-SPE) as a Clean-up Step for Phenolic Compound Determination of Myrciaria Cauliflora Peel. *Food Anal. Methods* **2020**, *13*, 155–165. [CrossRef]
62. Aguiar, J.; Gonçalves, J.L.; Alves, V.L.; Câmara, J.S. Chemical Fingerprint of Free Polyphenols and Antioxidant Activity in Dietary Fruits and Vegetables Using a Non-Targeted Approach Based on QuEChERS Ultrasound-Assisted Extraction Combined with UHPLC-PDA. *Antioxidants* **2020**, *9*, 305. [CrossRef] [PubMed]
63. Nicácio, A.E.; Rodrigues, C.A.; Jardim, I.C.S.F.; Visentainer, J.V.; Maldaner, L. Modified QuEChERS Method for Phenolic Compounds Determination in Mustard Greens (*Brassica juncea*) Using UHPLC-MS/MS. *Arab. J. Chem.* **2020**, *13*, 4681–4690. [CrossRef]
64. Gleichenhagen, M.; Schieber, A. Current Challenges in Polyphenol Analytical Chemistry. *Curr. Opin. Food Sci.* **2016**, *7*, 43–49. [CrossRef]
65. Fotovvat, M.; Radjabian, T.; Saboora, A. HPLC Fingerprint of Important Phenolic Compounds in Some *Salvia* L. Species from Iran. *Rec. Nat. Prod.* **2018**, *13*. [CrossRef]
66. Lei, Y.; Wang, Y.; Sun, Z.; Lin, M.; Cai, X.; Huang, D.; Luo, K.; Tan, S.; Zhang, Y.; Yan, J.; et al. Quantitative Analysis of Multicomponents by Single Marker Combined with HPLC Fingerprint Qualitative Analyses for Comprehensive Evaluation of Aurantii Fructus. *J. Sep. Sci.* **2020**, *43*, 1382–1392. [CrossRef]
67. Yang, F.; Chu, T.; Zhang, Y.; Liu, X.; Sun, G.; Chen, Z. Quality Assessment of Licorice (*Glycyrrhiza glabra* L.) from Different Sources by Multiple Fingerprint Profiles Combined with Quantitative Analysis, Antioxidant Activity and Chemometric Methods. *Food Chem.* **2020**, *324*, 126854. [CrossRef]

68. FDA. *Guidance for Industry Botanical Drug Products*; Center for Drug Evaluation and Research (CDER); Food and Drug Administration: Silver Spring, MD, USA, 2016; p. 34.

69. SFDA State Drug Administration of China. Requirements for Studying Fingerprint of Traditional Chinese Medicine Injection (Draft). *Chin. Tradit. Pat. Med.* **2000**, *22*, 671–675.

70. WHO. *WHO Traditional Medicine Strategy 2002–2005*; WHO: Geneva, Switzerland, 2002.

71. Yu, S.; Zhu, L.; Xiao, Z.; Shen, J.; Li, J.; Lai, H.; Li, J.; Chen, H.; Zhao, Z.; Yi, T. Rapid Fingerprint Analysis of Flos Carthami by Ultra-Performance Liquid Chromatography and Similarity Evaluation. *J. Chromatogr. Sci.* **2016**, *54*, 1619–1624. [CrossRef] [PubMed]

72. Viapiana, A.; Struck-Lewicka, W.; Konieczynski, P.; Wesolowski, M.; Kaliszan, R. An Approach Based on HPLC-Fingerprint and Chemometrics to Quality Consistency Evaluation of *Matricaria chamomilla* L. Commercial Samples. *Front. Plant Sci.* **2016**, *7*, 1561. [CrossRef] [PubMed]

73. Hawrył, A.; Hawrył, M.; Waksmundzka-Hajnos, M. Liquid Chromatography Fingerprint Analysis and Antioxidant Activity of Selected Lavender Species with Chemometric Calculations. *PLoS ONE* **2019**, *14*, e0218974. [CrossRef] [PubMed]

74. Bansal, A.; Chhabra, V.; Rawal, R.K.; Sharma, S. Chemometrics: A New Scenario in Herbal Drug Standardization. *J. Pharm. Anal.* **2014**, *4*, 223–233. [CrossRef]

75. Li, J.; He, X.; Li, M.; Zhao, W.; Liu, L.; Kong, X. Chemical Fingerprint and Quantitative Analysis for Quality Control of Polyphenols Extracted from Pomegranate Peel by HPLC. *Food Chem.* **2015**, *176*, 7–11. [CrossRef]

76. Liu, D.; Mei, Q.; Long, W.; Wan, X.; Wan, D.; Wang, L. HPLC Fingerprint Analysis and Content Determination of Extract with Anticancer Activities of Sedi Linearis Herba. *Pharmacogn. J.* **2017**, *9*, 128–134. [CrossRef]

77. Pan, H.-B.; Zhang, D.; Li, B.; Wu, Y.-Y.; Tu, Y.-Y. A Rapid UPLC Method for Simultaneous Analysis of Caffeine and 13 Index Polyphenols in Black Tea. *J. Chromatogr. Sci.* **2017**, *55*, 495–496. [CrossRef]

78. Viapiana, A.; Wesolowski, M. HPLC Fingerprint Combined with Quantitation of Phenolic Compounds and Chemometrics as an Efficient Strategy for Quality Consistency Evaluation of Sambucus Nigra Berries. *Nat. Prod. Commun.* **2016**, *11*, 1449–1454. [CrossRef]

79. Li, W.; Zhang, X.; Chen, R.; Li, Y.; Miao, J.; Liu, G.; Lan, Y.; Chen, Y.; Cao, Y. HPLC Fingerprint Analysis of Phyllanthus Emblica Ethanol Extract and Their Antioxidant and Anti-Inflammatory Properties. *J. Ethnopharmacol.* **2020**, *254*, 112740. [CrossRef]

80. Barreira, J.C.M.; Visnevschi-Necrasov, T.; Nunes, E.; Cunha, S.C.; Pereira, G.; Oliveira, M.B.P.P. Medicago Spp. as Potential Sources of Bioactive Isoflavones: Characterization According to Phylogenetic and Phenologic Factors. *Phytochemistry* **2015**, *116*, 230–238. [CrossRef] [PubMed]

81. Ojo, O.A.; Ojo, A.B.; Ajiboye, B.O.; Olaiya, O.; Okesola, M.A.; Boligon, A.A.; de Campos, M.M.A.; Oyinloye, B.E.; Kappo, A.P. HPLC-DAD Fingerprinting Analysis, Antioxidant Activities of *Tithonia diversifolia* (Hemsl.) A. Gray Leaves and Its Inhibition of Key Enzymes Linked to Alzheimer's Disease. *Toxicol. Rep.* **2018**, *5*, 585–592. [CrossRef] [PubMed]

82. Wu, L.; Wu, W.; Cai, Y.; Li, C.; Wang, L. HPLC Fingerprinting-Based Multivariate Analysis of Phenolic Compounds in Mango Leaves Varieties: Correlation to Their Antioxidant Activity and in Silico α-Glucoidase Inhibitory Ability. *J. Pharm. Biomed. Anal.* **2020**, *191*, 113616. [CrossRef] [PubMed]

83. Cacciola, F.; Farnetti, S.; Dugo, P.; Marriott, P.J.; Mondello, L. Comprehensive Two-Dimensional Liquid Chromatography for Polyphenol Analysis in Foodstuffs. *J. Sep. Sci.* **2017**, *40*, 7–24. [CrossRef] [PubMed]

84. Llorent-Martínez, E.J.; Molina-García, L.; Ruiz-Medina, A.; Ortega-Barrales, P. Quantitation of Selected Polyphenols in Plant-Based Food Supplements by Liquid Chromatography–Ion Trap Mass Spectrometry. *Food Anal. Methods* **2014**, *7*, 2177–2183. [CrossRef]

85. Huang, F.-Q.; Dong, X.; Yin, X.; Fan, Y.; Fan, Y.; Mao, C.; Zhou, W. A Mass Spectrometry Database for Identification of Saponins in Plants. *J. Chromatogr. A* **2020**, *1625*, 461296. [CrossRef]

86. Kang, J.; Hick, L.A.; Price, W.E. A Fragmentation Study of Isoflavones in Negative Electrospray Ionization by MSn Ion Trap Mass Spectrometry and Triple Quadrupole Mass Spectrometry. *Rapid Commun. Mass Spectrom.* **2007**, *21*, 857–868. [CrossRef]

87. Vlaisavljević, S.; Kaurinović, B.; Popović, M.; Vasiljević, S. Profile of Phenolic Compounds in Trifolium Pratense L. Extracts at Different Growth Stages and Their Biological Activities. *Int. J. Food Prop.* **2017**, *20*, 3090–3101. [CrossRef]

88. Zhao, X.; Zhang, S.; Liu, D.; Yang, M.; Wei, J. Analysis of Flavonoids in Dalbergia Odorifera by Ultra-Performance Liquid Chromatography with Tandem Mass Spectrometry. *Molecules* **2020**, *25*, 389. [CrossRef]

89. Tao, W.; Zhou, Z.; Zhao, B.; Wei, T. Simultaneous Determination of Eight Catechins and Four Theaflavins in Green, Black and Oolong Tea Using New HPLC-MS-MS Method. *J. Pharm. Biomed. Anal.* **2016**, *131*, 140–145. [CrossRef]

90. Cuadrado-Silva, C.T.; Pozo-Bayón, M.Á.; Osorio, C. Targeted Metabolomic Analysis of Polyphenols with Antioxidant Activity in Sour Guava (*Psidium friedrichsthalianum* Nied.) Fruit. *Molecules* **2016**, *22*, 11. [CrossRef] [PubMed]

91. Gao, X.; Wang, N.; Jia, J.; Wang, P.; Zhang, A.; Qin, X. Chemical Profiling of Dingkun Dan by Ultra High Performance Liquid Chromatography Q Exactive Orbitrap High Resolution Mass Spectrometry. *J. Pharm. Biomed. Anal.* **2020**, *177*, 112732. [CrossRef]

92. Demarque, D.P.; Crotti, A.E.M.; Vessecchi, R.; Lopes, J.L.C.; Lopes, N.P. Fragmentation Reactions Using Electrospray Ionization Mass Spectrometry: An Important Tool for the Structural Elucidation and Characterization of Synthetic and Natural Products. *Nat. Prod. Rep.* **2016**, *33*, 432–455. [CrossRef] [PubMed]

93. Schmidt, J. Negative Ion Electrospray High-Resolution Tandem Mass Spectrometry of Polyphenols. *J. Mass Spectrom.* **2016**, *51*, 33–43. [CrossRef]

94. March, R.E.; Miao, X.-S.; Metcalfe, C.D.; Stobiecki, M.; Marczak, L. A Fragmentation Study of an Isoflavone Glycoside, Genistein-7-O-Glucoside, Using Electrospray Quadrupole Time-of-Flight Mass Spectrometry at High Mass Resolution. *Int. J. Mass Spectrom.* **2004**, *232*, 171–183. [CrossRef]

95. Fabre, N.; Rustan, I.; de Hoffmann, E.; Quetin-Leclercq, J. Determination of Flavone, Flavonol, and Flavanone Aglycones by Negative Ion Liquid Chromatography Electrospray Ion Trap Mass Spectrometry. *J. Am. Soc. Mass Spectrom.* **2001**, *12*, 707–715. [CrossRef]

96. Pires, F.B.; Dolwitsch, C.B.; Dal Prá, V.; Faccin, H.; Monego, D.L.; de Carvalho, L.M.; Viana, C.; Lameira, O.; Lima, F.O.; Bressan, L.; et al. Qualitative and Quantitative Analysis of the Phenolic Content of Connarus Var. Angustifolius, Cecropia Obtusa, Cecropia Palmata and Mansoa Alliacea Based on HPLC-DAD and UHPLC-ESI-MS/MS. *Rev. Bras. Farmacogn.* **2017**, *27*, 426–433. [CrossRef]

97. Marczak, Ł.; Znajdek-Awiżeń, P.; Bylka, W. The Use of Mass Spectrometric Techniques to Differentiate Isobaric and Isomeric Flavonoid Conjugates from Axyris Amaranthoides. *Molecules* **2016**, *21*, 1229. [CrossRef] [PubMed]

98. Frański, R.; Gierczyk, B.; Kozik, T.; Popenda, Ł.; Beszterda, M. Signals of Diagnostic Ions in the Product Ion Spectra of [M − H]− Ions of Methoxylated Flavonoids. *Rapid Commun. Mass Spectrom.* **2019**, *33*, 125–132. [CrossRef]

99. Sun, Y.; Li, L.; Liao, M.; Su, M.; Wan, C.; Zhang, L.; Zhang, H. A Systematic Data Acquisition and Mining Strategy for Chemical Profiling of *Aster tataricus* Rhizoma (Ziwan) by UHPLC-Q-TOF-MS and the Corresponding Anti-Depressive Activity Screening. *J. Pharm. Biomed. Anal.* **2018**, *154*, 216–226. [CrossRef]

100. Simirgiotis, M.J.; Quispe, C.; Mocan, A.; Villatoro, J.M.; Areche, C.; Bórquez, J.; Sepúlveda, B.; Echiburu-Chau, C. UHPLC High Resolution Orbitrap Metabolomic Fingerprinting of the Unique Species Ophryosporus Triangularis Meyen from the Atacama Desert, Northern Chile. *Rev. Bras. Farmacogn.* **2017**, *27*, 179–187. [CrossRef]

101. López-Gutiérrez, N.; Romero-González, R.; Plaza-Bolaños, P.; Martínez Vidal, J.L.; Garrido Frenich, A. Identification and Quantification of Phytochemicals in Nutraceutical Products from Green Tea by UHPLC-Orbitrap-MS. *Food Chem.* **2015**, *173*, 607–618. [CrossRef]

102. Lee, Y.H.; Kim, B.; Kim, S.; Kim, M.-S.; Kim, H.; Hwang, S.-R.; Kim, K.; Lee, J.H. Characterization of Metabolite Profiles from the Leaves of Green Perilla (*Perilla frutescens*) by Ultra High Performance Liquid Chromatography Coupled with Electrospray Ionization Quadrupole Time-of-Flight Mass Spectrometry and Screening for Their Antioxidant Properties. *J. Food Drug Anal.* **2017**, *25*, 776–788. [CrossRef]

103. Abdulla, R.; Mansur, S.; Lai, H.; Ubul, A.; Sun, G.; Huang, G.; Aisa, H.A. Qualitative Analysis of Polyphenols in Macroporous Resin Pretreated Pomegranate Husk Extract by HPLC-QTOF-MS. *Phytochem. Anal. PCA* **2017**, *28*, 465–473. [CrossRef] [PubMed]

104. Rocchetti, G.; Chiodelli, G.; Giuberti, G.; Ghisoni, S.; Baccolo, G.; Blasi, F.; Montesano, D.; Trevisan, M.; Lucini, L. UHPLC-ESI-QTOF-MS Profile of Polyphenols in Goji Berries (*Lycium barbarum* L.) and Its Dynamics during in Vitro Gastrointestinal Digestion and Fermentation. *J. Funct. Foods* **2018**, *40*, 564–572. [CrossRef]

105. Wang, Z.; Qu, Y.; Wang, L.; Zhang, X.; Xiao, H. Ultra-High Performance Liquid Chromatography with Linear Ion Trap-Orbitrap Hybrid Mass Spectrometry Combined with a Systematic Strategy Based on Fragment Ions for the Rapid Separation and Characterization of Components in Stellera Chamaejasme Extracts. *J. Sep. Sci.* **2016**, *39*, 1379–1388. [CrossRef] [PubMed]

106. Ben Said, R.; Hamed, A.I.; Mahalel, U.A.; Al-Ayed, A.S.; Kowalczyk, M.; Moldoch, J.; Oleszek, W.; Stochmal, A. Tentative Characterization of Polyphenolic Compounds in the Male Flowers of Phoenix Dactylifera by Liquid Chromatography Coupled with Mass Spectrometry and DFT. *Int. J. Mol. Sci.* **2017**, *18*, 512. [CrossRef]

107. Ben Haj Yahia, I.; Zaouali, Y.; Ciavatta, M.L.; Ligresti, A.; Jaouadi, R.; Boussaid, M.; Cutignano, A. Polyphenolic Profiling, Quantitative Assessment and Biological Activities of Tunisian Native *Mentha rotundifolia* (L.) Huds. *Molecules* **2019**, *24*, 2351. [CrossRef] [PubMed]

108. Ma, X.; Guo, X.; Song, Y.; Qiao, L.; Wang, W.; Zhao, M.; Tu, P.; Jiang, Y. An Integrated Strategy for Global Qualitative and Quantitative Profiling of Traditional Chinese Medicine Formulas: Baoyuan Decoction as a Case. *Sci. Rep.* **2016**, *6*, 38379. [CrossRef]

109. Kang, K.B.; Woo, S.; Ernst, M.; van der Hooft, J.J.J.; Nothias, L.-F.; da Silva, R.R.; Dorrestein, P.C.; Sung, S.H.; Lee, M. Assessing Specialized Metabolite Diversity of Alnus Species by a Digitized LC–MS/MS Data Analysis Workflow. *Phytochemistry* **2020**, *173*, 112292. [CrossRef]

110. Chiriac, E.R.; Chițescu, C.L.; Borda, D.; Lupoae, M.; Gird, C.E.; Geană, E.-I.; Blaga, G.-V.; Boscencu, R. Comparison of the Polyphenolic Profile of Medicago Sativa L. and Trifolium Pratense L. Sprouts in Different Germination Stages Using the UHPLC-Q Exactive Hybrid Quadrupole Orbitrap High-Resolution Mass Spectrometry. *Molecules* **2020**, *25*, 2321. [CrossRef]

111. D'Urso, G.; Montoro, P.; Piacente, S. Detection and Comparison of Phenolic Compounds in Different Extracts of Black Currant Leaves by Liquid Chromatography Coupled with High-Resolution ESI-LTQ-Orbitrap MS and High Sensitivity ESI-Qtrap MS. *J. Pharm. Biomed. Anal.* **2020**, *179*, 112926. [CrossRef] [PubMed]

112. Heras, R.M.-L.; Quifer-Rada, P.; Andrés, A.; Lamuela-Raventós, R. Polyphenolic Profile of Persimmon Leaves by High Resolution Mass Spectrometry (LC-ESI-LTQ-Orbitrap-MS). *J. Funct. Foods* **2016**, *23*, 370–377. [CrossRef]

113. Simirgiotis, M.J.; Quispe, C.; Areche, C.; Sepúlveda, B. Phenolic Compounds in Chilean Mistletoe (Quintral, Tristerix Tetrandus) Analyzed by UHPLC-Q/Orbitrap/MS/MS and Its Antioxidant Properties. *Molecules* **2016**, *21*, 245. [CrossRef] [PubMed]

114. Zhou, J.; Li, Y.; Chen, X.; Zhong, L.; Yin, Y. Development of Data-Independent Acquisition Workflows for Metabolomic Analysis on a Quadrupole-Orbitrap Platform. *Talanta* **2017**, *164*, 128–136. [CrossRef]

115. Xu, L.; Liu, Y.; Wu, H.; Wu, H.; Liu, X.; Zhou, A. Rapid Identification of Chemical Profile in Gandou Decoction by UPLC-Q-TOF-MSE Coupled with Novel Informatics UNIFI Platform. *J. Pharm. Anal.* **2020**, *10*, 35–48. [CrossRef]

116. Guo, X.; Long, P.; Meng, Q.; Ho, C.-T.; Zhang, L. An Emerging Strategy for Evaluating the Grades of Keemun Black Tea by Combinatory Liquid Chromatography-Orbitrap Mass Spectrometry-Based Untargeted Metabolomics and Inhibition Effects on α-Glucosidase and α-Amylase. *Food Chem.* **2018**, *246*, 74–81. [CrossRef] [PubMed]

117. Ahmad, N.; Zuo, Y.; Lu, X.; Anwar, F.; Hameed, S. Characterization of Free and Conjugated Phenolic Compounds in Fruits of Selected Wild Plants. *Food Chem.* **2016**, *190*, 80–89. [CrossRef] [PubMed]

118. Marsol-Vall, A.; Balcells, M.; Eras, J.; Canela-Garayoa, R. Injection-Port Derivatization Coupled to GC-MS/MS for the Analysis of Glycosylated and Non-Glycosylated Polyphenols in Fruit Samples. *Food Chem.* **2016**, *204*, 210–217. [CrossRef]

119. Pakkirisamy, M.; Kalakandan, S.; Ravichandran, K.; Ravichandran, K. Phytochemical Screening, GC-MS, FT-IR Analysis of Methanolic Extract of Curcuma Caesia Roxb (Black Turmeric). *Pharmacogn. J.* **2017**, *9*, 952–956. [CrossRef]

120. Sharma, S.; Saxena, D.C.; Riar, C.S. Using Combined Optimization, GC-MS and Analytical Technique to Analyze the Germination Effect on Phenolics, Dietary Fibers, Minerals and GABA Contents of Kodo Millet (*Paspalum scrobiculatum*). *Food Chem.* **2017**, *233*, 20–28. [CrossRef] [PubMed]

121. Sagbo, I.J.; Orock, A.E.; Kola, E.; Otang-Mbeng, W. Phytochemical Screening and Gas Chromatography-Mass Spectrometry Analysis of Ethanol Extract of *Scambiosa columbabria* L. *Pharmacogn. Res.* **2020**, *12*, 35. [CrossRef]

122. Rohloff, J. Analysis of Phenolic and Cyclic Compounds in Plants Using Derivatization Techniques in Combination with GC-MS-Based Metabolite Profiling. *Molecules* **2015**, *20*, 3431–3462. [CrossRef] [PubMed]

123. Da Silva, F.M.A.; Hanna, A.C.S.; de Souza, A.A.; da Silva Filho, F.A.; Canhoto, O.M.F.; Magalhães, A.; Benevides, P.J.C.; de Azevedo, M.B.M.; Siani, A.C.; Pohlit, A.M.; et al. Integrative Analysis Based on HPLC-DAD-MS/MS and NMR of Bertholletia Excelsa Bark Biomass Residues:Determination of Ellagic Acid Derivatives. *J. Braz. Chem. Soc.* **2019**, *30*, 830–836. [CrossRef]

124. Der Kooy, F.V.; Venkataya, B.; Pearson, J.L.; Torres, A.; Li, C.G.; Chang, D. Sensitivity of NMR-Based Metabolomics in Drug Discovery from Medicinal Plants. *Eur. J. Med. Plants* **2015**, 191–203. [CrossRef]

125. Valli, M.; Russo, H.M.; Pilon, A.C.; Pinto, M.E.F.; Dias, N.B.; Freire, R.T.; Castro-Gamboa, I.; Bolzani, V.D.S. Computational Methods for NMR and MS for Structure Elucidation II: Database Resources and Advanced Methods. *Phys. Sci. Rev.* **2019**, *4*. [CrossRef]

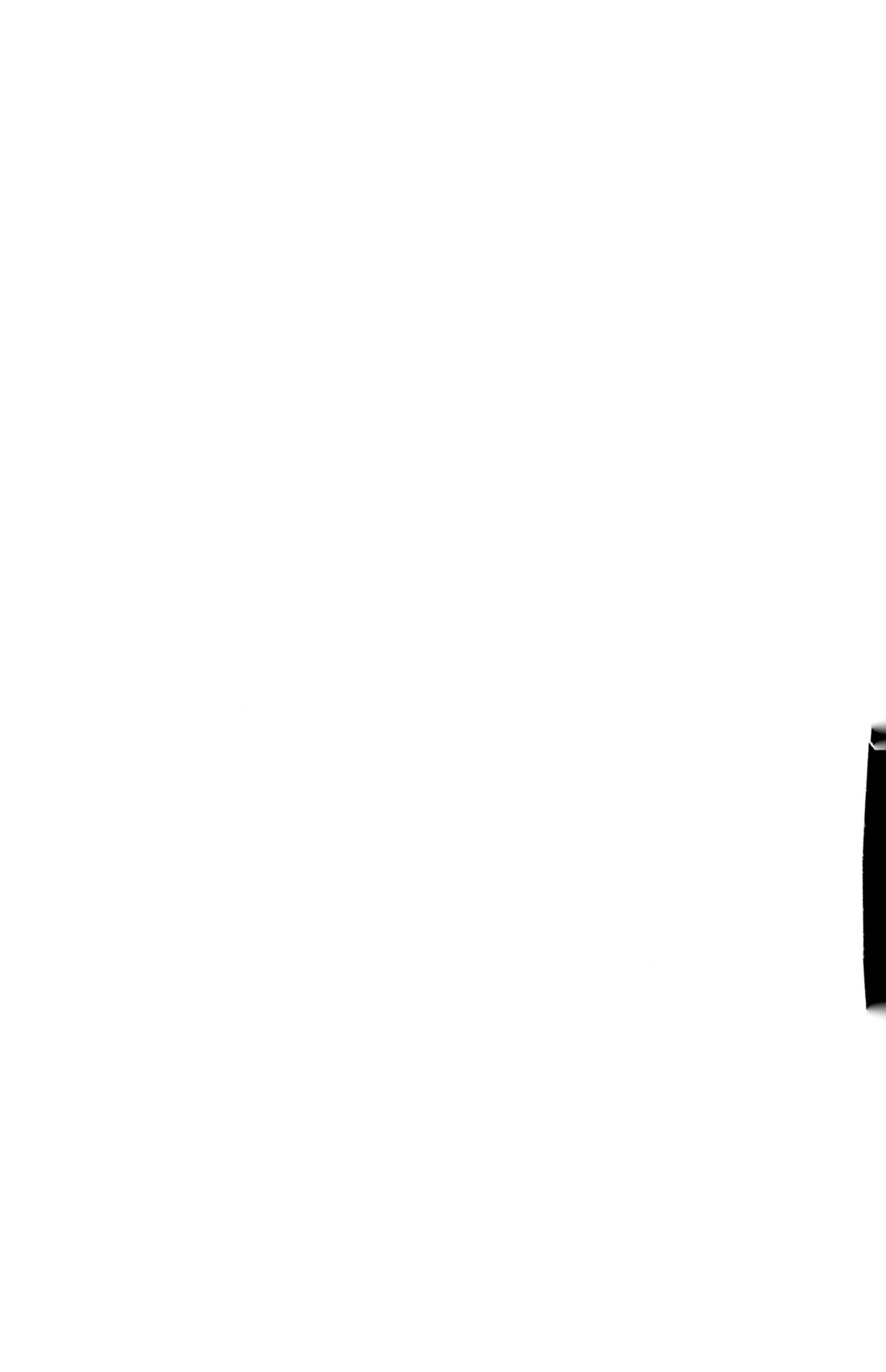

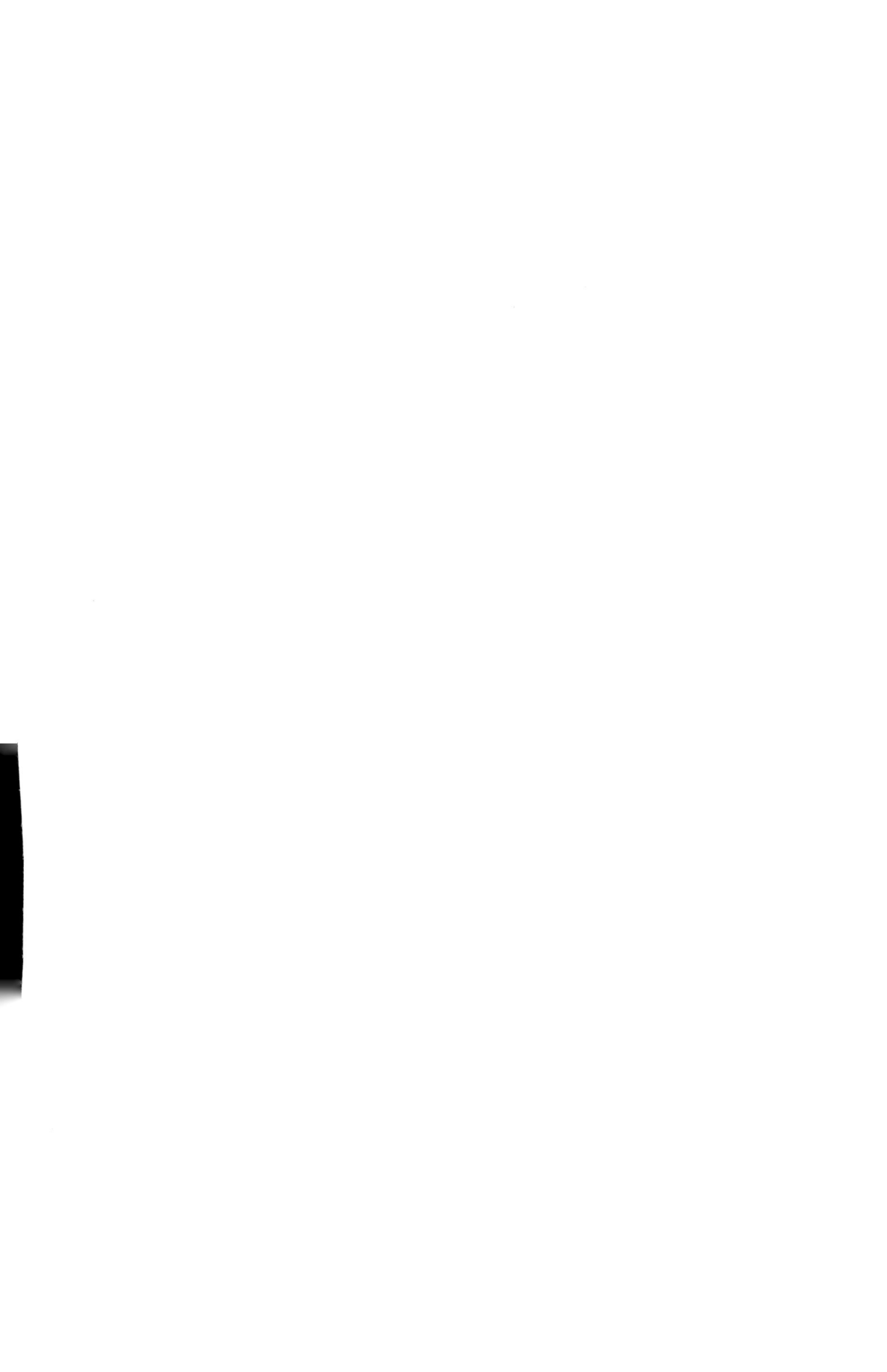

MDPI

St. Alban-Anlage 66

4052 Basel

Switzerland

www.mdpi.com

Separations Editorial Office

E-mail: separations@mdpi.com

www.mdpi.com/journal/separations

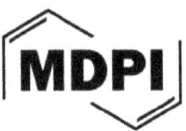